DEAD DOCTORS
DON'T LIE

DEAD DOCTORS DON'T LIE

Dr. Joel Wallach
&
Dr. Ma Lan

SMART HEALTH
619-788-7037
Mineralwellness.com

Other books by Dr. Joel Wallach & Dr. Ma Lan

Rare Earths: forbidden Cures
Let's Play Doctor
Let's Play Herbal Doctor
God Bless America

Cover design by Watts & Associates
Typography by Becky Earls

Request for bulk sales discounts, editorial permissions, or other
information should be addressed to the publisher:
> Wellness Publications LLC.
> P.O. Box 1812, Bonita, CA 91908
> 800/755-4656 (ph.)   619/420-2456 (fax)
> www.drjwallach.com   wellness@cts.com

ISBN 0-9748581-0-2
Printed in the United States of America

Dead Doctors Don't Lie, the book, is dedicated to the 60 million Americans who received the 90 minute audio-cassette tape, "Dead Doctors Don't Lie". The millions who listened, who understood, and who took positive action to enhance their own lives and the lives of others by supplementing with plant derived colloidal minerals.

When Dr. Joel Wallach began investigating the best way to educate people on the value of taking nutritional supplements, he looked at doctor's themselves. He assumed that they would be healthier than anyone else. However, what he discovered, in an 1895 edition of the *Journal of the American Medical Association* was that the average life of doctors was just 55 years. Anticipating this gap to be much closer today than 100 years ago, he researched it further. What he found was that today, the gap is closer–but only by three years.

A veterinarian for thirty years, Dr Wallach worked as a research veterinary pathologist with the National Institute of Health (NIH) at Emory University. Having discovered and identified the first animal models for cystic fibrosis in monkeys, he found that he could reproduce their condition at will because it was caused by a nutritional deficiency. His findings offered great promise for children suffering with the debilitating disease. The only problem he didn't anticipate was the reaction from the Institute. Within twenty-four hours after he made his findings public, he was fired. NIH wasn't interested in seeing their grants and other funding eliminated.

Dr. Wallach then made the decision to go to medical school so he could treat children for cystic fibrosis himself. Realizing that traditional medical school was likely to be as negative as the NIH, he accepted an invitation to teach nutrition at the National College of Naturopathic Medicine in Oregon. When he learned that he could be a primary care physician (which meant he could deliver babies, sew up chainsaw wounds, write prescriptions, and even get paid by insurance companies!) he decided to enroll as a full-time student.

Dr. Joel Wallach has been involved in biomedical research and clinical medicine for over forty years. He received the B.S. degree in agriculture from the University of Missouri with a major in animal husbandry (nutrition) and a minor in field crops and soils. In addition, he has the Doctor of Veterinary Medicine (D.V.M.) from the University of Missouri. He has also earned the N.D. degree (naturopathic physician) from the National College of Naturopathic Medicine in Portland, Oregon.

He has appeared frequently on network television and talk-radio programs as an expert on trace mineral and rare earth deficiency diseases. He is also the host of his own syndicated radio program. Additionally, he presents 300 free nutrition seminars to the general public and professional associations per year, and is the Editor-in-chief of the highly acclaimed alternative health magazine, *Health Consciousness.*

Dr. Ma Lan is vice-president of Wellness Lifestyle in San Diego, California. She earned her M.D. from Beijing Medical University and co-authored with Dr. Wallach the popular self-help book, *Let's Play Doctor*, now in its twelfth printing.

CONTENTS

PREFACE

Before written history, it took 100,000 years to double the earth's human population. After the dawn of agriculture, about five or six thousand years ago, it took seven hundred years to double the population of human kind. Today at the brink of the twenty-first century, it takes only about forty years to double our numbers. As a result of this avalanche of human flesh, the intercultural competition for our human bodily raw materials—the very basic stuff of life, optimal health, and longevity—has reached a cataclysmic pitch!

Unfortunately, the entire complement of the ninety essential nutrients required for optimal health and longevity of humans are either totally absent or their availability in food is so highly variable that your chances of getting them from food alone is more remote than winning the lottery.

Over the years, great cults have motivated zealous health disciples, propagating vegetarianism, macrobiotics, biofeedback, meditation, exercise, pure thought, and yoga. The lapdog followers of the allopathic cult have even called for free medical care for all, to the thrill of vote-buying politicians. Despite the "sermonizing," none of these practices have extended the human life span in America to more than 75.5 years—only 62 percent of our human genetic potential for longevity of 120 to 140 years.

Is allopathic medicine more cultish than science? Yes!

The greatest "scientific" thinkers—usually legends in their own minds—frantically search for ways to hang on to life until some serendipitous "miracle discovery" is made that will save the day, as long as it can be patented and it passes the Allopathic Inquisition, that is.

Allopathic Physicians (whether labeled MDs or DOs, allopaths who "crack backs") extol the virtues of vaccinations, the annual physical, eating from the four food groups, reducing your salt and fat intake and not smoking. Yet if these methods in themselves were sufficient to produce true health and longevity, doctors would live as long or longer than the average American. However, close inspection of doctors' health and longevity records show they are neither healthier nor do they live longer. And dead doctors don't lie.

Some with perfect faith in the allopathic medical profession prove their supreme devotion and pay a tremendous price to have themselves quick-frozen in liquid nitrogen (Cryogenic Suspension) to extend their "shelf life" until a medical cure can be discovered for their terminal disease and their faith is vindicated!

The "Immortalists," an anti-death cult, believe that if they disregard death and all of its trappings (i.e. cemetery plots, burial insurance, etc.) they will not die. Can we be "deprogrammed" in time? Only if we are willing to face the facts.

Frankly, all these false idols are killing us!

Both the 1936 U.S. Senate Document 264 and the 1992 Rio Earth Summit Report on mineral depletion graphically point out that our Earth's soils are anemic. Dozens of the sixty formerly-abundant soil elements—selenium, arsenic, tin, aluminum, chromium, vanadium, molybdenum, nickel, etc.—were just a short time ago thought by the medical profession to be totally toxic to humans if not completely non-essential for health. Don't look for these elements in your "scientifically enriched" food!

When the four food groups fail us (and they always do), surgeons sell us bionic joint replacements or "hawk" organ transplants. But this "bionic-parts service" and "flesh recycling" has not pushed back the curtain of death for Americans. The 75.5 year average life span for Americans places us seventeenth in longevity when compared with the other industrialized nations.

So bedazzled are we by the allopathic mantras that even our scientists remain befuddled! A two-year-long experiment in Tucson, Arizona, concocted by Roy Walford, placed six inhabitants (including himself) in a self-contained, self-perpetuating unit called Biosphere II (Earth being Biosphere I). The goal? To hedge against environmental disaster or perhaps set up a prototype for establishing a pioneer colony on a far-flung planet. The concept is romantic but hardly practical for the masses of we poor earth-bound sods.

Thanks to allopathy's incessant harping about "calories" and not a word about micronutrients, Walford erroneously believes—through faulty translation of animal data—that severely reduced caloric intake alone can extend human life spans by thirty to forty percent. A critical review of the data taken from the earliest reduced calorie/longevity experiments reveals that the level of vitamins, minerals, and trace minerals remained the same in all of the control and low calorie groups (calories reduced by thirty, forty-five, and sixty percent) regardless of their calorie level. It is not the reduced calories that extend life. It's a high nutrient density that extends life!

Walford was so obsessed with the low calorie theme that he downplayed the relative increase in vitamin and mineral concentration. Upon their exit from Biosphere II, after their two years self-imposed minimal caloric intake, five of the six Biosphere participants (excluding Walford) wanted only pizza and junk food. This was a clear manifestation of pica and cribbing. They also complained that the normally amiable group had broken down into argumentative behavior over every minor decision! In addition, two of the Biospherians, a short time after their exit from the dome, illegally broke into the Biosphere to steal records—criminal behavior! So much for that successful experiment.

We humans require the ninety essential nutrients in optimal levels in our daily diet to not only prevent debilitating developmental and degenerative diseases but also for normal sociability, for preventing criminal behavior (there are now 2,000,000 prisoners in American jails), and to reach our attainable life expectancy. We had better understand the basic mineral needs of our own emotions and bodies here on earth before we fly off to space stations and find ourselves having gone a bridge too far.

The 90s drive to patent genetically engineered crops ("Frankenstein Food"), enzymes, hormones, bacteria, cloned animals (*a' la* Dolly the cloned lamb), and even humans (identical humans can now be cloned at the embryonic stage: *"The Boys from Brazil"* are here!), has been a heroic, if not greedy, effort by our entrepreneurial scientists to further the cult of allopathy. But expecting genetically manipulated living cells to develop, maintain themselves, reach their genetic-potential for longevity, and perform without the basic stuff of life is to expect to drive a Mercedes Benz full speed from San Diego to Los Angeles—a distance of 150 miles—without any oil or coolant! Even the Mercedes engine, that German wonder of automotive engineering designed to go 300,000 miles without an overhaul will become a molten mass of expensive scrap before you've gone fifty miles.

Physicians who should know better are, in essence, recommending that their patients travel at maximum speed with only basic fuels. Yet when do they ever tell us to take in the ninety crucial nutrients that serve as humankind's "oils" and "coolants" that allow this fleshly masterpiece of engineering called our body to go its "300,000-plus miles?" Without those ninety nutrients, the human internal combustion engine never truly keeps from "burning up" physically, emotionally, or mentally. Bodily maintenance, repair, and ultimately life itself cannot go on!

Dead Doctors Don't Lie will give you facts, proven truths, and the knowledge and tools necessary to identify the elemental raw materials of life no longer found in our food. It identifies the raw materials necessary to turbo-charge and empower yourself and your families' and friends' lives with power-packed health and vitality.

Dead Doctors Don't Lie is hard ball. You'll be shocked as it reveals many facts and truths that are 180 degrees opposite from what the medical community has led you to believe! The reality is that the physicians who have brainwashed you for years cannot keep you healthy—nor can they save you. Nor can the practitioners of the other nutritional "cults" and "isms." Only those of us who take personal responsibility for maintaining and enriching our physical bodies with as much zeal as we maintain our expensive automobiles are going to make it! Your president, governor, mayor, councilman, postman, physician, or even your spouse can't do it for you. In most instances, they can't even help themselves! Only you can do it.

The good news is you don't have to wait for twenty years of expensive "double blind" studies to know how to start rescuing your health! We've already got the "control groups" who consistently made it to the end point of the human genetic potential for longevity (120 to 140 years) healthfully and with great vitality. They did it without "high tech medicine" or the "skills" of western physicians, and so can you. This control group of five ancient and highly diverse cultures share common denominators that include healthful, disease-free longevity, and unlimited access to adequate levels of all ninety essential nutrients required by humans. One of the secrets they shared includes access to unique natural sources of plant derived colloidal minerals. My promise to you is that if you plug into the thousands of years of accumulated knowledge of these long-lived peoples, you and yours can make it too!

Dr. Joel D. Wallach

1

SCIENCE WITH A CAPITAL "STOCK OPTION!"

Scientific research that began as the altruistic search for knowledge has increasingly become big business. The intrusion of money into science means "medicine" will never arrive at what truly works, unless they can patent it for maximum profits!

Pasteur brought about a revolution in medicine by associating bacteria or "germs" with disease. His work with vaccines to prevent bacterial and viral diseases like anthrax and rabies dominated medicine and health care until the 1930s when sulfa drugs and penicillin were discovered.

Prior to Pasteur's birth, nearly one third of the world's human population had been wiped out by a bacterial scourge known as the Bubonic plague. The plague was transmitted to men by fleas that were found on rats. When the exploding rat population was killed off, the hungry fleas simply jumped from the dead rats onto the nearest human, carrying with them the bacteria that was to be later identified as the cause of the deadly plague. The bacterium that was determined to be the cause of the Bubonic plague was originally named Pasteurella in honor of Pasteur's work.

During the nearly 200 years following Pasteur, it was believed that most diseases, including cancer and mental illness, were caused by bacterial "germs." The "Germ Theory of Disease" was considered the discovery of the century. Everything in medicine was then geared towards defeating this bacterial menace. "Aseptic" techniques were developed for surgery. Disinfectants, vaccines, and antibiotic after antibiotic appeared on the scene to save us from the "bacterial menace."

Tuberculosis sanitariums and "retardation" centers for the mentally ill sprang up all over America to isolate and treat the chronically ill felled by bacterial infections and those diseases mistakenly thought to be due to bacterial infections.

After World War II, Polio was the high profile viral disease that drove American medical research. This deadly virus attacked thousands of children in America and even crippled President Franklin Roosevelt. The March of Dimes was created and the cards for collecting dimes to defeat this new enemy dominated every schoolroom. This disease and other previously unknown viruses from the steamy far-flung jungles of the world challenged the idea that bacteria were the most important health threat. March of Dimes cards were given to each child to be returned to the school office when each slot was filled. School children became an army with the mission to raise millions of dollars in research funds to support basic viral research to save America from the scourge of Polio.

Virus "mania" gripped all of America. Repeating the overzealous mistakes made a generation earlier, every effort was made to attribute every disease from cancer to mental disease to viruses. The advent of the electron microscope which allowed researchers to actually visualize virus particles and the establishment of monkey colonies to develop a new generation of anti-viral vaccines were the medical research tools of the day. Viruses and the associated viral technology were "the discovery of the century."

During the 80s and 90s the development of genetic mapping techniques, genetic engineering, and cloning has now led "everyone" to blame all disease, including cancer and mental illness, on genetic "defects." The goal is to find a genetically engineered protein that, when inserted into the cell of a patient with a genetic disease, will unscramble the defective DNA and cure the disease. Today everyone "knows" that all disease has a genetic basis—certainly the mapping of the human genome, genetic engineering, and cloning are today's supposed "discoveries of the century." The March of Dimes has been reincarnated to help fight "birth defects" and their money collection techniques have been "cloned" a thousand fold to fight the "new menace" of genetic defects.

The terrible parallel between the medical "fever" over bacteria, viruses, and genetic engineering is that preceding each "discovery of the century" was the development of a new laboratory tool: bacterial stains, bacterial culturing, light microscope, cell culture, antibody identification, electron microscope, genetic mapping, amniocentesis, test tube babies, and the ultimate—cloning of mammals and humans.

See a pattern developing? The appearance of every new scientific tool brings with it the great scientific dance—grantsmanship. "Scientists" hit the rubber chicken circuit and TV talk shows to whip the public into a fever pitch of worry and fear so Congress can no longer refuse the research community the information and the tools necessary to find the answer *du jour* for better American health and greater longevity. A cynic might conclude that every new "public health menace" is preceded by the development of new laboratory tools on which to spend money. Perhaps we should be espousing the "Laboratory Equipment Breakthrough Theory of Disease" or the "Financial Incentive Theory of Disease."

In the case of the original bacterial investigations, the search was gloriously altruistic; it was a search for truth, knowledge, and understanding. The identifying feature of both the viral and genetic research hysteria is the enormous amount of hype and publicity which were generated purposely to raise huge sums of money from the government, from private coffers of pharmaceutical companies, and from the average American for research and development. Patents, stock options, and public offerings on the stock exchange flowed freely. Unfortunately, none of these genetically engineered answers have yet won the war on cancer or the war on other mineral deficiency diseases dubbed "genetic" diseases simply to cash in on the current "every disease has a genetic basis" climate.

A great example is the hype over "angiostatin" and "endostatin" as a cancer "cure." These substances are found naturally in shark cartilage, which has been used in cancer therapy by the Chinese for five-thousand years. The medical profession discounted the concept of using shark cartilage as a cancer therapy with the usual exclamation: *it's quackery!*

Now that the genetic engineering industry has found a way to produce angiostatin and endostatin in a patentable way, the hype is on. It is no longer "quackery"—it is "science" with a capital "Stock Option!"

Humans, like flamingos, angelfish, iguanas, cats, dogs, and elephants, do have a genetic potential for physical and emotional perfection and an upper genetic limit for height and longevity.

Attaining your disease-free genetic potential—the upper limit of what we can get out of life—for physical and emotional perfection and optimal longevity begins before conception. Without the intake of the proper amounts and constant flow of the full spectrum of the essential raw materials from pre-conception to our death bed, we are unable to attain these genetic potentials—we will fall short, we will get diseases, and will be dealt a shorter, disease-ridden life.

We have been cheated of a simple and healthful, essentially disease-free 120 year-long life by medical and pharmaceutical misinformation spoon-fed to us in daily doses by medical spin-doctors since Marcus Welby, M.D. first appeared on television.

2

SUPPLEMENTS FOR LIVESTOCK BUT NOT FOR US!

Raw materials are required by all living organisms. The obvious raw materials to sustain life, maintain and repair tissues and organs, support reproduction, and support longevity, are oxygen, water, and food. Clean oxygen and water, free of pathogens and pollution, are non-variables. Oxygen and water are the same in China, Germany, Brazil, Nigeria, Canada, and all fifty states in the United States.

Food is the variable. Whether prepared by mothers, hash slingers, pancake houses, or French chefs, and whether presented as a Reuben on Rye or a Spinach Souffle, all nourishment and all food comes from the soil, either directly or indirectly. The sun provides the energy to manufacture the carbon-based macronutrients (carbohydrates, fats, and proteins) and micronutrients like vitamins. The earth's crust—the soil— is the source of all our non-carbon based raw materials like minerals. Unfortunately, soil and its mineral composition does not occur in a uniform blanket around the crust of the earth. Soil is not homogenous but is a highly variable combination of raw materials. It is also a mixture of living organisms such as bacteria, fungi, protozoa, organic material (humus), and inorganic substances (minerals). People worldwide with the same basic genetic makeup do not have the same opportunity for health and longevity because of the wide variations in the chemical make-up of soil. And unfortunately, the endless pleadings from legions of nutritionists on the value of the "four food groups" cannot overcome the problem.

It wasn't the simple hunger for land that drove Americans west across the Great Plains. It was the hunger for good, well-mineralized soil that would support healthy families that drove them there. "Bottom" land or flood plains tended to be the desired land. The annual floods that inundated the bottomland brought a new supply of minerals and silt to replenish the exhausted soil.

As a result of this quest, Americans, as a culture, have historically enjoyed better diets than any other culture on earth. We have eaten higher quality food and certainly greater quantities per person than any culture in history for more than two hundred years. However, despite this fact, Americans are ranked seventeenth in longevity and nineteenth in healthfulness by the World Health Organization. Americans average a pitiful 75.5 years in longevity—only half of our potential longevity of 120 to 140 years. And according to the Centers for Disease Control, most Americans spend the last twelve years of their lives in misery, suffering from some combination of debilitating diseases. Obviously farming the best land has not been good enough because we're dying too soon.

The sad fact is, we have known this all along. The interface between the soil and human life is the farmer and rancher who raise the crops—grains, vegetables, fruit—and livestock, including cattle, hogs, sheep, poultry, and fish, which first consume the minerals and other raw materials from the soil. Since the beginning of time farmers and ranchers have universally been the first to suffer from, benefit from, and recognize the variations in the land's ability to produce crops and livestock as well as deficiencies of nutrients in the soil. Both natural and human-created mineral deficiencies in the soil prove costly in livestock disease and loss. To make farming, agriculture, and animal husbandry predictable and profitable industries, successful farmers and ranchers have learned to add vitamins, minerals, and trace minerals to animal feeds to make up for the difference of mineral deficiencies in the soil and standardize the nutritional value of livestock feeds.

I grew up in Missouri raising beef calves. The calves were only fed for four to six months before they were shipped off to be butchered or to other feeders. We always saved back the very best ones for ourselves. We knocked them in the head and butchered them—a simple cycle on the farm. I learned how to dress and skin a carcass and how to do an inspection of the internal organs to assure it was disease-free and safe to eat.

All four of my grandparents emigrated from the Ukraine just before World War I. They were tough yet simple rural people who worked hard. My maternal grandfather delivered his vegetables and corn to city dwellers with a horse and wagon. He died in his forties from tularemia that he contracted from the nick of a jagged bone while skinning a wild rabbit. He probably could have been saved with penicillin. Unfortunately, it hadn't been discovered yet. My maternal grandmother survived and raised her three children by gardening and by creating and operating a small farmers market and taking bets on the horse races.

My paternal grandparents raised five kids in a rural-suburban setting. They gardened and operated a recycling business, known in those days as the "junk business." My grandfather died in his eighties from the complications of alcoholism. My paternal grandmother was killed in a nursing home at age 97 from an overdose of insulin administered by one of the nurses.

We lived in a clapboard house in hay and corn fields of rural St. Louis county. The hay barn was four times bigger than the house. Our kitchen not only housed the wood stove we used for cooking and heating, it also served as a living room, office, and laundry room. There was a sagging brass bed at one end for grandma. We took baths in a galvanized oval wash tub in the middle of the kitchen near the warm stove.

The kitchen stove was fueled with wood and coal. From the age of six I was responsible for the wood supply. I walked the half-mile to the sawmill several times each day towing my Western Flyer wagon to bring home wood trimmings. In the winter, we used more coal in the stove for heating and cooking, and I was responsible for keeping the stove-side coal bucket full at all times.

The kitchen sink sported a hand water pump and the toilet was in the corner of the kitchen in what may have originally been a closet or pantry. There was also an outside "one-holer" as an added attraction in case two people needed to use the facility at the same time, or if one of us happened to be covered with mud or manure. The outhouse was hot, smelly, and always had a wasp nest in the ridge of the roof. There was rarely enough toilet paper, so we always carried a small roll in our overalls.

You could say this kind of living made us fairly self-reliant. We never worried about going without things. Back then, if we didn't know how to do something, we learned how to do it. If we didn't have something we really wanted, we had to make it, or earn enough money doing chores to buy it. The "difficult" was that which could be achieved with relative ease. The "impossible" simply took a little longer. This is not bravado or ego—it was just practical. It's how the west was won.

Raising and feeding livestock involves a lot of details and intimacy with work, responsibility, schedules, trucks and tractors, machinery maintenance, manure, the land, and fertilizer. Not to mention weather, hay, grain, harvest, feed pellets, vitamins, minerals and trace minerals, reproduction, birth, disease, death, and veterinarians.

Even as a teenager, it was fascinating to me that we went to a great deal of trouble to make sure that livestock had optimal amounts of vitamins, minerals, and trace minerals in their feed. No one seemed too worried about the need to give humans these same vital supplements, even though we ate out of the same fields! The reason we paid such close attention and exerted such energy for our livestock was to prevent disease, eliminate infertility, prevent birth defects, reduce losses from death, and reduce veterinary bills, all of which were expensive and counterproductive to a profitable livestock operation. This incongruity was driven home to me in several unique ways.

There are two parts to a basic cow/calf cattle operation. The first is the breeding herd that produces calves. The second is the feeding and raising of the calves for sale to other feeders or shipment of the cattle to be butchered. During the summer, calves have access to the pasture, and during the winter when the pasture is dormant they are fed hay and corn silage.

When the calves are weaned off of the cow, the bull calves are castrated and made into steers. This makes for better efficiencies in feeding and for a better quality of meat. Calves are normally fed for six to nine months before they are ready to ship. Short horn and horned Hereford calves are de-horned to prevent them from damaging other calves during shipping. The calves to be kept for breeding were identified with numbered and color-coded ear tags, tested for TB and orucellosis, and vaccinated against "black leg" and "shipping fever."

When we slaughtered a calf we made sure that nothing was wasted. In addition to the meat and bones, we ate the liver, heart, kidneys, brain, pancreas, stomach, and we even used the ten gallons of stomach contents as fertilizer for the garden. The horns and hooves were thrown to the dogs.

As a family, we ate out of the same fields that the calves did. Five rows of corn were saved back for family use and at the end of the field we had a garden where we grew our peas, beans, squash, potatoes, carrots, onions, and tomatoes. We wanted to live to be a hundred with no aches and pains, yet we didn't give ourselves the same vitamins, minerals, and trace minerals that we gave the calves and chickens.

We thought we were eating the finest of foods but in just a few years the nutritional deficiencies began to catch up with us. When I was fourteen years old my eyelids twitched so violently you could hear them click.

One day I came to recognize the fact that the twitching and clicking were somehow connected, so I called my mother to ask her what she thought was happening. I figured that if Mom didn't know what the answer to the problem was, it was time to get worried.

My mother saw the twitching and heard the clicking but she didn't know what to make of the situation, so we jumped into the car and drove the eighty miles into St. Louis to visit Dr. Mary Jane Skeffington, an eye specialist. For some unknown reason, she had me strip to my underwear for the eye exam. Back then I was just a red-necked kid from the farm. It didn't bother me to strip in front of the doctor so I stripped. Today, if an eye specialist asked you to strip down to your underwear you could appear on Oprah and say that you were sexually harassed by your eye doctor!

For two hours Dr. Skeffington ran in and out of the examining room to look into my eyes with her ophthalmoscope. I said, "Doc, I play junior varsity football, I am the captain of the wrestling team, and I lift weights. You can do whatever is necessary to solve the problem, including amputate my eyelids." She got the message that I was getting frustrated, so she disappeared into her office to find the answer.

When Dr. Skeffington emerged from her office, she handed me a Maybelline mascara eyelash brush and a hand mirror and said, "The only problem I can find is that your eyelashes are so long that they've grown forward and they hit your glasses, curling back and tickling your eyeballs. That's what's making your eyelids twitch!"

"Doc, let me get this straight, you want me to sit on the football bench with twenty-five guys weighing over 200 pounds each, and you want me to play with my eyelashes with a mascara eyelash brush? Fifty yards across the field are another twenty-five guys weighing over 200 pounds and they don't like me!"

I got dressed and went to the high school library looking for what I thought should be more serious answers for cramping and spasms of the eyelids. I found two health books written by nurses and looked in the index under muscle cramps and muscle twitches. Sure enough, they listed the cause as a calcium deficiency. Now this sounded logical to me!

I knew where we had calcium. The calf pellets stored in the barn were loaded with calcium. I ran home and filled the pockets of my shirt, jeans, and jacket with calf pellets. The next day in school while everyone else was eating jellybeans and M & M's, I was, without shame, eating calf pellets. In four days the cramps and twitches in my eyelids went away. I realized that day, at age fourteen, that doctors knew little or nothing about nutrition.

Thanks to the calf pellets, I went back to school and played high school football, was the captain of the wrestling team, and lifted weights. I only weighed 123 pounds, but my mental attitude allowed me to play center, offensive guard, and middle linebacker well enough to letter in football. No opposing player was too big for me. I just got lower and quicker off the line of scrimmage. On passing plays my job was to sack the quarterback on a linebacker blitz because I could get into the backfield before the offensive line even stood up to block. The same success and vibrant health followed me in wrestling and every other activity as long as I had the right nutrition.

Looking back, I should have known that I would have had to find the answer apart from the standard care the medical community offered. Prior to my high school athletic success, I was a sickly child. I was laid up every summer with a disease known to me only as "serum fever." Medicine offered no relief. When I was six my dad took me to see my uncle who was a chiropractor. That was his night job. His day job was delivering mail for the U.S. Postal Service. He dispensed vitamins and minerals for me from two quart-sized bottles. The first was a bottle of vitamins that were as large as horse pills and smelled of rancid cod liver oil. The second was a bottle of giant oblong multi-mineral tablets.

I was forced to take the vitamin and mineral supplements under the threat of death if I didn't comply. The task of making me take the vitamin and mineral pills was a grim daily battle, but today I'm glad that I was forced to take those horrible pills.

No one else in the family took vitamins, minerals, and trace minerals as a supplement. After all, they were "healthy!"

Sadly enough, because of these experiences we began using veterinarians, their medicines, and their advice for our own health maintenance over the "conventional" wisdom of the medical doctors.

When I was growing up, my ultimate goal was to become an Eagle Scout. I completed all of the various ranks necessary to be eligible to achieve the Tenderfoot, Second Class, First Class, Star, and Life ranks. I earned almost all of the required and elective merit badges including camping, cooking, hiking, forestry, agriculture, poultry keeping, soil conservation, wildlife management, engineering, first aid, reading, writing, bookkeeping, book repair, bird watching, fishing, reptile keeping, taxidermy, archery, marksmanship, and citizenship.

The only required merit badges I didn't have that were needed to become an Eagle Scout were swimming and life saving. I was sixteen years old and couldn't swim. The odds in favor of Joel Wallach becoming an Eagle Scout without these two merit badges were zero.

My father and scoutmaster, Sydney Jacobs, joined forces and signed me up for swimming and lifesaving courses at the YMCA. They told me not to come back to a weekly scout meeting and not to go on any troop campouts until I had accomplished the necessary requirements to earn the swimming and lifesaving merit badges and ultimately the rank of Eagle Scout. Three months later I became an Eagle Scout—the impossible had been accomplished.

In those days, Eagle Scouts were honored every year during national Eagle Scout Day. One of the perks of becoming an Eagle Scout was being allowed to take an active part in a profession or trade of your choice for a day. I wanted to work with veterinarians. (You can probably understand why I didn't want to spend the day with an "eye specialist"—I already had!) I was assigned to the Ralston Purina feed company in St. Louis which included tours of their feed formulation laboratories and their Gray Summit Research Farm.

At the Ralston Purina Gray Summit Research Farm, new formulations and diets were tested on colonies of dogs, cats, mice, rats, rabbits, sheep, pigs, horses, cows, pigeons, chickens, turkeys, ducks, pea fowl, mink, ferrets, fox, and trout. They actually tested diets on hundreds of generations of each type of animal to be sure the diet would prevent diseases and birth defects before the diet was released for general use.

The purpose of the extensive diet testing by Ralston Purina was to make sure there were sufficient amounts of all of the known micronutrients to prevent infertility, birth defects, degenerative diseases, and reduced life spans. Special rations were designed by Purina to prevent and cure specific diseases such as heart disease and arthritis. The incredible thing was that they worked!

The obvious question to consider is this: Was there a nutrition company that created the same type of complete nutritional products for humans as were being created for animals?

To some, the possibility that human nutrition would ever be given such attention seemed impossible. But by then, my life on the farm had taught me to believe the impossible just takes a little bit longer.

3

A Carrot Is Not a Carrot!

I worked at the St. Louis Zoo during the summer of my first two years in high school. The highlight of my zoo experience was to work with Marlin Perkins of the original "Mutual of Omaha Wild Kingdom" television series. I first became aware of Mr. Perkins when he served as director of the Lincoln Park Zoo. He was also the host of the weekly television show, *Zoo Parade.*

When I applied for the summer jobs at the St. Louis Zoo, I assured the interviewer that I could and would do anything necessary just to be able to work with Marlin Perkins. I was hired for several reasons—one, because of my experience with livestock, second, the fact that I was an Eagle Scout, and third, because of my zeal and enthusiasm. I was assigned to a job in the elephant barn and then later to the children's zoo, two of Mr. Perkins' favorite haunts.

My elephant barn responsibilities were very basic. My employer took me at my word when I said that I would do anything to work with Marlin Perkins. The eleven Asian elephants were trained show animals. During the summer they performed three times each weekday and Saturday, and four times on Sunday. My job was to manually remove the manure from each of their rectums before each show to prevent them from creating a mess on the stage and from throwing the bowling-ball-sized droppings into the audience.

To relieve the elephants of their manure supply, they were chained by one front leg and one rear leg to iron rings set in the floor. I stripped to the waist, lubricated my bare arm with liquid soap water and went to it just as I had been instructed. They did not use the disposable plastic gloves that I had used for artificial insemination of mares and cows. The bare arm technique for removing manure from the elephant was the way it had always been done by generations of elephant trainers, and I was not about to risk losing the job by making any suggestions.

I removed about a bushel of manure from each animal before each show. Needless to say, it was a very humbling experience. As crude and humbling as it was, however, I did not shrink from my duty, and as a reward for my diligence I was asked to expand my work responsibility into the children's petting zoo. There, at least, the animals disposed of their manure without my assistance.

Great care was given to the food preparation and supplement programs designed for the hand-raised zoo babies. I personally bottle-fed and helped raise Florence and Pearl, two baby elephants who came to St. Louis when they were only a week old. They were so young that they still had their umbilical cords attached.

Hours were spent in preparing their milk and supplement formulas three times per day under the watchful eye of Floyd Smith, the legendary St. Louis Zoo elephant trainer.

Floyd gave me a notebook and had me record every ounce of formula, every piece of celery, every carrot, every bean, every grape, and every mouthful of fresh summer grass consumed by the two little elephants. The most interesting part of Smith's nutritional program for the two babies was the daily inclusion of several handfuls of blue clay. To my amazement, they eagerly ate the balls of clay as if they were candies, and, according to Floyd Smith, the clay was extremely important as a source of trace minerals for the very survivability of the two little pachyderms.

I listened to Floyd intently because he was one of the few people in America who had ever successfully hand-raised baby elephants. The two elephant babies grew up to be show girls at the Baraboo, Wisconsin Circus World Museum, and, of course, I was the proud godfather.

I went to the high school library and checked out the only book I could find that contained veterinary information on exotic animal species, *Circus Doctor* by Dr. Henderson, the veterinarian for the Ringling Brothers, Barnum and Baily Circus. There were wonderful stories of capturing escaped animals and treating lions, tigers, and bears for toothaches and worms, as well as raising orphaned baby animals in the kitchen. I began to dream about being a circus, zoo, or a wildlife veterinarian myself one day.

A fact that high school students frequently overlook until it has become a *fait accompli* is that after they graduate they get kicked out of class, whether they like it or not. About ten per cent of our class went to college. For the rest, the first few weeks were a vacuum. Some rambled down to the school building and sought permission to sit in on classes. A few did it purely for the lack of anything else to do.

Fortunately, for me there were choices; at least I thought so. One alternative, if all else failed, was to stay put, work a farm, and eke out whatever existence I could. Second, the Korean War was heating up, so I thought of joining up and becoming a Marine like my scoutmaster, Sydney Jacobs, who served with General MacArthur in the Pacific. Mr. Jacobs had run our scout troup as if it were the Marine Expeditionary Force. My third choice was to go to college. As is frequently the case, the greatest advocates of education are those who have never had access to that privilege themselves. My parents made it very clear to me that the only choice I had was to go to college, or, in the immortal words of my dad, "You will be dead meat."

I graduated high school with a C-minus average, only because my biology teacher had given me an A. Neither my mother nor father had graduated high school, but they encouraged me to keep going and do whatever it took to get into veterinary school, even with my C-minus average. So, number three it was. I was off to college.

The accepted path to veterinary school in those days was agricultural school, so that's where I headed. There was never any question of me going to any of the big and famous universities. They were just simply too expensive. The University of Missouri was only $500 per semester, which, in comparison to other universities, was very inexpensive. However, five hundred dollars was a lot of money to Mom and Dad, so tuition money would have to be raised the old fashioned way—hard work.

I traveled to Columbia, Missouri, in June of 1958, interviewed and negotiated with advisors, checked into a dormitory, and within days had a regular seven day a week job feeding and milking one of the university's experimental dairy herds and feeding the beef department's Angus herd. These chores had to be done each day before breakfast. The main goal of the dairy experiment was to regulate the bull calves' hormones so that they could produce economical amounts of milk. We never were able to produce more than a teacup of milk from any bull calf. The project was not cost effective so I guess you could say that a failed experiment made me skeptical of "scientific geniuses" forever.

The milking, feeding, halter breaking, and grooming of calves for show and judging classes, the manure, the silage, the hay, and the highly supplemented feed pellets were all too familiar, so the summer went by without incident or the need for major mental adjustments. College didn't seem too hard after all.

By the time classes had started in the fall, I was an old hand at my jobs, feeding and milking the herds and halter breaking calves for livestock judging classes. Certainly nothing was new here. I would get up at four a.m. to milk and feed silage to the cows. When I went into class afterwards there was never any difficulty in finding a seat. Everyone just moved away, because I reeked of silage and cow manure. I always ended up with a huge "clear zone" around me.

Unfortunately, the two jobs were not enough to pay for the tuition, books, room, food, and incidentals, so I had to add a third one. This time I stayed indoors and worked in the Crowder Hall dining room as a busboy where my nutritional education continued "informally". There were a variety of food ideas and preferences in that dining hall. There were no more rules set by Mom and Dad. If a student wanted to eat only mashed potatoes, he could do just that. If he only wanted to eat Jell-O, that was fine, too. I ate everything available and continued to take my daily handful of vitamins, minerals, and trace minerals.

The only trouble was the busboy job required that I stay back in the dining hall and clean up after dinner, and that intruded into study time and, consequently, into my sleep time. The problem was, I needed all the sleep I could get to be able to wake at four a.m. each day. This schedule was alright during the summer, but now that classes had started I was reduced to just a few hours of sleep per day.

My major was in animal husbandry and nutrition and my minor was in field crops and soils. I learned the basics of soil chemistry, geology, and how to grow the maximum yields in terms of tons and bushels per acre of ground. What was exciting was that I also learned how to design vitamin, mineral, and trace mineral supplement programs for livestock and agricultural economics. I even tried out for the university wrestling team and nailed down the 123-pound slot, the same weight division I wrestled in high school.

Not knowing how to budget my study time along with three jobs and a wrestling schedule created a near disaster for me. At the end of my first semester, I had earned a letter in wrestling and a C or B grade in almost every course—algebra, history, soils, and animal husbandry—English composition and inorganic chemistry were the two exceptions. I earned an A in English and a D in inorganic chemistry. The five-hour inorganic chemistry course was a pivotal one used specifically to weed out weak pre-veterinary and pre-med students in the first semester.

My advisor looked at my first semester B-minus report card, shook his head, and pronounced a death sentence over my dreams of ever becoming a veterinarian. He assured me that the competition for veterinary school was keen. There were only thirty freshman slots for 300 to 500 veterinary program applicants. I was devastated when he told me that an applicant with a B-minus average with a solid D in inorganic chemistry was not exactly going to be at the top of the list. He recommended that I go home and save the future tuition fees.

My first reaction was shock—total and speechless shock. I had worked hard, never missed a class, and studied as much as humanly possible with the grueling work schedule I had. It was then that I realized that I had worked very hard, but not very smart. This was the turning point where I decided that playtime was over. I desperately wanted to be a veterinarian and I was going to do whatever it took to become one.

I kept the jobs because I had to. I stayed on the wrestling team, but everything else disappeared—the Friday night dances, the girls, and the movies. They all went the same direction—out of my life.

My roommate had gotten an A-minus average. He knew how to study. He knew how to budget time, so he agreed to take me under his wing and show me how to do it. We took our thirty semester hours of course work and sorted and ranked each class according to its hourly value. We took the available study time and divided it up into relative hourly and half-hourly allotments. The plan worked like a dream.

There were courses in history, English composition, government and constitution, field crops, soils, fertilizer, animal husbandry, zoology, experimental zoology, genetics, poultry science, livestock judging, nutrition, entomology, algebra, ROTC, biochemistry, agricultural bio-chemistry, and organic chemistry. The courses that provided the greatest insights into my questions and chosen career as a veterinarian were soils, nutrition, agricultural biochemistry, and organic chemistry. The study of organic chemistry was essentially the study of carbon, carbon compounds, and carbon chains of various configurations, along with the kaleidoscope of cellular enzyme reactions that they were involved in.

Organic chemistry teaches you the actual physical structure of amino acids, proteins, carbohydrates, fats, oils, triglycerides, cholesterol, vitamins, hormones, and enzymes, and how they interact. Even though the course was called organic chemistry, we learned that every reaction and interaction of organic molecules required inorganic mineral catalysts and cofactors to complete. Without these mineral catalysts and cofactors, biochemical reactions can't reach their end point.

Think of it: vitamins, enzymes, hormones, every sub-cellular bio-chemical reaction, every metabolic cycle required mineral cofactors and catalysts, even oxygen itself could not be utilized without mineral cofactors. I learned that two-thirds of the essential nutrients, sixty out of ninety, were minerals.

Boyd Odell, affectionately known as "Digger Odell" after the radio funeral director character, was my professor in agricultural biochemistry. His research dealt with mineral deficiencies during pregnancy and the resulting congenital birth defects. He created spina bifida in laboratory animals in 1956 by feeding the pregnant mothers with diets deficient in zinc, vitamin B12, and folic acid.

It was exciting to know that we could prevent up to ninety-eight per cent of the birth defects in animals by supplementing the female with the proper nutrients prior to conception. The question we pondered was whether we could prevent birth defects in humans with nutritional supplements.

I studied dozens of congenital birth defects in laboratory and farm animals and what nutritional deficiencies produced them. What we found was that, in most instances, "genetic defects" are simple mineral deficiencies that leave a repeatable "fingerprint" on a specific gene, in a specific location, on a specific chromosome. They are no more compli-cated in concept than a deficiency of zinc resulting in a cleft palate or spina bifida in a farm animal. These minerals attached to the DNA molecule are known as "metallic fingers" and are essential to the function and repeatability of DNA to RNA to structural or enzymatic protein. As simple as it sounds, mineral deficiencies are the root cause of most diseases mistakenly thought to be "genetically transmitted."

Nutrition class taught us how to ensure that all of the essential nutrients, energy, and protein requirements were in each ration and that every mouthful was as nutritionally perfect for the submissive animal as it was for the dominant animal in the herd. We learned the nutritional requirements for optimal disease resistance, fertility, normal embryonic development, growth development, and milk and wool production for many different species. We learned the many deficiency diseases that occur when single and multiple nutrients were missing from a ration.

Calcium deficiency alone could result in as many as 147 different diseases ranging from osteoporosis, osteoarthritis, osteomalacia, degenerative athritis, Bell's Palsy, tinnitis, trigeminal neuralgia, and spinal stenosis to name a few.

4

WE CURED DISEASES IN ANIMALS WITH NUTRITION!

Agriculture school was a four-year course. The majority of students worked their way through and then headed back to the family farm armed with all kinds of high tech information for increasing yields, conserving the soil, reducing costs, and becoming more profitable. Those intent on going to veterinary school generally made application in their second year of Ag school, hoping to be accepted after graduation with a four year B.S. degree in Agriculture. A select few Ag students with superb grades entered veterinary school at the start of their fourth year. A tiny group of elite students had made it into veterinary school at the start of their third year.

Richard, my roommate, and I applied for veterinary school in 1960, mid-way into our second year of Ag school. We figured we'd at least practice the application and interview with the admissions committee. There was at least a reasonable hope of obtaining a veterinary student slot after our third year of Ag School. To our great surprise and joy we were accepted for entrance into veterinary school at the end of our sophomore year in Ag school—unheard of! Our Ag school classmates were agape with disbelief. Richard and I felt like we were the few, the proud, the Marines! Both just twenty years old, we'd been accepted into veterinary school with students who were in their thirties and forties, thanks to our grades and the sincere, lengthy letters of commendation we'd received from the husbandrymen of the university beef and dairy herds.

Once admitted to veterinary school, we weren't required to finish the two remaining years of Ag school. In fact, we were discouraged from attempting it because of the enormous first year veterinary school class load. Despite the warnings, Richard and I decided to go for broke and finish the last two years of Ag school simultaneously with the first two years of veterinary school. Not being quitters, we had started Ag school with the real goal of earning the B.S. degree. Not to finish was not only unthinkable—it was not even a possibility in our minds. With that same determination we attacked the courses in veterinary school just like we did in college; anatomy, histology, pathology, parasitology, microbiology, physiology, embryology, nutrition, pharmacology, clinical laboratory, and clinical diagnosis filled our days.

The most important lesson from veterinary school was learned early on. ***The reason that we put the vitamins, minerals, and trace minerals into animal feeds was because we don't have health insurance policies for livestock!*** If we used a human type health care system for them it would be "sticker shock" for you when you went to the store to buy meat, dairy, poultry, and eggs. Hamburger would cost you $275 per pound, boneless, skinless chicken breasts would be $450 per pound and a dozen eggs would be $50 just to pay for the health care. We learned that by significantly reducing or totally eliminating health care costs for animals we could keep the price of animal products low enough for the average American to afford them.

While the other vet students played bridge and threw horseshoes after class, I spent my extra time in the library and pathology departments studying nutrition and the diseases that resulted from nutritional deficiencies. I was so excited, I was beside myself; the pieces of the puzzle were coming together!

The fact that veterinarians could prevent and cure diseases in a whole herd or flock with nutritional supplements was a great fascination to me. If this concept of herd health could successfully be applied to humans we could eliminate an enormous amount of unnecessary misery, add many health-full years to people's lives, and save individuals and governments gobs of money!

While I was learning that vitamins, enzymes, and hormones were important to health, my studies kept pointing me to one basic fact: the plants livestock eat can't make minerals. Mineral deficiencies caused expensive diseases and livestock losses. To ensure optimum levels of all known essential minerals to prevent disease, we supplemented animal diets and rations with them; we did not leave the presence of these essential nutrients in the livestock feed to chance! So why weren't we doing that with the "human herd?"

For example, the mineral selenium was universally thought to be toxic until 1957 when it was found to be an essential nutrient in trace amounts in laboratory animals and livestock. Selenium deficiency causes infertility, miscarriages, cystic fibrosis of the pancreas, Sudden Infant Death Syndrome in animals, liver cirrhosis, stiff lamb disease, white muscle disease, muscular dystrophy, anemias, encephalomalacia (Alzheimer's disease), cardiomyopathy heart disease, and mulberry heart disease. In each case, selenium supplementation prevented the disease and in many cases reversed or cured existing diseases, which were all significant causes of animal losses to the livestock industry.

Muscle is meat. Muscle disease costs farmers money. In livestock we prevent and reverse these diseases with a few pennies a day of selenium because we don't have health insurance to pay for symptomatic treatment or to pay for the losses of meat production.

In humans we deal with fibromyalgia, muscular dystrophy, liver cirrhosis, and cardiomyopathy by treating the *symptoms*—not the deficiency, with muscle relaxants, prednisone, liver transplants, pacemakers, and heart transplants.

Another early symptom of selenium deficiency in older humans is the appearance of "liver spots" or "age spots." When one has ten age spots on their skin they have millions of them in their brain, eyes, thyroid gland, heart, lungs, liver, kidneys, intestines, bone marrow, and muscle. This "pigment of aging," scientifically known as *ceroid lipofucsin*, is a collection of rancid fat known as "free radicals" that interferes with cell function and increases one's risk of cancer, Alzheimer's disease, and heart disease many times.

Selenium supplementation along with the elimination of margarine and fried foods from the diet will make liver spots and age spots disappear on the outside. When they are gone on the outside they are going away on the inside. Once the pigment of aging goes away on the inside, people can add five, ten, twenty, and maybe even fifty extra health-full years to their life.

During the 1950s, we learned that copper deficiency would cause aneurysms. Turkeys raised on pasture for market will "finish" at different times over the summer. That's bad news for the farmer in terms of efficiency. To solve the problem, turkeys were placed on complete feed pellets with the goal of getting them ready for market within a few days or a week of each other. In the first thirteen weeks on the original complete pellet ration, fully half of the turkeys on this ration died. Farmers were picking them up by the bushel baskets full and taking them to the state diagnostic lab to see what they died from.

At autopsy, it was obvious that almost all of the dead turkeys had died from a ruptured aortic aneurysm. One clever pathologist said, "This has got to be due to a copper deficiency, because copper is required to manufacture the heavy elastic fibers found in arteries." The next year the amount of copper was doubled in the feed pellets and not a single turkey died from a ruptured aneurysm.

Copper deficiency in human beings presents itself first as white, gray, or silver hair. Copper is required as a cofactor to manufacture hair pigment for blond, red, brown, or black hair. Additional symptoms of copper deficiency include crow's feet, skin wrinkles, spider veins, varicose veins, hemorrhoids, liver cirrhosis, iron storage disease, and iron resistant anemia.

All of the copper deficiency diseases have been eliminated in the animal industry with commercially prepared pellets. In humans these copper deficiencies are treated symptomatically at great expense, unnecessary misery, and even death. When humans supplement with plant derived colloidal copper, their original hair color can come back, spider veins, varicose veins, and hemorrhoids can go away and some aneurysms can heal.

If an animal has arthritis, it has pain, lies down, and won't spend time at the feed box. As a result, it won't gain weight. Skinny animals don't sell for much. That's why the animal industry learned hundreds of years ago to prevent and cure livestock arthritis by supplementing with clay, bone meal, and lime stone. As veterinary science progressed, nutritional formulas to cure arthritis in pigeons, turkeys, dogs, cats, sheep, pigs, horses, cows, lions, tigers, and bears have become common place. Any number of feed pellets or other supplements exist to cure arthritis by rebuilding cartilage, ligaments, tendons, connective tissue, bone foundation, and bone matrix.

The prognosis is not so good for the human victims of arthritis. Wear and tear arthritis, osteoarthritis, degenerative arthritis, and ankylosing spondylitis make up 85 percent of all human arthritis. Seventy-five percent of all Americans over the age of 50 get arthritis of one type or another and to one degree or another. The Centers for Disease Control predict that 35 million to 50 million "Baby Boomers" will get arthritis in the next seven to ten years, and yet there's not a single medical treatment designed to prevent or fix it.

Painkillers and anti-inflammatory drugs are the arthritis treatment of choice in humans, though they're dangerous—even deadly side effects are rarely mentioned. None prevent or cure arthritis.

Aspirin doesn't fix arthritis and can cause gastric bleeding and death. **Tylenol**™ doesn't fix arthritis and causes 50,000 cases of kidney failure each year. Ten percent—five-thousand—of these cases of kidney failure are severe enough to require a kidney transplant. Ibuprofen, Advil™, and Aleve™ don't fix arthritis either, but they can cause liver damage in up to ten percent of users, some even requiring a liver transplant. Methotrexate™ and gold shots don't cure arthritis and they depress the bone marrow so it can't make normal platelets and white blood cells. Prednisone and cortisone don't fix arthritis and they *suppress* your immune system, leaving you open to diseases far worse than arthritis. Prolonged steroid use also accelerates demineralization of your bones.

When these over-the-counter and prescription drugs don't work anymore to relieve pain and inflammation, the only thing left for you medically is joint replacement surgery. These surgeries rarely work out well; they always have to be tinkered with. Elizabeth Taylor had three hip surgeries. How many hips does Elizabeth Taylor have? Two years after her last surgery she developed compression fractures of four vertebrae!

Treating arthritis' symptoms instead of the problem causing the pain is like cutting the wires to your dashboard warning lights so they don't annoy you anymore. Any responsible person knows the solution is to fix the problem that caused the warning light to go on . . . not ignore the light and burn out the engine. Killing the pain of arthritis without rebuilding the joints themselves is the same as cutting the wire to the red warning light!

Trace mineral depletion in animals and humans starts by causing the body to compensate for the shortage of a particular trace element. Increased intestinal absorption efficiency and/or reduction of excretion and gradual diminishment of body reserves take place. This phase of trace mineral deficiency returns to normal very quickly with a return of normal intake. There is little or no disturbance of biological structure or function; it is certainly not detectable by means of standard medical tests.

The compensated metabolic phase follows if the deficiency continues. It's characterized by a reduction of certain specific biochemical functions, such as trace mineral dependent enzyme reactions or receptor sites. The "homeostatic" mechanism becomes ineffective in maintaining the normal trace element concentrations at receptor sites causing a reduction in biochemical function (i.e. low blood sugar, irregular heart beat, white hair, hypertension, etc.).

The decompensated phase of trace element deficiency follows with the appearance of symptoms or defects. The body can no longer make up for the shortages. Trace mineral deficiency appears metabolically (prediabetes), cognitively (learning disabilities, ADD, ADHD), emotionally (panic attacks, anxiety, depression, Dr. Jekyll/Mr. Hyde), developmentally (dyslexia, gay behavior, cleft palate, Down's syndrome), and structurally (noisy joints, arthritis, bone spurs, aneurysms). A noticeable lack of stamina and longevity result.

The clinical phase of trace mineral deficiencies is characterized by the onset of full-blown disease states and even death—i.e., cardiomyopathy, diabetes, cancer, liver cirrhosis. Most trace mineral deficiencies in the clinical phase, though, are never diagnosed as such by the "orthodox" physician. The "cure," however, is often simply a matter of replacing the missing trace element. Positive clinical responses using this method can occur in as little as 48 hours to 30 days. Only those very few people whose deficiencies have caused permanent biochemical, chromosomal, or gross physical damage will not return to normal health.

Amazing as it sounds, relief for many apparently ill people is as little as a month away if the missing essential minerals are supplied in the proper amount. We can cure animals with nutrition, now let's take care of the "human herd!"

5

THE STUDENT BECOMES
THE TEACHER

I worked nights in the veterinary anatomy department preparing dogs, cats, sheep, goats, pigs, horses, cattle, and poultry as cadavers for dissection. Arteries were filled with red latex for easy tracing. Some mature specimens were prepared as articulated skeletons, which required long hours of simmering and cleaning the flesh from the bones. Each leg was placed in its own nylon stocking to keep all of the small bones of the foot properly assigned while the remnants of flesh were boiled away in a large steel drum. It was long, lonely, and stinky work, but the pay was good and I could study nutrition, nutritional deficiencies, and pathology while the bones simmered.

The summer between my freshman and sophomore years in veterinary school I began to take graduate courses in animal and human pathology and worked as a student pathology assistant performing autopsies on pets, livestock, laboratory animals, and wild species. The graduate pathology courses were the most interesting because I was introduced to human pathology through slide sets of human autopsies. I began taking three-hour and five-hour courses with a goal of earning a Ph. D. in comparative pathology down the road. One needed 21 hours of course work for a Masters degree, and over 38 hours for a Ph.D.

As a student veterinary pathology assistant I worked under the watchful eye of Dr. Loren Kintner. He was an artist with the physical and mechanical techniques of the autopsy room. Accurate and skilled in microscopic diagnosis, he was a real expert in culturing microorganisms too. Kintner's hidden asset was his power of observation and ability to listen and to hear bits and pieces of important clues provided unknowingly by the animals' owners, students, and clinicians.

Kintner taught me how to sharpen knives so sharp, they could cut a paper towel. He taught me how to remove the intact brain from the skull of a pig with three deft blows of a cleaver and a cow's brain with three blows of an axe—the years of cutting wood and learning axmanship was paying off. The mechanics of getting into the body cavities, skulls, and joints of dozens of species of animals and humans was an art in itself. I had to learn how to use skinning knives, scalpels, saws, shears, cleavers, and axes in a new way.

Each day after 3:00 p.m. I would go to the autopsy room, look in the cooler, and remove the pile of bodies. Once the bodies were matched with the autopsy request form, they were weighed, photographed, measured, and the body cavities opened up for examination. For a budding pathologist, it was like Christmas everyday.

Organ colors, shapes, weights, textures, and density were noted. Photographs were taken for the record, publications, and teaching. A standard approach to doing the autopsies for each species was established to avoid overlooking valuable anatomical clues. Samples were taken for microscopic examination and for culturing bacteria. Hemorrhages, abscesses, pneumonia, goiter, fractures, aneurysms, arteriosclerosis, and cancer were properly identified and photographed. The presence of parasites and abnormal lesions or structures was noted on the autopsy sheet. The cause of death on the autopsy record was left blank and filled in after the slides were viewed, toxicology results were available, and cultures were evaluated unless the cause could be immediately determined.

Many long nights at the microscope studying the hundreds of tissue samples and bacterial cultures generated by the autopsies taught me the secrets of life, disease, and death. Determining the time of death by examining the body temperature, relative state of digestion of stomach contents, and the presence of fly eggs and nibble marks on the lips and ear by mice was one early lesson. Recognizing and confirming the presence of bacterial diseases, viral diseases, parasitic diseases, poisoning, lightning strikes, trauma, cancer, tuberculosis, diabetes, multiple sclerosis, osteoporosis and the most interesting of all—nutritional deficiency diseases—was another. Comparing slides from veterinary and human autopsies, I noted another fascinating thing: human diseased tissue looked just like animal diseased tissue. Liver slides easily revealed the creature's sex. Red blood cells told other stories: boat shaped red blood cells came from camels. Red blood cells from birds, frogs, or reptiles have nuclei in them.

Diseased tissue—human or animal—presents a three-fold signature or finger print: anatomical changes that can be observed with the human eye ("gross anatomy"), microscopic changes, and biochemical changes. I soon learned to love the simple logic of pathology. With the mathematical precision of $2 + 2 = 4$, the answer in pathology is always there if you know the language and the questions to ask. Physical change "X" plus microscopic change "Y" and biochemical change "Z" equals one unique disease. I loved it! It was like classical Sherlockian deduction, "After you have eliminated the impossible, Watson, that which remains, no matter how unlikely, must be the truth."

Large animals were brought to the autopsy room on the bed of a truck. The overhead door was opened and the truck backed into the gymnasium-sized room. A stainless steel obstetrical chain was attached to a leg and the animal lifted off of the truck onto the tile floor by means of an electric power hoist. After hosing down the bodies of larger animals to eliminate mud and manure from the skin, the body cavities were opened up the same way each time and the positional relationships of organs were noted before the actual autopsy began. A grate-covered trench drain in the room's center caught the stomach and bowel contents, blood, and the large amount of water that was used to maintain cleanliness. Smaller animals—sheep, deer, small pigs, dogs, cats, turkeys, ducks, chickens, rabbits, rats, and mice—were autopsied on a small table with running water and a drain at one end to carry off blood and other fluids. Knee high gumboots were the uniform of the day to keep our shoes clean and to prevent slipping in the blood and water that were always on the floor.

Kintner was the most revered veterinary pathologist in the state of Missouri. Equally respected by academics, practicing veterinarians, and farmers alike, Kintner was sent the most difficult cases. Ninety-nine point nine percent of the time he could figure out what had caused the death when others had failed.

Performing 10 to 25 autopsies per day, the sheer volume of work taught me the basics of pathology. In a few weeks, I felt very well versed in the basics of animal pathology. My optimism would soon be tested. Shortly after arriving in the pathology lab, Dr. Kintner was scheduled to go on vacation for a week. His parting words were, "If you have any problems, just call Dr. McGinnity, the head of the large animal clinic; he's a pretty good pathologist." Murphy's Law clearly states, "If something can go wrong, it will. And if it can go wrong at a bad time or a worse time, it will go wrong at the worse time!" That's what happened to Joel Wallach. At 3: 00 p.m. on the Monday afternoon just hours following Dr. Kintner's departure, an army of farmers began arriving at the lab and backing up trucks loaded with dead animals into the autopsy room. There was literally a traffic jam.

Suddenly, there were carcasses of pigs, horses, sheep, and cattle lying in piles all over the autopsy room floor. Farmers stood by their pile of dead animals with autopsy request forms in hand. Used to Dr. Kintner's good and efficient services, they were impatient and stared at me with that look that said, "Well get on with it! Don't just stand there."

I dove into the piles of bloated bodies with gusto. Though I went through the mechanics of opening them up for examination, I didn't find any familiar tissue changes or easy answers like, "hit by car." I went through the piles searching for some familiar landmarks, and the animals very quickly began to look alike. Panic was mounting. I was supposed to be holding up the reputation of Dr. Kintner's pathology lab, but the tangible and vocal impatience of the frustrated farmers only made matters worse.

I sent another student to alert Dr. McGinnity. He was beside me in moments and recognized immediately that I was swamped with pathology cases and needed help. He quickly brought organization, calm, and focus to the chaotic situation. He drew my eye to a slight discoloration here, a tiny pinpoint hemorrhage there, a reduction in normal size or a change in organ texture. Bit by bit, Dr. McGinnity led me and taught me where the rubber met the road when it came to finding useful information at the autopsy table and adding it together to come to a useful collection of information known as a diagnosis. Between the two of us, we went through the whole forest of carcasses in a matter of hours. To use an analogy, I ended up flying the plane, but with the comfort of knowing that the flight instructor was in the right-hand seat beside me. We provided the service that the farmers were expecting. I had landed safely and learned early on, that when you don't know, it's best to ask for help from those who do know.

It is difficult to assess the contributions made to a pathologist's level of expertise and competence by each individual autopsy, but I know that it is enormous. Even when the process of growth and level of wisdom is not necessarily expanded due to repeated autopsy of the same type of disease, the lack of variety of disease exposure is more than compensated for by the depth and intensity of the experience. Pilots who safely coax

747s through numerous "touch and go" landings accomplish wondrous things even if they never leave the vicinity of the airport. Practice makes perfect.

On one occasion a farmer brought in a large Holstein cow that he had buried in a ditch for a week before he got curious as to why the old girl had died. He dug her up and brought her bloated purple carcass in for an autopsy. The cow's belly was distended and as tight as a drumhead. I hooked the chain to the decomposed cow's rear leg and lifted with the power hoist. Her rear leg tore loose like the drumstick of a well done turkey and a hundred gallons of putrid purple fluid noisily gushed out of her abdominal cavity under great pressure—most of the fluid seemed to find it's way into my boots. I wound up throwing those boots away because the smell never left. I learned to wear a rubber apron that reached my ankles so nothing could get into my boots as well.

A farmer brought in a pickup truck full of a dozen Hampshire lambs. Superficially, the lambs looked well nourished but dead—many with hay still in their mouths. Autopsies of all the lambs revealed nothing too exciting. They were all in perfect shape except that they all suffered from obvious goiter. Their thyroid glands were an angry purple color and enlarged ten times the normal size. Their blood had a slight chocolate color. In questioning the farmer, he claimed he had lost almost his entire flock of 500 lambs on one cool night. He had dutifully provided the lambs with a trace mineral salt block that contained iodine.

Chocolate discoloration of the blood indicated a problem with nitrates, a common fertilizer and pollutant from feed lots. I learned that it was a dry year in his county and the corn that they used for silage was heavily laden with nitrates as a result of the drought. Nitrates act as a goitrogen, a substance that depresses thyroid activity and creates a goiter, even when iodine is present in the diet. All the lambs had nitrate-induced goiter and hypothyroidism. They died during the cool fall nights, because they couldn't control their body temperature. This flock of lambs with nitrate-induced hypothyroidism became the subject of my first peer review, refereed journal article. I was published!

By the time I graduated veterinary school in 1964, I was an accomplished comparative pathologist. The combination of courses in basic veterinary pathology, advanced veterinary pathology, two summers of graduate courses in human and animal pathology, and the practical experience of thousands of autopsies in Dr. Kitner's autopsy room had trained me well. My peer reviewed article along with my studies in histopathology were the "icing on the cake." It didn't hurt that during my last two years of veterinary school I lived in a church parsonage in Roachport, Missouri. The rent was exchanged for providing veterinary services to the farmers of Roachport.

After graduating veterinary school, Richard Montrey, my roommate, and I headed off into different directions. He took a commission as an officer in the army veterinary corps. I took a position at the Iowa State Diagnostic Laboratory in Ames, Iowa doing service pathology for the veterinary school, laboratory animal facilities in the medical school, regional farmers, practicing veterinarians, and the wildlife department. Soon I was back to my old routine of doing as many as ten to 25 pathology cases per day by myself. A single case might include a 2,000-pound bull, a bucket full of dead rats, a pickup truck filled with 200 dead baby pigs or 20 turkeys in a trash can. On occasion I was blessed with the carcass of a deer, fox, coyote, raccoon, bobcat, snake, fish, turkey, or pheasant from the wildlife department. The sources of the wild animals ranged from road kills and wild animals baled in hay to animals killed in people's basements.

I quickly learned that wild animals were rife with nutritional deficiency diseases too. Dependent on the land and plants grown on the land for minerals, they were lucky if they found natural salt licks, clay beds, creek banks, coal deposits, or some other source of minerals. Many weren't lucky and suffered from infertility, congenital birth defects (spina bifida, cleft palate, heart defects, cerebral palsy, and extra or missing limbs), and degenerative diseases (arthritis, osteoporosis, kidney stones, diabetes, muscular dystrophy, and encephalomalacia).

Teaching filled my "spare" time as I taught veterinary pathology to senior veterinary and graduate students. To do that, I had to create a tissue and organ museum. While creating that museum and taking still more graduate courses in human and veterinary neuroanatomy, neuropathology and advanced pathology, I literally looked at thousands of tissue, bacterial, and parasitology slides each month and continuously expanded my own knowledge.

But for what great purpose was I expanding my knowledge? I'd soon learn. Jim Howard, a fellow veterinary pathology graduate student, and I shared an office in the diagnostic lab. We studied together a lot and became good friends. Jim was scheduled to leave Iowa State University at the end of the spring term and go to South Africa to do autopsies and parasite studies in hippos killed in population control programs. I had pangs of envy! Jim was going to be a wildlife veterinarian in Africa. The combination of being a wildlife veterinarian and a forest ranger in Africa was the dream career of many veterinary students. Jim suddenly canceled his trip when his daughter developed asthma.

Because we were friends and I had followed Jim's African project from the very beginning, I asked if I could fill his slot. I hoped the fact that I had worked with Marlin Perkins and that I was already an accomplished comparative and wildlife pathologist would qualify me. Letters were sent off to make the request official. My stint at the St. Louis Zoo and my association with Perkins carried the day. The fact that I was already an accomplished pathologist and that I was ready, willing, and able to go were the final qualifications. I resigned my post at the diagnostic lab and prepared to leave in two weeks for the new African adventure. The staff of the lab gave me a going away party with all kinds of favors of an African theme. In the midst of the festivities, I received a telegram informing me that my appointment in Africa was put on hold because of political problems with the U.S. They couldn't justify the money for an American to work the hippo project.

I decided to go anyway, figuring that they could hardly refuse me if I was there looking them in their eyes. I figured they could refund the cost of my tickets later. I flew to Johannesburg to take the first step. I wasn't going to let an international fuss interfere with my African adventure. Jim Howard and I had a mutual friend from South Africa by the name of John Marie. John made arrangements for his father to pick me up from the Jon Smuts Airport in Johannesburg and take me to the offices of the game and parks department. John's father had been the president of the National Wool Board Coop and knew everyone in the South African government.

By the time I had arrived in South Africa, the U.S. was at serious odds with the South African government. A trade embargo had been implemented to prevent export of American goods to South Africa. Americans were not too popular. At first the South African government wanted me to agree to a cancellation of my appointment, so I cooled my heels in a hotel for about a week. A week in Africa is very hot and very slow.

Finally a government veterinarian contacted me at the hotel. He said they had an assignment if I wanted it. I was to be shipped to the border of South Africa to do disease control of wildlife coming in from Botswana. I was supposed to work with rangers who would shoot any animals that came into a double-fenced kill zone. I'd then autopsy the animals, take blood samples, and look for foot and mouth disease, Renderpest, heart water, and black water disease.

"Why am I suddenly eligible for work?" I asked. They couldn't get anybody else to take the job. When I pressed for more details, the veterinarian responded, "We've already sent three veterinarians to do the work and only one came back alive." "What did they die from?" I asked. "I'll be very honest with you—Bilharzia—blood flukes," he said. I visited the lone survivor. He was my age but looked yellow and a thousand years older. He talked in hushed tones, eyes flitting, "They all die! They all die!"

I checked out several parasitology books from the library and learned everything there was to know about Bilharzia. Infected people or animals pass the eggs into the urine and then into water. The larval stages hatch from the eggs and then enter snails. A second intermediate stage then leaves the snail into the water. From the water the final larval stage enters humans through the skin and then into the blood stream. After a thorough literature search I concluded, "Simple! Avoid water! Just keep away from pools, ponds, streams, and water troughs. Resist the understandable temptation to take off your shoes and socks and stick your feet in a pond to cool off. Just bear with the 120 degree temperatures of the Kalahari Desert!"

I found myself in a government veterinary office in the small town of Vryheid. I lived in a small confining hotel room, but I was on the road a great deal of time and wasn't bothered too much by the sparse accommodations. Vryheid was an Afrikaaner-speaking town. The white population spoke 14th century Dutch; the black population spoke Zulu. If anyone could speak English, they chose not to do so. I picked up grade school primers and began to learn Afrikaans and Zulu. I checked out history books and learned the dual histories of the Afrikaan and Zulu cultures.

Early in the mornings, I was picked up by rangers. We patrolled the border area. Kudu, impala, eland and other animals were shot and autopsied. Slides were made of blood and spleen smears to look for parasites; blood was collected to test for viral diseases. Once each week, I held a small animal clinic to administer rabies vaccine to dogs and cats. Once per month I was required to give a small animal clinic in the town of Dundee. The driver who came to collect me was a slight Indian man by the name of Mukherjee. Surprisingly, the town was made up mostly of Indian merchants. With a name like, "Dundee," I was expecting a clan of Scotsmen!

I soon learned that in South Africa, rugby was more of a religion than a sport. The sports boycott was a bigger thorn in their side than any economic sanctions. Inevitably, the rugby fever got to me too. I was already in great physical shape from my wrestling and weight lifting, and I began to show up at rugby practices for the Vryheid police team. Being the new guy on the block, the first team coach asked me to fill in a red-shirt slot, as they were a man short. Rugby players were as big as university football players from America and as fast and as agile as soccer players. They never wore padding and were very aggressive. Never intimidated by a big guy, when they ran at me I took them out with a football block to the knees, whether they had the ball or not. I was elevated to a member of the first string for the next three months.

I guess you could say that I found the secret to surviving the Kalahari and the rugby field was no fluke.

6

OPERATION RHINO

After three months in Vreyheid as a State Veterinarian, I was contacted by the same government veterinarian and asked to take up another position. This next adventure was to be with the Natal Game and Fish Department on a project known as "Operation Rhino," tracking, catching, moving, and studying the rare and endangered white rhino. They were using a new experimental drug identified only as M-99—later known as etorphine. A derivative of morphine, M-99 was 25,000 times more potent than morphine. It was very effective as an immobilizing drug for large animals, but they had to have a veterinarian work on the project to handle the drug because it was a controlled narcotic.

I was transported to the Umfolozi Provincial Park in Natal, the home of the largest herd of free-ranging white rhino. The herd of 500 rhino migrated between the Umfolozi and a second park known as Hluhluwe Game Reserve. The connecting strip of Crown Land between the two parks was known as "the Corridor."

My responsibility was to control, administer, and deliver M-99. M-99 was a major advance in capture drug technology. Because of it's great strength in small concentrations, accurate darting equipment could be used to deliver the drugs. The breakthrough drug had another advantage: it had an antidote. Instead of having to wait for long unpredictable periods of time for a drugged animal to recover as with the original capture drugs, one could administer the antidote intravenously, and the rhino would wake up when you wanted it to. It would be conscious and could be safely crated in a matter of minutes. The crated rhino is then winched up a set of steel rollers hooked onto the bed of the truck. The boxed rhino could then be released in other areas or taken to the training *bomas*, the Zulu word for corral. Young and medium sized rhino were kept in the *bomas*, where they would be accustomed to being locked up in shipping boxes for long oceanic voyages or long, scorching overland trips.

Operation Rhino was just getting into full swing in August 1965. They chose me reluctantly for the high profile and romantic Operation Rhino project for two reasons. One, I was immediately available to go through basic game ranger training. Two, no local veterinarians wanted to be on foot in the desert tracking and capturing rhino using the new experimental drugs and dart gun delivery system. For a farm boy, a one ton rhino is no different than an angry one ton shorthorn bull. I respected them but I wasn't afraid. Additionally, the elephants at the St. Louis Zoo were much bigger than the rhino, and for this job, I wouldn't be getting so "up close and personal."

Ironically, by 1961, fifty plus years of conservation efforts on behalf of the endangered white rhino had created a relative overpopulation because of the land's limited ability to annually recover and support large numbers of rhino. Between 1812 and 1896, the southern race of white rhino dwindled because the incessant northward spread of agriculture which from the Cape greatly reduced the suitable grassland available to the white rhino, a specialized grazing animal. Little by little, the grass cover of the *veldt* was burned and replaced with crops and orchards. There was still plenty of land unoccupied by man, but it invariably had a dense cover of acacia and other bush. The white rhino was not a sufficiently flexible animal to make the adjustment. As late as 1890, small battalions of armed Zulu poachers were commissioned to collect rhino horn, a commodity much in demand in the Orient. They relentlessly hunted the scattered individuals of a once grand population of white rhino, decimating their ranks further. By 1896, the white rhino was officially thought to be extinct.

In 1927, surprisingly a small herd was located in a minute triangle of land framed by the White and Black Umfolozi Rivers in Zululand near the eastern coast of Natal Province, the lush mideastern province of the Republic of South Africa. Only twenty individual white rhino were counted. This unexpected discovery led to the establishment of Crown Land to protect the animals. Mr. Vaughn Kirby and Captain H.B. Potter, the original conservators, led small squads of loyal Zulu game scouts in fending off poachers. Continued protection by the Natal Parks Board over the years saw the white rhino numbers swell to a respectable five hundred head by 1960.

A corridor existed between the two reserves where the white rhino lived. In addition to overpopulation problems, the corridor between the two reserves was coming under serious political scrutiny. Some wanted the corridor land turned over to Zulu tribesmen for subsistence farming.

There were two possible alternatives to solving the rhino problem: (1) begin a systematic program of cropping and controlling the rhino numbers by a shooting program; or, (2) carry out the seemingly impossible dream of moving a significant portion of the Umfolozi herd to other reserves and establish satellite herds. The Natal Game and Fish Department opted to set up the satellite herds and establish captive herds of white rhino in game parks all over the world—"Operation Rhino" was born.

Skills from my Eagle Scout days already qualified me as an experienced tracker and hunter, so the concept of getting close to the rhino for a shot with the tranquilizer gun was no great mental leap for me. The original delivery system for the tranquilizer drugs was primitive and unique. The first delivery system for immobilizing drugs was simply a standard target dart with a needle that was dipped in pure nicotine. The darts were shot into the animal by means of a CO_2 powered "tranquilizer gun," or "dart gun."

Injected nicotine temporarily paralyzes the animal's nervous system so the immobilized animal can be caught with a lariat, cowboy style. This primitive darting system was limited to deer-sized animals because the volume and dose of drug was limited to what would adhere to the needle. Only the appearance of powerful immobilizing drugs like M-99/etorphine allowed a project like Operation Rhino to be carried out. Etorphine is 25,000 times more potent than morphine, so only a one milligram dose was required to immobilize an adult white rhino weighing 6,000 pounds or a small cow elephant—a thimble full of etorphine, one c.c. of the liquid drug. That small amount could easily be contained in a small "syringe" that could accurately be shot through the dart gun. And unlike previous immobilizing agents, etorphine had a quick acting antidote, nalorphine, which could revive the rhino at will. The completed dart fit neatly into the barrel of a 20-gauge shotgun. A rubber plunger lubricated with petroleum jelly was placed halfway up the length of the dart tube. The appropriate dose of liquid M-99 was loaded into the front end of the tube ahead of the plunger; then a hollow needle with a barb screwed into place at the front end of the dart.

The rhino to be captured was identified and approached from down wind to within the accurate darting range of 10 to 25 yards. To assemble the dart, a steel ball bearing was placed in the rear cavity of the tail assembly of the dart, and a baking soda pellet was placed on top of the ball bearing. The whole assembly was the size of an "AA" battery and was then covered with wax paper that was held in place with clear nail polish. This much of the dart could be assembled in advance. Just before the dart was to be fired through the tranquilizer gun though, white corn vinegar was poured into the rear of the dart behind the plunger. The tail assembly of the dart was screwed into place and the completed dart was fired at the rhino. The final assembly of the dart just prior to firing it at the rhino was kind of like firing a second shot at an animal with a flintlock. Quick loading had to be done to be successful. When the dart hit its target, momentum carried the ball bearing forward driving the baking soda pellet through the wax paper barrier into the vinegar, resulting in the generation of carbon dioxide. The expanding carbon dioxide gas then forced the plunger forward, injecting the M-99 into the rhino.

The whole injection process might take just seconds if the weather was hot and if the delivery assembly had been constructed perfectly. On a cold day when the plunger lubricant was thick and cold, the injection process might take as long as several minutes—if the needle barb held in place for the entire dose of M-99 to be dispensed. On occasion the dart mechanism would prematurely fire in mid-flight, uselessly spraying out the drug.

The next generation of dart injection assemblies were placed directly in the rear cavity of the plunger. The new injection technology was a primer cap with a floating firing pin held in place with a weighted spring. When the dart hit the target, the weight of the firing pin compressed the spring to set off the primer. The resulting gas from the exploding primer pushed the plunger forward in a tenth of a second. In addition to the greater injection speed, this new delivery system could effectively inject volumes of drugs—up to ten milliliters of a liquid drug—so a wild adult elephant weighing fifteen thousand pounds could now be tranquilized!

The primer injection system raised the darting process from the realm of an art form to a more predictable level and a technology.

There were two types of tranquilizer guns. The original was the classic factory production Daisy CO_2 pellet gun mechanism hooked to a .20 gauge shotgun barrel. The gun was powered with a Daisy brand compressed CO_2 cartridge. A charge of CO_2 drove the dart in a flat trajectory accurately for about fifteen to twenty yards. The slow speed and large size of the dart made the whole process iffy—wind, brush, grass, and temperature all affected accuracy. The second version of the tranquilizer gun was a .20 gauge single shot breech-loading shotgun. Twenty gauge shot gun shells were opened up and the shot removed, the dart with arrow style feather fletching was then inserted tail first into the shell. The shot shell and the dart were put into the breech of the gun. This system was used with small darts, on occasion, for long shots of fifty yards and the larger darts used for elephant.

A negative feature of the shotgun shell delivery system was that the feathers on the tail of the darts would melt from the heat of the powder blast. If the basic dart body and tail survived the powder blast and the impact that resulted from hitting the rhino, the tail had to be refletched as if one was making an arrow. My archery merit badge paid off in refeathering darts too.

The second generation of shotgun dart delivery system was a special insert that went into the breech of the shot gun that held the dart and was powered by a .22 caliber Ramset charge used to drive nails into concrete. This little Ramset charge would drive a standard one-millimeter rhino dart accurately for 75 to 100 yards under ideal circumstances.

Once a rhino was darted, a team of Zulu scouts mounted on horses followed the disappearing animal, keeping visual contact until the animal became immobilized. The scouts were protected from injury during the chase by crash helmets and heavy leather gauntlets. Thick canvas aprons shielded the horses from three-inch-long, sharp, ripping acacia thorns and coronet guards protected their hooves from rocks and cactus thorns.

When the downed rhino's position was fixed, the horsemen relayed the message by walkie-talkie to the waiting truck crew and the catching team.

The truck crew would back up to the nose of the tranquilized rhino, and the one ton transport crate was dumped on the ground in front of it. A two-inch-thick manila rope was lashed around the animal's head, behind the posterior horn, passed forward through the crate and out a three-inch hole in the opposite end door. When the rhino was given the antidote, it would recover from the affects of the M-99 in a moment or two, stand up and was pulled and pushed and guided into the crate, the rear door was closed and we had a rhino.

We braved blistering desert heat over 100°F, deadly cobras, and the life-threatening charges of Cape buffalo and the rhinos themselves. We lived off the land, eating wart hogs that were deemed to be grazing competitors with the rhino. We stayed in the field for as long as a month living in tents and cabins. In addition to the wildlife work, I also took care of two hundred head of horses and mules used by the park service. Fuel was expensive and horses could run on grass and hay.

I observed that rhino, elephant, and other animals spent a great deal of time breaking apart and eating clay termite nests and crushed limestone road beds for calcium and trace minerals. Wild animals obviously required minerals, too. To confirm this observation, soil, vegetation, and water analyses were made in various areas of the parks. These studies proved that the healthier and larger animals came from areas that were mineral rich. Wild animal populations avoided mineral poor water, forage, and soils—the same behavior as my soils professor, Bill Albrecht, had pointed out in domestic livestock!

The heavily mineralized water holes were used to the point that all plant life surrounding the water was devastated and completely consumed down to the roots. The water holes were surrounded by great bare dustpans. By contrast, the soft water holes, the ones that lacked minerals, had brush and grass growing right up to the waterline because the mineral deficient plants and water held little or no interest to the animals as food.

One invariably saw more small animal life while stalking rhino than when taking a casual stroll through the grass. On many occasions, while concentrating on the approach to a rhino, a family of warthogs would be flushed from their dust baths. Their thunderous exit can make one think one has stumbled upon a buffalo, and result in the appearance of a nervous sweat, followed by a deep sigh of relief.

The general principles for stalking rhino are the same as for stalking other animals. Sudden encounters are to be expected, but on many occasions I couldn't avoid being rattled a bit. Early in my training period, John Clark, the reserve's main rhino tracker, and I were stalking a rhino on the open veldt when I flushed a cobra! We were on our bellies in rather short dry grass about fifty yards behind a lone bull rhino, when I heard a faint rustle in the grass to my right.

Moving just my eyes, I saw the flared hood of a *Ringhal* cobra not ten inches away from my face. The shiny black snake had been caught unaware by our silent approach. Alarmed, it had reared up with its hood spread in a typical cobra warning. John was only two feet away from me but was so intent on stalking the rhino that he was unaware of my predicament.

Fortunately, the Ringhal is not an aggressive snake, and when it realized that I was not a source of immediate danger, it lowered the front part of its body into the grass and moved off. Unlike most species of cobra, the Ringhal, which literally means "ring-necked" in Afrikaans, gives birth to live young. These interesting snakes prefer to feign death when approached, by turning over on their backs; however, if handled or accidentally trod upon they will bite vigorously or eject a fine venom spray at their tormentor's face.

Following the snake's departure, I rolled on my back sweating profusely for a few minutes before John realized something had happened. We shared a chuckle and then went on and caught our rhino.

I had been lucky that day, for if I had been bitten, it would have meant an hour's ride to the camp and the refrigerator that held the lifesaving antivenin. It was impossible to keep antivenin in the Land Rover, since the temperature in the vehicle climbed above 80 degrees at midday during the winter, and over 120 degrees in the summer.

For me, the thirst to use a new skill is insatiable, and I was anxious to get as much experience as I possibly could tranquilizing rhino. We were out driving in the hilly southwestern portion of the reserve near the Madhlozi River, when we caught sight of a young cow rhino that met our requirements. We pulled off of the road and motioned for Moses and his truck crew to wait.

Moses and his five-man crew climbed out of the truck and perched on top of the rhino crate to watch the proceedings. The rhino saw us get out of our vehicle and walk casually towards her. The wind was in our favor, but when we came within fifty yards of her, she snorted, turned, and trotted off into the wind, tail up in typical rhino fashion.

Sometimes a bold approach on the part of the hunter is less disconcerting to the rhino than a sneaky approach in open country. The huge animal has difficulty in recognizing vertical objects, and as long as the hunter approaches from the perpendicular to the rhino's gaze, the rhino is usually mesmerized and will hold their ground.

Failing on our first approach, we stubbornly trotted upwind after our shy cow. Our next attempt up the side of one more hill was also useless. In a last desperate effort to avoid failure, I used "Kentucky windage," aimed the tranquilizer gun about four feet above the cow's shoulder in-line with her leg, and lobbed the dart downhill over a distance of sixty yards. I saw the dart hit the grass at the young cow's feet and thought the day's catch was officially a flop.

As the cow retreated up the succeeding hill, I noticed that she was showing an unusually springy "hackney" gait—typical of the early stages of being tranquilized. Watching for a few additional moments, I realized that she must have gotten the drug somehow. We dashed back to the Land Rover and circled around to the hill's ridge, where the cow was quite comfortably asleep in the shade. At a glance, we could see that the dart had struck her in the foot, needle first. It held fast, allowing the drugs to be injected.

Every now and then an incident occurred which reminded us that rhino are wild animals, and that becoming blasé or overconfident about them could be extremely dangerous.

We were looking for a young bull to fill the only empty pen in the *boma*. The day was far from perfect for catching operations because of a twenty-five-mile-an-hour wind that was occasionally gusting up to sixty. Most wildlife had sought cover from the driving wind and the chafing sound of the sand being whipped up from the veldt. After an entire morning of searching, we had caught only a brief glimpse of three black rhino as they covered the open veldt, their tails held high in the air and their rumps to the fierce wind.

A troop of about fifteen Chacma baboons occupied our attention for a few moments, as they began quarreling over some delectable scorpions at the edge of a water hole. While we watched, we took a short rest to eat sandwiches and cookies and then continued our drive east along a little-used vehicle track. Before long we came upon a bachelor herd of five young bulls taking shelter from the wind in a shallow pan. Making a stalk on these animals was fairly easy, because they were battened down in the mud with the roaring of the wind in their ears and the constant blast of windblown sand on their skins.

Getting within fifteen feet helped reduce the wind's deflecting effect on the tranquilizer dart. After picking out the most likely looking bull, I darted him in the shoulder just above the waterline. The rhino herd, caught completely unaware, jumped to the alert at the report of the dart gun. They milled around and shouldered each other for a moment, then thundered from the pan as a unit with mud and water flying.

The game scouts that we normally used for horsemen were on another assignment, so we tagged after the rhino alone on foot. Trotting steadily about twenty yards apart, we kept our eyes to the ground so as not to lose the rapidly fading windblown tracks.

Suddenly, I realized there was a large mass on the path in front of me. I came to a slow-motion stop and saw an old cow rhino with an unusually straight horn staring intently at me. Behind the cow was a one thousand pound bull calf turning first to the left, then to the right in blind confusion.

I whistled to let the old girl know I was a human, hoping she would turn and trot off. Only then did I realize I was on her windward side, but it was too late! Out of reflex she ran straight into the wind towards me.

I was stumped for a moment, since I hadn't been in this predicament before. But when she came within ten feet and continued to disregard my shouting, I pulled myself up into a handy acacia tree, just before the bull calf arrived and whacked the trunk of my tree with his horn, displaying a certain degree of devilish gusto.

Moses, the driver, pulled up with the truck shortly afterwards, a broad grin beaming on his face—he and his crew had seen the rhino chase me up the tree. After I broke down and returned the smile, he let out a hearty base James Earl Jones laugh. Now I had truly been initiated into the capture team.

We picked up the drugged bull with anticlimactic ease and deposited it at the *boma* only to find an urgent message waiting for me to contact Nick Steele, the senior ranger as soon as we returned.

By the time I reached Nick Steele's office, he was tense and tight-lipped. After inviting me to sit down he related a chilling story. A Zulu woman collecting firewood had been killed by a white rhino in the Biyala native location while returning to her *kraal*. Her eight-year-old daughter had witnessed the tragedy and ran back to the *kraal* for help. To complicate matters, the poor woman had an infant strapped to her back in traditional Zulu fashion. Fortunately, the woman's would-be rescuers found the infant miraculously unharmed, silent and wide-eyed! This story took the humor out of the day's earlier events.

The dead mother and the children had met a lone rhino on the path to the *kraal* on many similar occasions. The normally docile white rhino had simply left the path at the appearance of the villagers. This time, for some unknown reason, the rhino chose to hold its ground, flared its nostrils, and let out great chuffing and snorting sounds. The woman was still unafraid, so she picked up clods of dirt and threw them at the determined rhino.

The rhino had apparently been baffled by this action, because it was allowed to go on for several moments without reaction. Finally, the rhino decided it had had enough and came straight at the woman, who stood her ground, shouting and waving her arms until the aggravated rhino struck. The animal's horn struck the woman in the groin and passed through her body to reappear between her shoulder blades, narrowly missing the child on her back. Only then did the older child, until then frozen with fear, run weeping back to the *kraal.*

Steele was only waiting for official permission from the Native Trust for us to enter the location and capture the offending rhino. The Biyala were justifiably upset and seemed to think that the Parks Board was responsible for the animal's action. The headman of the *kraal* was very worried, because most of the young men had armed themselves with spears and a few handmade shotguns and disappeared into the bush. The proud people were not poachers, but cattlemen. In the past, they had been fined for permitting their cattle to graze in the game reserve and cause damage to the veldt. To the Biyala, the parallel was simple—if they were responsible for the actions of their cattle, we were responsible for the actions of the game animals!

Steele felt that there was now a serious threat to the ninety-five rhino in the various native locations, as well as to the rangers who hoped to rescue them.

Five days passed before we received permission from the Native Trust to enter the Biyala location. We were now officially sanctioned to take in a squad of SAP (South African Police) for protection during our hunt for the killer rhino. It took three more days to organize and coordinate the Biyala operation. When we finally left the main camp, we were in full-dress Parks Board uniforms and fitted with side arms. Our Land Rover was fitted with a field radio set on a frequency with the Mpila main office in the Umfolozi game reserve and the SAP vehicles. This was the only time we were ever required to carry arms on rhino operations during my stay with the Parks Board. We drove to the Madlozi camp, where we picked up John Tinley, the regional ranger, and his head tracker.

John was the Parks Board's gentle giant—he was six-foot-seven, soft-spoken, and very likable. He was also one of the Parks Board's best rifle shots. It was a good feeling to have John's rifle backing us up on this expedition.

Our small safari of two Land Rovers and two trucks reached the police outpost at midmorning. The Biyala headman was there, and he was shaking his head woefully, as he explained to the sergeant that the *kraal's* young men were still upset and bent on seeking revenge for the woman's death.

After a quick cup of tea and going over the game plan, the safari left with the addition of three Land Rovers full of SAP. On the way to the Biyala Trust where the woman had been killed, the headman explained to us that there were more than ten white rhino in the area, and there was no way to identify the killer with any degree of certainty. When we arrived at the kraal, we found small groups of silent women and hushed children watching us with somber eyes. The only men in camp were the headman and a half-dozen elders. With the armed young men in the bush, it was readily apparent that we not only had to be concerned for the rhino's safety, but also for our own.

A check of the area immediately surrounding the kraal revealed the fresh tracks and steaming manure of many white rhino. Steaming dung piles and sharp tracks in the dust let us know that there were several rhino of different ages in the area. The eight-day delay in getting to the scene had allowed the offending rhino's trail to grow cold.

After a more thorough look around, we radioed Mpila to ask just how many rhino we were supposed to catch and relocate to Umfolozi under the circumstances. The message came back to catch at least one by nightfall. Failing to do this, we were to find an old bull, shoot it and give the meat to the village; hopefully, this assertive act of killing one rhino would satisfy the villagers' hunger for revenge and save the others from reprisal.

After loading up the dart guns, we spread out and gingerly began a criss-cross search through the dry bush. Suddenly, a lone bull was flushed from his hiding place in the dense thorn and nearly ran down Tinley's head tracker. Deftly stepping aside with the grace and confidence of a matador, the ever-alert scout allowed the bull to pass by in its frenzied escape.

We followed the tracker for nearly a mile, before he pointed to the bull's ears sticking over some low bush about a hundred yards away. We were downwind, but the dry leaves on the ground prevented a silent stalk and placed the odds in the bull's favor.

Ever alert to our presence the bull kept a constant distance of forty yards. On the open veldt, one could easily sink an accurate dart shot at that distance, but in heavy bush, it might as well be a hundred miles. A blade of grass could deflect the dart's flight enough to cause a miss. I had to get closer.

As we reached the base of the slope, where John had a vantage point, he signaled violently to me to turn on the walkie-talkie. John radioed the location of a cow and a calf. The two rhino had barely avoided me by standing still in a heavy screen of cover, allowing us to pass within a few yards of them on our way into the fields. Fanning out, we turned back with our dart guns cocked. A cow appeared in the small clearing to my right, snorting and crashing through the bush. Just before firing my dart gun, John shouted that his dart had already struck the rhino. We waited a few minutes before trailing her and found her lying down in a small open acacia thicket with her calf nudging her in an effort to get her up and escape. The squealing calf was bewildered by it's mother's sudden desire to sleep in the face of immediate and obvious danger.

I unloaded my dart gun and poured out half of the M-99 from the dart to make the dose appropriate for the calf. It was then a simple matter for me to walk up and dart the calf from about ten yards. The young bull went down quickly next to its mother. After anchoring the animals to trees with ropes, I radioed to Moses to bring up the trucks and the police.

While the vehicles were grinding their way towards us over the rough terrain, ten old women and about twenty-five chattering children appeared in the area to see and touch the rhino that the "uniforms" had "killed." Big John kept the women and children entertained with jokes and stories in fluent Zulu until the truck arrived.

The SAP stayed near the drugged rhino and probably by their presence prevented the kraal's young men from venting their rage on the immobilized animals.

The crate was put in place in front of the cow. The Biyala children closed around us with intense curiosity, as the rope was placed on the rhino's head. Their curiosity was brought to a greater peak when I put the needle containing the antidote into the cow's ear vein. John explained in Zulu that we were wizards and were going to wake up the "dead" rhino and take them home with us.

When the cow stirred to get up, a huge sigh of awe was released from the crowd. As the cow was guided nimbly into the crate, torrents of approving laughter could be heard from the children. The calf was able to get up without the antidote and was ushered into the second box.

We had plenty of help with the massive rollers that afternoon. The older children volunteered to help lift them into position on the tailgate of the truck. The loaded crates were winched onto the trucks, and we happily left the Biyala location just as darkness fell. The squad of SAP left us at the boundary fence to the Umfolozi. Thankfully, it hadn't been necessary for them to come to blows with the Biyala, for they were normally good neighbors.

While we drove straight through the Umfolozi on the main tourist road, we radioed Mpila and Steele was informed of the successful events in the Biyala location. The scouts and rangers on alert could now stand down and relax.

At the Black Umfolozi River crossing we continued north through the corridor to Hluhluwe. The cow and calf were released into the safety of the reserve in the darkness. They trotted off, uncertain in their new surroundings and unaware of the drama that had taken place on behalf of their kind.

The Parks Board was determined to remain good neighbors with the surrounding Zulus in the various locations. To show our thanks to the Biyala for their restraint and cooperation, we shot six wildebeests and sent the meat to their *kraals*.

After six months of working on the Operation Rhino project I was presented with an orphan white rhino that had been found alone and dehydrated. The small female calf was only a few days old, about ten inches of its umbilical cord was still attached to its belly. No one had ever been successful in raising such a small baby rhino before. However, I had raised two baby elephants and I was a veterinarian, so I took on the project with great optimism.

Canned milk had been tried as a formula for previous attempts to raise rhino calves. All had subsequently died from diarrhea and dehydration. I used very diluted powdered milk designed for calves that had been fortified with vitamins and minerals. Giving very small amounts at each feeding, I left the rhino baby a little bit on the hungry side. The conservative approach worked and the infant rhino flourished.

Measurements of her height, weight, length, horn growth, and dental eruptions were faithfully recorded daily—basic information never before recorded for the early development of the white rhino was now available. The resultant growth and dental records and the enriched milk formula were written up as an original article for the International Zoo Yearbook. When the baby was six months old she was shipped to the zoo in Natal, where she was very popular because of her fondness for humans.

I was also assigned to do hundreds of autopsies on antelope, zebra, hippo, and wart hogs killed during population control programs. I also examined the white and black rhino found dead or killed because they had been injured by tourist cars. Arthritis, osteoporosis, goiter, heart disease, parasites, and birth defects were common, just as I had seen in domestic animals, captive zoo animals, and North American wild animals. Wild animals exhibited pica and cribbing, that behavior of eating non-food items when they are mineral deficient. I've seen giraffe eat antelope bones; elephants eat termite nests containing trace minerals brought up from hundreds of feet underground by the tireless insects. All wild animals preferred highly mineralized and muddy water to clear soft water.

Even here in the bosom of a pristine natural habitat, I was constantly reminded that plants can't manufacture minerals. If there are no minerals in the soil, they're not in the plants. If there are no minerals in plants, the plant-eating wild animals will get mineral deficiency diseases. It's elementary, Watson!

There was no human hospital or clinic within a hundred miles. For the Zulu on foot, it might as well have been a thousand miles. It didn't take long for the word to get around that I was some kind of doctor. The local people started dropping by for advice, minor surgery, and treatment. I delivered babies, cleaned infected wounds, sewed lacerations, drew blood samples, and handed out aspirin and cough syrup to kids with the croup.

Nutritional deficiencies were very common. Vitamin A deficiencies in children caused keratitis, corneal ulcers, and blindness. Calcium deficiency caused osteomalacia in children and arthritis and osteoporosis in adults. Iodine and copper deficiencies caused goiter in adults and miscarriages. Infants born with spina bifida and serious cleft palates as a result of folic acid or zinc deficiencies did not survive the primitive environment. Simple protein deficiency was not uncommon and revealed itself as bloated edematous children with Kwashiorkor. Beriberi with resultant congestive heart failure was common, the result of a thiamin or vitamin B1 deficiency. I handed out multiple vitamin-mineral tablets that I picked up in the rare excursions to Durban.

From these experiences on the farm, in the laboratory, and in the wilds of Africa I quickly learned that it doesn't matter whether one is a creationist or a student of evolution—our immediate mutual problem is that the Earth, our planet, is a limited finite resource for the raw materials that are the basis of all plant, animal, and human life as we know it. Living organisms procure their raw materials of essential elements and minerals for reproduction, development, growth and maintenance and for longevity from a thin, fragile blanket of organic and inorganic matter and gas on or just above the Earth's crust.

7

EVERY ANIMAL AND EVERY HUMAN

THAT DIES OF NATURAL CAUSES, DIES OF A NUTRITIONAL DEFICIENCY DISEASE

Excursions to Southern Rhodesia (now Zimbabwe) to deliver captured wild and *boma* trained white rhino to Kyle Dam Game Reserve and Wankie National Park were a common part of Operation Rhino. While there, I was invited to participate in elephant capture projects designed to brand and mark them for population and migration studies.

The permanent elephant population was facing a crisis in the Wankie National Park. Civilization and agriculture were crowding them on every side. The normal elephant migration formerly gave the park four months to recover during the rainy season. With man staking a claim on every side, the migrations stopped. Overgrazing stripped the grasslands and young trees bare. Doom was on the horizon for the elephant—nobody wanted them. They were neither rare nor endangered, and they were destructive.

While we had a social beer "off the shelf" on the patio of the Kyle Dam Pub to savor our success in replanting a white rhino population in Rhodesia, we began to design our plans for Operation Elephant. The Rhodesians didn't have the money, the trained personnel, the darting equipment, or the drugs to bring Operation Elephant to reality by themselves. I promised to get the darting equipment, the M-99, and the money and to personally see that the project in fact happened.

In the spring of 1966, my mentor, Marlin Perkins sent me a telegram inviting me to leave the Operation Rhino project in South Africa to join him in a large research project in the United States.

Perkins, along with Barry Commoner, a professor of botany at Washington University in St. Louis, Missouri had gotten a $7.5 million grant from the National Institutes of Health to study the world ecology, the environment, and the impact of pollution on the plant and animal populations of the world. The program combined the facilities of Washington University's biology department, the Shaw's Botanical Gardens, and the St. Louis Zoological Gardens into a new university department known as The Center for the Biology of Natural Systems.

I thought about the invitation for about a week and initially wrote a polite thank you but no thank you letter which I placed on the mantel. A month later I realized the letter was still there, unmailed. I reread the letter, then tore it up. Marlin Perkins had personally written the invitation, and Perkins was not the sort of person you could turn down. I had said that I would do anything to work with Perkins; besides, I would be working with a greater variety of animal species!

At Perkin's request I became a postdoctoral fellow in comparative pathology and comparative medicine at The Center for the Biology for Natural Systems. I was given an office in the zoo hospital, a fully equipped pathology laboratory, and an autopsy room with a walk-in cooler and an electric hoist for lifting and moving large animals. There were knives, cleavers, axes, saws, and sample bottles filled with formaldehyde waiting for me to fill them.

The facilities and tools were all too familiar. My liaison at the zoo was Robert Frueh, assistant curator of mammals, Charlie Hoessle, assistant curator of reptiles and Mike Flieg, curator of birds. My advisor and supervisor for human pathology and autopsies was Dr. Malcom Peterson, a human pathologist at the Barnes Hospital, Washington University School of Medicine.

The mechanics of human pathology were the same as the mechanics of veterinary pathology. The skull and body cavities are opened up with knives, saws, and bone shears so the organs can be viewed. Tissue and blood samples are routinely collected for microscopic and chemical analysis. Extra care had to be taken to prevent blood, body fluids, or urine from getting into one's eyes, nose, or mouth. The human pathologist had to be doubly careful not to cut himself with an instrument or bone splinter to avoid injecting himself with potentially deadly organisms.

The differences between human pathology and veterinarian pathology are blatant. First of all, just about every clinical veterinarian will do a courtesy autopsy as a learning experience and to answer the questions of the animals owners. However, autopsies are only done on five percent of people who die in hospitals primarily to avoid the collection of data that would support malpractice suits.

The human pathologist looks for pneumonia, trauma, ruptured aneurysms, blood clots, perforating gastric ulcers, heart attacks, cancer, and might do a chemical or drug screen if the clinical case history suggests a need. The human pathologist limits the data on the autopsy report to the size and color of organs, gross findings, microscopic and laboratory findings and a "cause of death." The human pathologist *never* lists the nutritional deficiency which causes aneurysms, diabetes, blood clots, heart attacks, cancer, Alzheimers, even osteoporosis. As a result of this frequent omission of information, clinical nutrition in human health never progresses. My job included changing this huge oversight!

Twenty to 30 postdoctoral fellows were attached to the center at any given time. We were an eclectic bunch of graduate students that included botanists, biologists, environmental engineers, biochemists, computer experts, forestry experts, water experts, geneticists, geologists, anthropologists, astronomers, meteorologists, and myself, a comparative pathologist. To solve problems quickly without having to redo research that some other group had already done, each team member was required to learn the scientific language of the other disciplines represented at the Center. Time was too short for delays caused by semantics. After all, there was an environmental crisis in the world and we were chosen to *identify and solve* the looming world problem.

While there, I continued my graduate studies in pathology and now, subcellular biology. I was also responsible for doing complete autopsies on animals that died in the St. Louis Zoo. This of course included all of the attendant tissue and laboratory analysis, the goal being to identify pollution and environmental problems. I was supposed to find a modern day "canary in the mine," a species that would act as an early warning system for impending environmental doom, much like the old coal miners used canaries to warn them of the presence of deadly suffocating and explosive gases.

I did complete postmortems on every snake, fish, alligator, turtle, parrot, duck, pigeon, ostrich, zebra, antelope, llama, fox, wolf, pig, monkey, and ape that died in the zoo. Dr. Peterson and I then compared the causes of death in the zoo animals with similar disease in humans, looking for common threads that might be caused by pollution.

The first revelation I ran into was that the responsibility for the zoo animal dietary supplement programs were not controlled by any central authority. If an animal were the curator's pet project, it got lots of scrutiny for its nutritional program. Animals that weren't that exciting or part of a herd or flock might have its diet program left to the whims of individual keepers. Some keepers concocted homemade vitamin mineral supplements by grinding up pills designed for humans. Some believed animals could get all their vitamins and minerals by eating high quality food. As a result, zoo animals developed nutritional deficiencies just like domestic animals, wild animals, and humans.

Though the stated goal of the zoo was protecting and propagating endangered species, the nutritional deficiency diseases proved something was lacking in the pursuit of that goal. I saw marmosets, alligators, and shrews that died of diabetes, a chromium and vanadium deficiency. I autopsied dozens of alligators and a Cayman that died of steatitis, a vitamin E and selenium deficiency. I diagnosed ostriches and aoudads suffering from muscular dystrophy, a selenium and vitamin E deficiency. I recorded many wild sheep, llamas, kudus, pheasants, and monkeys with cardiomyopathy heart disease, a selenium deficiency. I came across pheasants, ostriches, gorillas, and squirrel monkeys with ruptured aneurysms, a copper deficiency. There were lions, wolves, woolly monkeys, alligators, iguanas, and parrots with osteoporosis, a calcium and magnesium deficiency. There was arteriosclerosis in vegetarian animals such as pheasant, parrots, kangaroo, a magnesium deficiency. There were even sheep, monkeys, rhino, and kangaroos with osteoarthritis, a calcium and magnesium deficiency. Congenital birth defects that could be attributed to nutritional deficiencies in the mother during early pregnancy were prevalent as well: cerebral palsy in a llama, a copper deficiency; spina bifida in a monkey, a folic acid or zinc deficiency; cleft palate in arctic foxes, a vitamin A or zinc deficiency; ventricular septal heart defect in a kangaroo, a vitamin A or zinc deficiency. Diets were evaluated. Vitamins, minerals, and trace minerals were calculated and adjusted to prevent disease and promote fertility and normal pregnancies. Sometimes we could use existing rations as a base to start with: rabbit pellets for kangaroos, dog food for wolves, laboratory monkey biscuits for monkeys and baboons, turkey pellets for pheasants, duck pellets for ducks, swans, and geese, horse feed for zebras, and elephant and cattle pellets for llamas and buffalo. More complicated diet programs had to be made from scratch for shrews, marmosets, and iguanas.

The tissue bank I started provided frozen and preserved tissues and organs of rare and endangered species to investigators studying anatomy, anthropology, biochemistry, and pathology. I consulted with other zoos, universities, hospitals, the National Science Foundation, and the National

Institutes of Health as a member of a NIH site visit committee that approved or disapproved funding for research done using exotic species as the animal model. Starting the *Journal of Zoo Animal Medicine* was a natural outgrowth of these labors, and I remained the editor-in-chief for three years. As a result of these associations I was constantly traveling and was a regularly featured speaker at medical, veterinary, zoo, and nutritional seminars. Along the way, I worked for and consulted with the world's foremost zoos in the Bronx, Denver, Detroit, Jacksonville, Kansas City, Los Angeles, Madison, Memphis, Miami, Milwaukee, St. Louis, San Diego, Topeka, Tucson, and Washington, D.C. Overseas I served the zoo populations in Frankfurt, Tel Aviv, and New Dehli, to name a few.

It wasn't all hum-drum lab work. On occasion, I got to practice the darting skills sharpened in South Africa.

My first personal experience with a zoo escape came about when a spectacled bear climbed out of its moated grotto. The young male had been a resident of the exhibit with a female of his species and six sun bears for more than two years. The bear had arrived as a cub and in the beginning was easily contained by the walled moat. The now adult bear had calmly crawled out of the moat when he accidentally discovered he could reach the top of the wall with his front paws.

Several keepers kept the bear in the vicinity of the moat by rattling long bamboo poles on the asphalt in front of him. I darted the bear. After the dart struck him, he dashed back into the security of the grotto. After the bear fell into a deep sleep, he was placed on a piece of plywood and dragged into his grotto, where he was kept until the outside wall was raised an additional two feet.

A year later I was asked to immobilize a female spectacled bear and collect a milk sample. My first reaction was to think of the old Eskimo joke, "To become a man one was required to sleep with a woman and catch a polar bear." The joke continues that the "mauled initiate got the commands mixed up; he caught a woman and tried to have sex with a polar bear." I initially thought that the request to collect a milk sample from the bear was a "snipe hunt!"

In actuality the milk sample was required because the first-time mother had abandoned her cub. We were going to hand rear the rat-sized cub.

Robert Freuh and I went to the service area in the rear of the den where the female bear had been separated. I carefully measured out the dosage of the M-99 and darted her through the cage bars using a CO_2 pistol. After about five minutes the bear collapsed with her back to the cage door and began to snore loudly.

After an appropriate amount of time had passed, I used a bamboo pole to tap her on the nose to make sure that in fact she was in fact out cold. The tapping got no reaction, we opened the door and entered the cage. The dart was on the far side of the bear. To remove the dart and collect the milk sample, we stepped over the recumbent bear, placing her between the open door and us.

To remove the barbed needle, one has to rotate the needle in a 360-degree circle about four times to lay the barb down on the needle; it is then an easy pull to remove the needle from the animal.

As I began to rotate the barbed needle the female bear lurched upright into a standing position on her hind feet and let out a blood-curdling growl. I placed my foot on her hip and shoved her out the door into the service aisle and pulled the door closed. The bear was out in the keeper's service aisle and we were locked in the bear's cage!

As the bear tottered out into the aisle, the bear keeper bringing her bucket food met her. I yelled at him to back out of the hall and run to the hospital for the drug box and a rope. While we waited for our supplies the bear became animated and paced up and down the hall growling and grunting.

The keeper returned in short order and lowered the drug box and the rope into the cage through a ventilation duct in the roof. After a few unsuccessful attempts, I was able to lasso the bear and Robert and I were able to pull her up to the bars so I could give the additional drugs necessary to get her to sleep.

With the bear finally immobilized, we got our milk sample and we pulled her back into the cage. The orphaned cub was raised successfully on the resultant formula, and the recipe was written up as an article in the International Zoo Year Book.

After spending 12 plus years doing autopsies on 17,500 animals of over 454 species and 3,000 humans for a comparison, it was apparent that every animal and every human who dies of natural causes dies of a nutritional deficiency disease.

The autopsy findings were so obvious and so profound that they stood out like a beacon. At the cost of $7.5 million I had been trained to make observations and quickly convert the raw material to useful and problem solving information.

The nutritional awareness in humans during the sixties was focused on vitamins. Theron Randolph emphasized the relationship between niacin (B3) deficiency and schizophrenia. Linus Pauling promoted vitamin C for preventing cancer. Vitamin E was touted for people's sex life and longevity. The focus on vitamins resulted in most zoo animals receiving supplemental vitamin A, vitamin C, vitamin E, and niacin. It was only in the livestock industry that was dependent on nutritional supplements for optimal fertility, growth, longevity, and profit, where minerals were the focus and fads did not dictate the supplements used.

The basic functions of life itself cannot be performed without minerals, either as a major part of the function or as a catalytic cofactor. No biological process is exempt. The concept holds true for RNA, DNA, subcellular and digestive enzymes, biochemical reactions, hormone function, energy use and to utilize oxygen and vitamins. Nothing in a living system works without one or more mineral co-factors.

Minerals and mineral supplements to our meals are in fact a necessity of a long and healthful, disease-free life. Since before recorded history, man craved and consciously consumed minerals including the major minerals, trace minerals, and rare earths in the form of clays, salts, animal tissue such as bones and meat or colloidal mineral-rich plants. Simply said, minerals are the currency of life. The medical profession ignores this truth to the point of absurdity.

The Center for the Biology of Natural Systems encouraged publication of findings that resulted from our studies. Some 70 peer review and refereed journal articles and fifteen chapters in eight multi-author textbooks resulted from my own comparative pathology research. I was also a member of the ad hoc committee of the National Science Foundation that authored the Animal Welfare Act of 1968. The act outlined the nutritional and housing requirements for laboratory and zoo animals.

A direct result of my work was that several animal feed companies including Ralston Purina and Hill's Packing Company developed special diets for zoo animals and captive wild species. The immediate pay off was that fertility of captive zoo animals was more consistent from the smallest of zoos to the largest and most sophisticated zoos. Captive rare and endangered animals lived longer and developed fewer degenerative diseases.

8

THE BOOK

While still at the Center for the Biology of Natural Systems and the St. Louis Zoo I interacted almost daily with the St. Louis Zoo's long time clinical veterinarian, Dr. Alfred Moller. I had a lot of experience immobilizing large animals with tranquilizers in Africa, so he would frequently ask me to do the anesthesia on a zoo animal while he did the necessary procedure or surgery.

Dr. Moller, also the clinical veterinarian for the Clydesdales belonging to Anheiser Busch, convinced the W.B. Saunders Publishing Company that a scientific reference book covering every known health and normal physiological data and disease of every known animal needed to be written. W.B. Saunders is the largest publisher of medical and veterinary textbooks in the world, and it was considered to be a great victory and asset to have them as our publisher. The book would consist of 28 chapters written by 28 experts from zoos and universities. It would take an estimated five to eight years to complete. Each chapter of the book was to focus on a specific group or classification of animals. Everything known about each group was to be assembled in the appropriate chapter. If important information was not available, we were supposed to do the studies necessary to get it.

The tome would be the equivalent of a modern day Noah's ark of health information, the most complete reference ever compiled on exotic animals both wild and captive. All the normal blood, urine and spinal fluid values, gestation periods, recorded longevity, known diseases and causes of death (including bacterial, viral, parasites, degenerative, and nutritional) would be included. Every known anesthesia, vaccine, and antibiotic for exotic animals were included in each separate chapter. It would be a huge undertaking.

Because I was considered the junior member of the project, I was initially given the chapter on bees, fruit flies, and mealworms. I only knew what I had learned about these insects in zoology and entomology in agriculture school. Undaunted, I immediately did a library search for everything known about them. Within a month, I was an expert on the nutrition, diseases, and life cycles of bees, fruit flies, and mealworms. I dutifully set about to write my assigned chapters.

In 1965, personal computers didn't exist. I started with your basic black Underwood upright typewriter and a ream of 8 1/2 x 11 white bond paper. Many paragraphs and tables were typed, cut, pasted, and repasted. Quarts of correction fluid were employed. The mechanics of writing in those days were slow and tedious, but I was on a mission and my cup was half full not half empty.

All of the authors were assembled in Philadelphia in the penthouse belonging to W.B. Saunders to kick off the project. The publisher provided a project editor, Carroll Cann, who was to be assigned to guide the project along. Carroll also chaired the meeting. We were wined and dined and given a tour of the publishing facility.

Carroll Cann warned the gathered contributors that over the years some of them would never finish the project. Some would fall ill, some would die, some would get divorces, and some would just quit because of fatigue related to the enormity of the project before it is finished. But, Carroll said, finish it we will!

Six months into the project, I received a call from Moller saying that one of the contributors had already quit. Would I please take over his project—the chapter on fish? Saying yes, I did the necessary literature research in various libraries. Within a month, I was an expert on the diseases, parasites, anesthesia, environmental requirements, nutrition, and reproductive cycles of fish. Every flat surface in the house was covered with paper, reprints, journals, monographs, reference books, and the early drafts of chapters. Finishing my assigned chapters became an obsession that drove me day and night seven days each week.

Some months later, the same scenario repeated itself and I was asked to write the chapter on waterfowl. The tried and true process was repeated. I did the research and collected what was known about the normal laboratory values, parasites, diseases, nutrition, and reproduction of domestic and wild waterfowl. The creation of each chapter for the book was attacked in the same way that course work was attacked while I was in veterinary school. "If it ain't broke don't fix it!"

About half way through the development of the book I was offered a position as the pathologist of the Brookfield Zoo in Chicago—it would be a jump from a 50 acre zoo with a population of 2,500 animals to a 200 acre zoo with a population of 4,500 animals. The pay was double at the Brookfield Zoo and the facilities were considerably larger and more advanced, so I accepted the offer and was off to Chicago.

A real factor in my decision to take the Brookfield position was the presence of five trained bottle-nosed dolphins in a giant salt-water tank. Just down the road, the Shedd Aquarium had fresh-water dolphins and a world class fish collection and a complete library on marine mammal and fish diseases.

I arrived at the Brookfield Zoo to learn that the clinical veterinarian, Weaver Williamson, had been severely mauled by a big male chimpanzee. From my first day I had to take double duty as a clinical veterinarian as well as the pathologist. This meant that I started each day two hours earlier to make clinical rounds, look at every animal, talk to the keepers about their charges and answer their questions about nutrition, injuries, parasites, reproduction, or disease problems:

There was the male African elephant, Pete, who was given 20 tranquilizer pills each morning in a banana so the keepers could handle him.

There were the antibiotics that had to be given to a lion with an infected tooth by means of a dart and a blowgun.

There was worm medicine to give to a polar bear cub in the belly of a fish.

There was the pining of a hawk's fractured wing.

There were conversations with the curators for future exhibit plans or nutritional programs.

I wasn't even totally moved into my new zoo hospital office when two of the zoo's biologists inquired if I knew anything about genetics? Initially I smiled and said that I knew the basics of genetics, but by no means was I an expert. I learned later in the conversation that they had been working with a pair of Arctic foxes and that for five years in a row the pair had produced smaller than normal litters with 100 percent fatal birth defects.

Arctic foxes normally have large litters of 10 to 15 kits. This pair of foxes had litters of three to five kits. Some of the litters were born dead; others born alive but with hydrocephalus; some were born with no eyes, and some were born with diaphragmatic hernias. The last litter was born with all four kits having cleft pallets. The biologist felt that the parent foxes were from incompatible gene pools, and that the only way to solve the problem was to put together a major expedition to the Arctic to catch wild foxes to assure a broader gene pool in the zoo population.

After about an hour of listening to the biologists' theories, I knew the foxes' problem was a nutritional deficiency rather than a gene problem. Naively I said, "You're in luck, this is not a gene problem." Looking like they had been slapped in the face with a decomposed fish, the two biologists fired right back, "How do you know? You're admittedly not an expert in genetics and you just got here!"

My response was, "If there was a genetic problem, the birth defects in kits in each litter would be the same year after year. In this case each litter had different birth defects than the others." It's very obvious that the problem was a nutritional deficiency in the mother early in pregnancy— congenital birth defects, not genetic. Of course, they chuckled and said, "That's the most absurd thing we have ever heard of."

My next comment was to ask for the pair of foxes to be transferred to the zoo hospital for observation. After all, they wouldn't want these poor pitiful genetically defective specimens on display, would they? They turned the foxes over to me.

Investigating the diets of the foxes, I learned that the basic diet for the last five years was ground up horse heart "sprinkled" daily with powdered vitamins and minerals at the discretion of the keeper. The amounts of vitamins and minerals delivered to the foxes were highly variable. Sometimes they were fed too much. Sometimes they weren't fed enough depending on how the keeper's favorite football team fared and whether or not he had a "bad hair day."

I went to the grocery store, bought some off-the-shelf Gaines Burgers, semi-moist dog food patties, and began to feed the pair of foxes. Four months later, they had a normal litter of 11 kits. Within the year, I inbred the mother with a son, the father to his daughters and brothers to sisters. If there were a genetic defect and a defective gene pool, the intense inbreeding would bring it out into the open. All the resultant litters were normal and had 10 to 15 kits.

There were so many Arctic fox kits that resulted from the inbreeding experiment that the zoo curators created a special display for them to illustrate color phases but they begged me not to pull the same stunt with elephants.

The work on the book continued. If there were no normal blood values for Siberian Ibex, a type of wild goat, I would enlist the help of the curators and catch the zoo's flock of 21. Using my round-up skills learned on Angus, Hereford, and shorthorn calves, I caught them one at a time with my lariat. I would weigh, identify, and tag them for the curators, and take the blood samples for my book database. An original article resulted and was published in a peer review journal. The data was used for the book. The zoo got a feather in its cap for the original study that would help all zoos that kept Ibex, and I got the basic data for the book. This was repeated with Dahl sheep, havalinas, monkeys of all types, bears, kangaroos, pheasants, parrots, ostrich, snakes, turtles, and fish. It felt like I was the veterinarian for Noah and the animals in his ark.

The autopsies continued; the same pattern of nutritional diseases I observed at the St. Louis Zoo was also evident at the Brookfield Zoo. All animals dying of natural causes died of a nutritional deficiency disease. For example, kidney stones in tortoises and iguanas were a universal problem. The standard diets of captive tortoises and iguanas were based on fruit, eggs, raw meat, and lettuce with little or no minerals, certainly no calcium. Where did the calcium come from that was in the turtle and iguana kidney stones? It came from the bones of the iguanas and the bones and the shells of the tortoises when they had raging osteoporosis. The fact that kidney stones resulted from too little calcium in the diet was well known in domestic animals so it was easy to find appropriate references for a refereed journal article and for the book.

By this time, I was on a roll. I rarely saw a new disease, but I did see lots of familiar diseases in different animal species. Selenium deficiency, calcium deficiency, copper deficiency, zinc deficiency, magnesium deficiency, and iodine deficiency were common. Vitamin and protein deficiencies were less common. The clinical symptoms and the gross, microscopic autopsy signs and the biochemical finger prints in a snake, fish, alligator, ostrich, wombat, yak, lion, wolf, Ibex, Dahl sheep, llama, dolphin, and humans were the same!

The completeness and value of any theory depends on the number and accuracy of the facts one assembles to arrive at those conclusions. Darwin, the naturalist, arrived at his controversial theories on evolution and natural selection while on an unprecedented continuous world journey, island and continent hopping on the *H.M.S. Beagle.* No one before him had personally observed the contiguous stream of facts necessary to see the concept of natural selection.

Prior to my nutrition and pathology studies in captive and wild exotic animals, no single individual trained in comparative pathology and comparative medicine had studied the degenerative diseases from so many different species of animals from all over the world and compared the results with information on diseases of human beings with the single goal of finding common useful threads. I found the threads and wove them into a tight fabric of truth—every animal and every human being that dies of natural causes, dies of nutritional deficiency diseases! The medical profession didn't accept the truth because they didn't have the $7.5 million worth of training that I had benefited from. They weren't stupid, and I wasn't any smarter than they were. They were, however, ignorant of all the facts and therefore they are universally unable to see the truth.

9

THE GREAT BEAR ESCAPE

The Seven Seas Panorama at the Brookfield Zoo featured bottle-nosed dolphins, walrus, seals, sea lions, penguins, and dozens of species of fish and invertebrates. The clinical care of these marine animals was also part of my responsibility. Each day I spent an hour checking the animals to ensure they were in the peak of health to participate in their daily performances. I would inspect the fish, squid, and mussels that were fed to these animals.

Examining the dolphins required time in the water with them, which in turn required that I learn how to use SCUBA equipment. My pursuit of the swimming and life saving merit badges for my Eagle Scout rank had taught me how to swim very well and how to function efficiently in the water. Three days each week I would get on my SCUBA gear and get into the giant 250,000 gallon salt water tank with the zoo's 5 dolphins. The time with the dolphins allowed me to observe their feeding habits and ability to move and check their pulses, temperature, and respiration on a regular basis. Time in the tank was a chance to exercise and a wonderful break from the daily clinic rounds and the intensity of the pathology lab and the autopsies.

Each dolphin had it's own personality. Some were aloof and would only let me hang on if they were commanded to do it by their trainer. Most liked human contact and would invite me to hitch along for a ride by rubbing against me like a cat looking for attention;—the fun began by grabbing onto their dorsal fin and away we would go at top speed. Soon enough however I'd be back at work collecting blood and stool samples for routine tests and to check for parasites. Skin inspections were also important for detecting parasite, fungus, or bacterial problems. Deficiency diseases plague even the playful dolphins (and whales), though they're subject to arthritis, osteoporosis, and kidney stones, especially if they feed almost exclusively on the soft bodied squid.

A fresh-water dolphin on exhibit at the Shedd Aquarium died. Because of my experience with marine dolphins at the Brookfield Zoo, I was called upon to do the autopsy with the goal of getting enough information to save the other fresh water dolphins in the display. The survivors weren't looking too well at that point for good reason. The autopsy revealed congestive heart failure to be the cause. The liver, kidneys, and lungs had no sign of organic disease. Nevertheless, a microscopic examination of the peripheral nerves revealed a demyelinating process characteristic of *Beriberi*—a thiamin or vitamin B-1 deficiency.

The dolphins' diet consisted exclusively of frozen smelt. Smelt muscle tissue contains a significant amount of *thiaminase* enzyme that was more than canceling out any thiamin the dolphin received from their daily vitamin supplement. While cooking deactivates the enzymes of raw meat, obviously dolphins don't cook their food. Solving the deficiency state involved immediately changing the diet to include a variety of fish that were free of the *thiaminase*. They also received a 100 mg. of thiamin daily in addition to their current vitamin-mineral supplement. Thankfully, the remaining fresh water dolphins responded well, immediately ending the crisis at the Shedd Aquarium.

Some zoo emergencies transpire more quickly though. It was seven a.m. on Thursday, July 17, 1970, when I got the call. "Doc, this is a security guard at the zoo—we have an emergency, the bear moats are flooded, please come to the front gate quick!" The guard hung up before he told me what the emergency was, but I assumed it was serious. It was obvious from his voice that he was under a great deal of stress. All attempts to call back were futile—all the lines were busy.

Sluggishly, I pulled on a pair of old jeans and a work shirt in anticipation of a wet environment. As an afterthought I picked my 12 gauge shot gun with a half-full box of shells with #6 bird shot and left for the zoo without shaving. My station wagon pulled into the street before I realized the street was flooded. I'd been remotely aware of the rainstorm during the night, but the thunder had never fully awakened me. Fully awake now, I realized that the storm could be wreaking havoc with the bear moats. At the lowest part of the Brookfield Zoo, the bear grottos consist of five separate outdoor enclosures housing from east to west, ten black bears, four polar bears, three polar bears, two brown bears, and three spectacled bears. Each of the enclosures are separated from the public space by a 20 foot wide 12 foot deep moat and finally by a four foot high public barrier chain-link fence.

The zoo generated revenue by selling large plastic bags of marsh-mallows that could be fed to the bears. The bears became legendary for their antics of waving and clapping like a human to entice people to throw them the spun corn syrup marshmallows. The resulting accumu-lation of discarded empty plastic bags was cleaned up the following morning by ground crews. Before the plastic bags could be removed this morning, the rains had come. Normally the slanted concrete moats are kept dry by a six-inch drain at the bottom. The storm brought five inches of rain in just a few hours. The entire day's collection of plastic marsh-mallow bags were swept into the moat and plugged the drain. Immediately, the moats began to fill with millions of gallons of water.

It took 15 minutes to arrive at the zoo even though I only lived 5 blocks away. Five inches of rain in 90 minutes had flooded the streets. Many early risers were swamped in their stalled cars. At the zoo, the entrance gates were closed, and all the early shift employees were still outside the perimeter fence. The guard failed to recognize my sleepy unshaven face and didn't want to let me in the zoo because, "The polar bears were out!" My pass key opened the gate for my station wagon. I told the guard through my open window that if he wanted the bears back in the pens, he would have to let me in the zoo.

Relaxing at my grin, he now told me that the bears had been loose for several hours. Because the phone had been out of order, he was only able to get the call out at 7:00 a.m. No one else was allowed in the zoo until I had a chance to fully evaluate the situation.

I arrived at the zoo hospital to find one of the zoo's associate directors had already arrived. Obviously under great stress, his eyes were bulging, and he was as red as a beet. Seeing me, he blurted the order to, "tranquilize the bears and get them back in the moats!" At first I started to comply with his order; I made up three fully loaded tranquilizer darts, picked up two dart guns, two lariats, and now more seriously the shotgun and shells. Dewey Garvey, the bear keeper, drove up to the zoo hospital in a dump truck to pick up a bushel of fish with the hope that he could coax the bears back into their moats with the promise of fish.

The trip to the grottos was unusually quiet. Dewey and I were striving to see ahead through the tags of morning mist to catch a glimpse of the escaped bears. My first view of the bear grottos was that of a polar bear standing on it's hind legs, hock deep in the water on the public walk with both front paws poking in the refreshment stand through broken windows. The great white bear was deeply intent on scooping out ice cream cones and berry flavored snow cone syrup in gallon plastic jugs as fast as he could, eating the cones and biting holes into the plastic jugs so he could get at the sweet syrup. Before our arrival the bear had pulled out the cash register and cuffed it about, leaving it floating with the other debris.

Looking further up the line of grottos it was obvious that all seven of the polar bears had been able to swim out of their flooded enclosures. We spotted a second polar bear sitting in front of the children's zoo delicately playing with the store of helium bottles meant for inflating balloons. He was busy entertaining himself with the noises he produced by clanging them against one another. Two other polar bears were swimming in and out of the east grottos with the grizzlies. One polar bear was in with the ten black bears. The remaining two polar bears were swimming back and forth in the deeper part of the flooded public space, belly-flopping and using their front legs to push the thick mat of flood debris ahead of themselves like kids do with bubble bath in their tubs. The sight was captivating and for an instant we could only appreciate the humor of the scene. Then the awful weight of the situation crept into my mind.

Polar bears are listed as rare and endangered. Worth thousands of dollars each, the zoo polar bears have no fear of man and are among the largest of the land carnivores. Their fluffy white fur, broad head, prominent Roman nose, and begging antics make them one of the most appealing zoo attractions. For curiosity's sake or simple hunger for marshmallows, these bears would readily approach any human. I couldn't risk anyone being mauled or killed even for such zoological prizes.

On the other hand, the polar bears' grottos were still flooded with the water in the moats well over the tops of the four foot high public barrier fence and water at the center of the moats more than 20 feet deep. Tranquilizers were not the answer for this situation, since the immobilized bears would be helpless in the deep water. It would be next to impossible to safely render any aid to a tranquilized bear because of the presence of the other escapees and the depth of the water. My African experience had taught me that drugged animals that were near water holes or rivers would invariably head for the water and drown. After a few moments of internal debate, I decided that it would be best not to tranquilize the polar bears, but rather rely on the theory that they were in unfamiliar territory and if intimidated, given the opportunity and choice, they would choose home sweet home!

I dropped Dewey off with his bushel of fish at the utility entrance to the bear grotto, hoping to catch them in their dens by baiting them with the fish. The associate director had circled to the rear of the moat and positioned his car at the East End of the grottos, honking his horn to help deter the bears from escaping into the general zoo grounds. I drove the dump truck back and forth in the public space of the moat area and by backfiring the engine I was able to drive all of the polar bears into one moat or the other. Two were with the grizzlies, one was with the black bears, and the four remaining polar bears were swimming back and forth between the two polar bear grottos.

Dewey slapped fish against the wall of the rear dens hoping to entice the bears back into the den where he could lock them up. The bears were having a wonderful adventure. By now they were full of ice cream cones and snow cone syrup, so why would they want to go home?

Dewey next tried to toss fish to the bears. Being in a playful mood they picked up the fish and threw them into the flooded moats and dove in after them. Positioning the truck at the west end of the of the public area, I abandoned it but left the engine running to act as much as a barrier as possible. I took the shotgun with me and stepped into the waist deep water. I was surrounded by floating marshmallows, plastic bags, leaves, paper, and empty trashcans. A polar bear intent on frolicking swam towards me. When he swam up to ten feet of me I fired a load of # 6 bird shot into the water about two feet in front of his nose. To my relief, the theory actually worked and the fluffy bear abruptly wheeled around like a dolphin and hurriedly swam back into the safety of the familiar grotto. This process was repeated several times as each bear tried to get a second helping of the new found freedom.

By 8:00 a.m., Wally Buegel, the captain of the zoo security patrol, and Pete Price, the foreman of the maintenance department, had arrived with their men and equipment. A gasoline operated water pump was set up and the process of emptying the millions of gallons of water from the moat was begun at the snail's pace of 380 gallons an hour. While the men toiled with their pump, the curious bears made several excursions up to the fence, curiously swimming up to the noisy pump for a look. Each time the bears would advance the men would scatter to their trucks. I positioned myself between the men and the bears and each time that the bears would approach, I could send them back to their moats by firing into the water in front of them.

Once when I attempted to fire, the trigger pull was met with the audible click of the firing pin falling on an empty chamber and the bear kept coming. The ground crew scattered while I attempted to pump another shell into the chamber—but the magazine was empty. Miraculously, the bear had quickly been conditioned to expect a loud report after hearing the distinctive sound of the shotgun's pumping mechanism. Hearing that sound again, the bear quickly turned to escape the expected explosion and swam back to the grotto with its tail tucked well between its legs.

Despite extra water pumps, runoff was continuing to pour into the grotto area. We were making no real progress to evacuate the water. Unfortunately, the bears were now completely intermingled and their tempers were starting to flare. Perhaps the sugar binge with the snow cone syrup was making them argumentative! Once again, Dewey and I had to position ourselves between the firemen and the bears to keep the animals where they belonged. After pumping 45,000 gallons of water from the larger east polar bear moat, the water level had still only dropped three feet. At least the regular bear keeper had arrived and had been able to slam the grizzly den door on one surprised polar bear. The remaining polar bears, curious to find their buddies, swam out of the moat into the now dry public space and walked back towards their regular moat. Shotgun in hand, safety off, I walked parallel with the bears keeping them between the moats and myself. With anticlimactic irony, the bears simply climbed over the public fence rail voluntarily and belly flopped into the partially flooded moat.

The high water problem continued. I donned my SCUBA harness and jumped into the flooded moat. The zero visibility and flood debris made finding the drain difficult. Groping around the bottom of the moat, I eventually was able to relieve the drain of its many marshmallow bags until the water flowed freely out. We had to repeat the process several times because the drain would become plugged from new debris, but soon the water was gone.

Although the individual bears in the various groups were not the same species, we didn't care since we could now safely transfer them at our leisure later on. The primary objective to return the bears to the security of a den had been accomplished without anyone or any bear being injured or killed.

By now the visitors were being allowed into the zoo. I had to smile as I overheard the comment of one person who was unimpressed with the bear exhibit: "How boring! The polar bears looked so lazy!"

10

THE MUNCHIES AND MINERAL DEFICIENCIES

Work on "the book" continued. I took a leave of absence from the Brookfield Zoo and spent three weeks of isolation in Hawaii entering four years of accumulated data into the book. The work was finally beginning to take shape. By this time, all but two chapters of the book had wound up in my lap. What I didn't know from personal experience I gleaned from published articles in veterinary journals, wildlife journals, zoo records, and laboratory animal journals. The two co-authors still left in the book project were responsible for the chapters on caged birds and reptiles. One was asked to write the chapter on caged birds. His busy private practice in New York left him promising his work but never completing it. The other co-author was a veterinarian and MD who taught public health at Harvard Medical School. His claim to exotic animal fame was an article he'd once written on ameobic infections in the Komodo dragon. It wasn't exactly Komodo Dragon Dysentery, but you get the picture. Extremely arrogant, he wanted half of the book royalties "to lend his name to the project," even though he was only contributing one chapter. When he threatened to leave the project if he didn't get his way, Carroll Cann the project editor at W.B. Saunders told him to jump in the lake. The contract he'd signed only entitled him to royalties based on his percentage of the work. Obviously I would soon end up with the reptile and caged bird chapters and I quickly became pre-occupied with my new venture.

After a four year stint at the Brookfield Zoo, I wound up at the Yerkes

Regional Primate Research Center in Atlanta, Georgia. The primate center was administered by Emory University and funded by a variety of agencies including NIH and NASA. Physically the center was located across the street from the Centers for Disease Control, a dream position for a comparative pathologist.

The researchers I assisted used New World and Old World monkeys, chimpanzees, gorillas, and orangutans in their studies of nutrition, pharmacology, breeding colonies, and behavioral studies. Sometimes the animals were killed at the end of the study, sometimes they died from the effects of the drugs or nutritional deficiencies, and sometimes they died of natural causes. My job was to help the investigators know everything possible about their primates, their diets, and—if necessary— their deaths. Nutritional deficiencies in monkeys, great apes, and humans were studied closely.

The basic diet of the Yerkes primates was commercially prepared complete "monkey biscuits." The monkey biscuits contained all of the vitamins, minerals, trace minerals, amino acids, and essential fatty acids known to be required by monkeys and apes. This information had been gathered from literally thousands of basic nutrition studies in monkeys and the great apes. The monkey biscuits were supplemented with cabbage, citrus fruits, bananas, alfalfa hay, spinach, ground meat, onions, beets, nuts, carrots, eggs, and rolled oats to keep the animals busy browsing. These add-on foods were either sprayed with salt water or a trace mineral salt block was tied to the outside of the cage where it could be licked.

Nutritional studies were done by creating special pelleted diets that had one or more nutrients missing to map out the various symptoms and diseases that resulted. In the early days of zoos and primate laboratories, bone problems such as osteomalacia in baby primates and osteoporosis in adult primates were commonplace as their diets were almost exclusively grains, vegetables, and fruit with little or no regard for their mineral needs. The advent of the commercial monkey biscuits pretty much eliminated the problems in modern zoos and primate colonies unless nutritional deficiencies were being created for study purposes.

There were as many as ten pathology cases per day at the Yerkes facility. We looked for viruses, bacteria, parasites, degenerative diseases, nutritional deficiencies, and complications of surgical interventions and drug studies. Microscopic slides were made of all tissues and organs, chemical analysis was made of blood, urine, and spinal fluid and samples were taken for viral and bacterial cultures. The ultimate goal was to find and develop an animal model for the study of some human disease in hopes of producing a prevention program or a cure. A real advantage of the position at Yerkes was the proximity to the Centers for Disease Control and their weekly pathology study programs for human diseases. The world's experts on these diseases provided unknown cases in the form of histories, microscopic slides, and sometimes lab results. In many cases the slides were made with standard stains and we had a week to figure out what the disease was.

At the presentation, the attendees including myself played a game of "pin the label on the disease." Presenters would use a review of the clinical history, the pathology results, and special stains on the microscopic slides to reveal the identification of the mystery disease. It was a great opportunity to advance my study of human disease and the technique to diagnose them. Those who had made the right diagnosis got all excited and pumped, made victory signs and confirmed, "I knew it, I knew it!" The rest varied from, "I was going to say that, and changed my mind," to, "it had me baffled from the beginning." What the exercise did for everyone, of course, was to hone that person's skills, so that regardless of exhilaration or disappointment, all emerged winners at the end of the day. This weekly challenge went on for several years, and at each successive meeting my Sherlockian deduction skills became sharper and sharper. The truth was getting clearer. It was elementary Watson— *when an animal or human dies of natural causes, they die of a nutritional deficiency disease.*

To me the most interesting primate and human cases were the ones that involved nutritional deficiencies. Despite my interest, the golden age of critical and detailed research projects for the essentiality of various minerals in animal nutrition occurred between 1920 and 1978. Any remaining curiosity about the role of mineral deficiencies in human pathology was dealt a crippling blow by the discovery of penicillin in 1938 and a second body punch by the isolation of cortisone in 1942. The *coup de grace* came in the ranks of the medical community in the 1980s during the heady drive to find patentable genetic engineering techniques to treat everything from bowel gas to cancer. While the basic studies of nutrition have become the neglected stepchild of 21st century science, the unquestionable basic mineral needs of our human flesh cry out for attention from the waiting rooms of physicians' offices, hospital wards, and morgues.

Obesity and overweight problems are synonymous with Americans. Nibble, nibble, nibble all the way home. Pica is a seeking, a craving with licking and chewing behavior that has its genesis in mineral deficiencies. No known vitamin, protein, or calorie deficiency initiates this behavior. Nor will supplementing the diet with vitamins or eating sugar, carbohydrate, fat, or protein quench it! Cribbing is a name given to a particular form of pica in domestic animals. Cribbing occurs when animals chew or gnaw on a wooden feed box, fence, hitching post, or barn door. A good farmer knows that when a horse cribs, the animal really has a craving for minerals. The farmer or rancher supplements the animals diet with minerals to save the animal's life, save on veterinary bills, and save from having to rebuild the fence, because a mineral deficient animal will literally eat the fence looking for minerals.

Essential minerals never occur in a uniform blanket around the crust of the Earth, they occur in veins like chocolate ripple ice cream. Whatever essential minerals might have been in the Earth's crust have been depleted. It's no surprise that the animal pica, cribbing, and cravings humans know as the "munchies," dominate the American scene. "Salt appetite" or the "munchies" is very striking in both pregnant animals and pregnant humans. Our search for the "munchies" is a plague that shows America as a whole is now minerally deficient—dieters, athletes, vegetarians, meat eaters, embryos, fetuses, children, teen-agers, young adults, adults, and seniors alike are exhibiting symptoms of mineral craving once known primarily among expectant mothers.

From antiquity, the description of cribbing and pica in humans relates it's major incidence to pregnant women. The Hawaiian King Kamehameha's mother, Queen Kekuiapoiwa, had cravings for *eyeballs*. Although she specifically wanted chiefs' eyes, she was given the salty eyes of sharks to eat. The snack food and fast food industries are aware of this relationship between pica, cribbing, and cravings, sugar binges and salt hunger and they use it to their advantage by liberally salting or sweetening their products. Unfortunately for humans, our bodies temporarily interpret sugar and salt intake as a fulfillment of the cravings for essential minerals. Historically, the consumption of salt to satisfy a pica behavior was of value because salt was not processed and did often times contain small amounts of trace minerals and rare earths.

Today, contrary to popular belief, salt is not intrinsically harmful. It does present the problem of allowing our bodies to perceive that we are getting sufficient minerals when we eat salt. This is the mineral equivalent of the "empty calorie diets" concept. Just as processed white flour and sugar calories satisfy hunger while providing no protein, essential fatty acids, or vitamins, processed salt confuses the body into believing it is consuming adequate minerals. Farmers and husbandrymen use the salt hunger to ensure the consumption of trace minerals in livestock by incorporating trace minerals in salt blocks containing a minimum of 85 percent sodium chloride—anything less than 85 percent sodium chloride in a salt block will be ignored by the animals even if they have major mineral deficiencies. These animals never get high blood pressure, though they consume as much salt as they wish. For them, adequate salt intake guarantees proper mineral intake.

Most physicians would have you believe that you need little or no salt. They must think that the general public is dumber than cows, for the first food item a good husbandryman puts out for his livestock is a salt block. At the same time, the multi-billion dollar a year snack food industry is well aware of your need and craving for salt and other minerals. Even the USDA says that 95 percent of all Americans of all age groups, toddlers, teen-agers, adults, and seniors are minerally deficient.

In July of 1993, thousands of people in the upper Midwest and on the east coast of the United States were swooning and fainting during a sweltering heat wave that soared above 110°F. Seven-hundred-thirty-three, in fact, died during the heat wave. The effects of the heat wave on the population were so dramatic that the body count was published in newspaper headlines as though they were fallen American soldiers in a far off place. Seemingly, no one knew what to do. The state medical examiner of Pennsylvania said, "We don't know why so many have been affected by the heat—half of the dead and the hospitalized had air conditioners." That is especially odd when one thinks of the millions of people around the world who live in terrible deserts with temperatures of 120° in the shade. They don't have air conditioners, and they don't die from the heat. Could it be that some genetic shield protects them?

The cause of this disaster was screaming at the medical profession but no one heard, voiced, or printed the appropriate public warning. Having lived in the Kalahari Desert while in Africa, I had taken basic medical physiology, and I was already a pretty fair human pathologist. I knew the horrible toll of the heat wave was the result of a simple salt or sodium deficiency. It was basic heat stroke that any boy scout could diagnose, recognize, and remedy with water and salt. Yes, the cause of these thousands of American casualties was a simple salt deficiency. Almost all of those who died during the heat wave were on salt restricted diets. *It was a physician-caused disaster.*

The human tragedy of the heat wave of '93 was a direct result of the medical profession's paranoia of salt. They put their human charges on a low sodium or low salt diet for hypertension and heart disease. There is not a single double-blind study that shows significant benefit of a low sodium diet. About a week after the carnage the state medical examiners office again marveled from its pulpit, "the only common denominator we found in the dead and the affected during the heat wave was that they all had heart disease and high blood pressure." Yes, as predicted, their physicians had placed them all on low salt or no salt diets. Those who were successfully treated were given IV saline—salt water!

Yes, the medical profession must think that the public is dumber than a cow. Unfortunately, it is the medical profession itself which turns out to be *dumber than history*.

Aristotle noted in *Historia Animalicem* VIII, that "sheep are healthier when they are given salt." They never get hypertension and high blood pressure!

Where salt was rare, it was traded ounce for ounce for gold, brides, or slaves. Salt and salt-rich clays were the first mineral food supplements consciously used by man in the dawn of time. The Roman statesman Cassiodorus was quite observant when he said, "Some seek not gold, but there lives not a man who does not need salt."

Rome's major highway was called Via Salacia—the salt road; soldiers used it to carry salt up from the Tiber River where barges brought salt from the salt pans of Ostia. Soldiers "worth their salt" were paid a "salary" —the word salary is derived from salarium, a soldier's "salt ration."

Marco Polo reported salt coins and discs in Cathay. Salt discs in Ethiopia were "salted away" in the king's treasury. The production of salt as a food supplement for man and beast is as old as civilization itself. Salt was produced in shallow ponds of seawater through evaporation and by mining rock salt from large land-locked deposits.

The rock salt mines of the Alps (Salzberg, Halstatt, and Durrenberg) played an essential role in the development of cultures in ancient prehistoric Europe. The Hallstatt salt mine is one of the oldest commercial salt businesses on Earth—it is located 50 miles from Salzburg ("salt town"). Salt has been mined from the Salzburg mine since the early Iron Age. Salzberg ("salt mountain") contains a salt deposit 2,000 feet wide and 2,500 feet deep. Tools found in the salt mines date back to the Bronze Age (1400 B.C.). Early communities sprang up around salt springs as humans followed and hunted wild herbivores that were drawn to the springs by their craving for salt—a behavior known as pica and cribbing. I saw this same pattern in Africa—the water supply that had salt and minerals in it was heavily used by the game animals, while the water that was mineral and salt free was rarely used.

From the 9th to the 14th centuries, peat was soaked in sea water, dried, burnt, and the resultant ash was then extracted with sea water; many millions of tons of peat were harvested for this mineral/salt dietary supplement process for commercial trade.

Mesopotamian towns specialized in the salt production industry and transported salt up the Tigris and Euphrates Rivers. Jericho (8,000 B.C.), near the Dead Sea and the salt mountain of Mo are the oldest known agricultural communities that participated in the salt trade.

The merchants of Venice developed an elaborate salt trade and by the 6th century the salt trade from the villages surrounding the city was its main business. By 1184 Venice controlled the export of Chioggia salt, and by the 14th century was providing salt to Alexandria, Cyprus, and the Balearic Islands.

The salted herring trade developed in the 1300s. The Dutch perfected the process of salting fish as a method of preservation. At its peak, this industry produced 3 billion salted herring annually using 123 million kg of salt per year. In the beginning of the 20th century, salt pork and salt herring provided the main source of animal protein for most of Scandinavia with a daily per person consumption of 100 grams or a quarter of a pound. (Modern physicians want their patients to consume less than 3 grams per day.)

Perhaps the most famous and romantic modern day part of the salt industry occurred in Africa. Twice each year great camel caravans carried salt slabs from the Taoudeni Salt Swamp in the Sahara to Timbuktu in Mali. Two thousand to 25,000 camels (only 25% survived the journey) were used to carry over 300 tons of salt slabs more than 720 km.

In other parts of salt-poor Africa, humans developed the practice of drinking cattle blood or urine to obtain salt. The residents of the Sierra Leone coast gave all they possessed, including their wives and children, in exchange for salt, because salt is an absolute requirement for life. Salt is not equally distributed on Earth and is coveted by the have-nots. It is said by African tribesmen, "He who has salt has war."

The British imposed a despised salt tax on India. Ghandi (1924) published a monograph (*Common Salt*) in protest of the government monopoly. Ghandi pointed out that the grains and the green foods of India were very low in salt. Because of the vegetarian habit of the majority of tropical Indians, they required a significant salt supplement to their diet.

In 1930, Ghandi led 78 rabid supporters on a 300 km "Salt March" protest from Ahmedabad to the sea. He swam in the sea and picked up a crystal of salt at the beach and then walked back to Ahmedabad, where he was promptly arrested and thrown into prison. Angered, 100,000 Indians revolted against the salt tax and were arrested after they too picked up untaxed salt. The British salt tax was finally repealed in 1946.

Death of soldiers from sodium loss historically occurred during military operations in tropical countries. Soldiers in the desert could lose 24 pints of water per day as sweat, which included a loss of 70 to 100 grams or a quarter of a pound of salt per day.

Salt is known as the most universal and most widely used food supplement and condiment. So great is the human craving for salt, it is obvious that salt itself is in fact necessary to the health and even the life of man. Yet, it's claimed by modern medicine to be dangerous. As we've seen, that's only true to the extent that human salt consumption masks the absence of other essential minerals. The average salt requirement for man is about six to ten grams per day. If you are very good at following a doctor's advice to restrict salt to less than one gram per day, you will increase your risk of a heart attack by 600 percent.

In addition to the legitimate salt cravings medicine seeks to suppress, the human craving for minerals is also well documented:

A catalogue of bizarre instances of human pica is found in the doctoral theses of Augustus Fredericus Mergiletus (1701). In men, he recorded one individual who ate leather, wood, nestlings, and live mice. A second consumed woolen garments, leather, a live cat, and small mice. A third ate cat's tails and decomposed human flesh infested with maggots.

In women, Mergiletus recorded cannibals who ate human flesh, including one horrible lady who "lured children to her house with the promise of sweets, killed them and pickled them for storage and consumption at a later date"—a female version of Jeffrey Dahmer! The murders of the children were only discovered when the woman's cat stole the pickled hand of a child and carried it over to the neighbor's house.

Girls who ate their hair, cotton thread from their own clothes, raw grain, and lizards have also been documented.

Cooper (1957), in her classic report on pica, refers to several ancient and medieval writers who emphasized the occurrence of pica in pregnant women. Aetios noted pregnant women to crave various and odd foods, some salty and some acid, saying that "some crave for sand, oyster shells and wood ashes." He recommended a diet including "fruits, green vegetables, pigs feet, fresh fish and old tawny fragrant wine."

Boezo (1638) noted that pica occurred most often in pregnant women. Boezo saw pica as a physiological problem, and is the first to mention iron preparation as a treatment for pica. He suggested "one and one-half scruples of iron dross taken for many days as wonderfully beneficial for men and women."

Boezo also noted the case of "a virgin who was accustomed to devour salt in great quantities from which chronic behavior she developed diarrhea and wasting." She probably had Addison's disease.

Christiani of Frankfurt (1691) reported a woman who ate 1400 salt herrings during her pregnancy.

LeConte (1846) suggested that animals eating earth do so because of "want of inorganic elements."

The most common descriptions of pica and cribbing by Mergiletus were of women's desire for clay, mud, and mortar scraped from walls, just like modern children who eat caulking and lead paint. We have often said that children who eat lead paint are screaming for minerals for their mineral starved bodies—give them minerals and they won't eat lead paint.

Pica is no stranger today either. In modern times, the substances frequently reported as eaten as a result of pica behavior in humans includes paper, metallic gum wrappers, chewing gum, ice, dirt, coal, clay, chalk, starch, baking powder, pebbles, wood, plaster, paint, chimney soot, hair, human and animal feces, and cloth. Because of social constraints on our public behavior, most people under public scrutiny who display pica will chew gum, eat sugar, chocolate, snack food, or soft drinks when they crave minerals. Other socially popular ways to respond to the cravings of mineral deficiencies are smoking, alcohol or drug use. Ice eating, known as pagophagia, is also common, especially for iron deficient children and adults.

The research confirms this:

Henrock (1831) attributed pica to "paucity of good blood and lack of proper nutrition."

Waller (1874) reported that David Livingston observed many cases of clay and earth eating (geophagia), a form of pica frequently found in pregnant women in central Africa.

Orr and Gilka (1931) and de Castro (1952) recognized that "edible Earths might be rich in sodium, iron and calcium."

Gelford (1945) reported that pica was common in Kenya amongst African tribes (Kikuyu) living mainly on a vegetarian diet. Pica was absent in those people eating diets rich in animal flesh, blood, and bones (Massai).

Nicolas Monardes (1493–1588), a Spanish physician, published *Historia Medicinal.* In the second volume is a scientific dialogue on the "virtues" of iron; however, iron was not generally accepted for medical use until the 1600s when Nicolas Le'mery found iron in animal tissue ash.

In 1745, V. Menghini demonstrated the iron in tissue was found primarily in red blood cells. Dr. Willis' "Preparation of Steel" was iron fillings and tartar roasted and given in wine as syrup or pills.

Dr. Thomas Sydenham (1682) recommended for all diseases involving anemia treatment by "bleeding" (if the patient was strong enough) followed by a course of Dr. Willis' "Preparation of Steel."

In 1850, it was reported in a medical journal that a woman who had lost three premature pregnancies was given "iron scales from the smith's anvil, steeped in 'hard' cider during her entire pregnancy. The woman's appetite increased, her digestion, health and spirits improved. She delivered a full term boy and who was so strong that he could walk by nine months of age. At age five he was so tall and strong that he became known as the 'iron baby.' "

Dickens and Ford reported that 25 percent of all children ate earth. Cooper (1957) reported a 21 percent rate of pica in American children referred to the Mother's Advisory Service in Baltimore.

Lanzkowsky (1959) reported that 12 children with pica had hemoglobin that ranged from 3-g percent to 10.9 percent with a mean of 7.89 +/- 2.64. The institution of iron dextran "resulted in a cure for pica in one to two weeks." Again, if children have optimal intakes of nutritional minerals they will not eat lead paint.

McDonald and Marshall (1964) reported on 25 children who ate sand. They divided the group in half, giving one group iron and the other group saline. After three to four months 11 of the 13 children given iron were cured of their pica behavior compared with only three of the 12 given saline.

Reynolds et al (1968) reported that 38 people with anemia exhibited pagophagia, or ice eating, as the most common form of pica. Twenty-two of the 38 had their pica symptoms disappear after correcting the iron depletion.

Woods and Weisinger (1970) reproduced pagophagia experimentally in rats by withdrawing blood. The pagophagia in the anemic rats was cured when the anemia was cured. They also noted that pica and cribbing behaviors were not produced by vitamin deficiencies.

Two-thirds of the 153 pregnant women studied by Taggart (1961) developed cravings. The most common craving was for fruit, pickles, blood pudding, licorice, potato chips, cheese, and kippers. A craving for sweets, vegetables, nuts, and sweet pickles came in second place.

Phosphate appetite was described by LeVaillant (1796) as the anxious search by cattle in phosphate deficient South African pastures for discarded animal bones (osteophagia). Phosphorous deficient cattle also chewed on wood and each others horns.

Osteophagia has been reported in many wild species of herbivores including reindeer, caribou, red deer, camels, giraffe, elephant, and wildebeest.

It was demonstrated that calcium deficient weanling rats will consume large amounts of a lead acetate solution, even though it tastes bad, when compared with calcium fed controls.

Lithium was discovered in mineral water in 1817 by August Arfvedson in a Swedish Laboratory of Berzelius. Its use in mental illness dates back to 400 AD when Caelius Aurelianus prescribed lithium containing waters for mental illness.

In the 1840s, it was reported that lithium salts combined with uric acid dissolved urate deposits. Lithium was then used to treat kidney stones, "gravel," gout, and rheumatism as well as a plethora of physical and mental diseases.

Health spas picked up on the notoriety that lithium was receiving and marketed themselves with exaggerated claims of the lithium in their hot mineral springs, even going to the extent of adding the word "lithia" to their names to woo the public. Because of public access to lithium salts in spas, physicians looked for other arthritis therapies.

There are 75 metals listed in the periodic chart, all of which have been detected in human blood and other body fluids—we know that at least 60 of these metals (minerals) have direct or indirect physiological value for animals and man. Organically, not a single function in the animal or human body can take place without at least one mineral or metal cofactor.

"On an inorganic chemical basis little distinction can be made between metals. Both metals and non-metals enter actively into chemical reactions. The difference reveals itself in the physical properties. By common agreement, those elements that possess high electrical conductivity and a lustrous appearance in the solid state are considered to be metals," according to Bruce A. Rogers, metallurgist and physicist.

Minerals truly govern our lives whether we recognize it or not. Sadly, the current medical "wisdom" on salt and medicine's inability to recognize the many forms of pica that are exhibited in America show that we have failed to understand the true effects of mineral deficiency diseases.

11

MONKEY BUSINESS

Parasites were the specialty of Harold McClure, the head of the pathology department at Yerkes Regional Primate Research Center. My immediate supervisor, he'd been at Yerkes for fifteen years. To keep things fair between two published scientists, we had an agreement. Whoever made an unusual or exciting discovery would be the primary author of a resulting mutual effort. That understanding would soon be tested.

After getting into the swing of Yerkes' activities, Dr. McClure went on vacation for two weeks in November of 1977. That in itself should have been sufficient warning. Back at the University of Missouri, when Dr. Kintner, my pathology professor, went on vacation, the dead and dying appeared in droves. Dr. McClure was not gone three days when a six-month-old rhesus monkey was presented for autopsy.

The baby rhesus had snow-white hair instead of gray-green, was half the normal size, and suffered from anemia. I checked the monkey into the system and went through the usual routine. The infant monkey was weighed, measured, and identified by tattoo number. Blood and urine were collected for cultures and biochemical evaluation. Every tissue and organ system was examined. Stomach and intestinal contents were collected for culturing bacteria and viruses and chemically analyzed for poisons.

Anemia made the tissues and organs small and pale. The changes in the pancreas stood out, making it more interesting than the other organs. Not only was it small and pale, it was round in cross section instead of flat and was as hard as a rock. It was supposed to be flat and soft like raw bacon. In cutting through the pancreas it felt gritty and made noise like cutting through sand. Tissue samples were taken for microscopic examination. Twenty-four hours later the tissue sections were ready to be read. The pancreas, liver, heart, and lungs showed changes I had never seen before. I made notes and ran to the library and had the computer pull all of the articles related to such changes in animals—I got literally hundreds of articles describing a trace mineral deficiency. All the changes in the monkey were compatible with a selenium deficiency.

The next step was habit. Since the days of working with The Center for the Biology of Natural Systems I would always check diseases from two points of view—animal pathology and human pathology, the same diseases, but different languages! Veterinary terms for a disease were descriptions of the tissue changes themselves. Human terms for a disease tended to be named after the first person to describe them, or a clinical description of symptoms. I entered the question of selenium deficiency into the human computer software and got a big fat zero. No matter how I asked the question I got a big fat zero. It was like not having the right code word to enter into the program.

Before working at Yerkes, I had unearthed all my references and studies by hand. It was time consuming but very effective and accurate, so I went back to work. I went to the shelves in the medical library and began to look up diseases of the pancreas and liver of humans. The response was uniform: cancer, pancreatitis, cystic fibrosis. I must have gone through a dozen texts before I gave up. I got tired of seeing the same short paragraph written almost word for word in every text under the same heading—"cystic fibrosis of the pancreas." The texts went on to describe cystic fibrosis as "the most common human genetic disease, the genes for which were found in one in four Americans." According to the literature, this disease was transmitted by a simple Mendelian genetic defect. The child born with it failed to thrive, had a positive "sweat test," and if they survived for a few years they developed lung disease and they usually died before the age of twelve.

Within the veterinary literature for cystic fibrosis there was a terse, recurring statement saying cystic fibrosis didn't occur in animals and that an animal model did not yet exist. The investigation began to pick up speed and intensity! I began to feel that I had a winner, that I might have stumbled onto the first case of cystic fibrosis in an animal—not too surprisingly in a primate. I asked the computer for everything on human cystic fibrosis and got literally thousands of articles. There were photographs of the CF pancreas, livers, and hearts. Then there was the lung disease. Those same organs in the specimen monkey were a dead-ringer for human cystic fibrosis.

The next logical step was to sit down quietly and go through the two sets of information and log the matches—the microscopic features of cystic fibrosis and selenium deficiency matched. Bingo! I have no idea how long I was there. All I can remember is being so immersed in what I was doing, an express train could have passed through the library at eighty miles an hour and I would not have noticed. I just sat there, my mind racing crazily, papers all around me, some on the table, some on the floor.

Great moments in which truths are first recognized are difficult to describe for two reasons. First, they occur so rarely that few get much practice. Second, it's not always possible to isolate the precise instant at which the mind achieves lucidity. Sometimes, discovery just flows gradually like water filling a tank. Other times it strikes suddenly but takes a while to assume coherence and blossom to awareness, making the precise moment of realization tricky to define.

The more I looked, the more I saw the same pattern—congenital and neonatal selenium deficiency in animals equaled cystic fibrosis in humans. I had a great dilemma—what to do. First I had to pinch myself to make sure that I hadn't made a mistake, and then go through the whole thing again and make sure. It didn't take me long to realize that the biggest problem would be to prove it to people who were cystic fibrosis experts and convince them that CF was a congenital deficiency disease. How could I get them to listen and not tell me, "No, that's impossible, cystic fibrosis is a genetic disease" before I got five words out of my mouth? My first major obstacle would be to get a serious hearing of informed but objective listeners.

Keeping a low profile and feigning ignorance, I made quiet, discreet inquiries. I contacted the surgical pathology board at Grady Memorial Hospital, the teaching hospital for Emory University. I told them that I wanted to bring over a set of slides from an anemic, six-month-old infant. I didn't dare mention the word monkey. Armed with the appropriate slides of the pancreas in a cardboard holder, I presented myself at the Grady Memorial Hospital the following day. I made sure that the slides that I brought had all of the identifying landmarks of the pancreas to save time and unnecessary debate that I had seen in the CDC Thursday night sessions. The twelve members of the surgical pathology board view frozen slides from surgical cases and determine whether the pancreas, lung, breast, prostate, or testicle is cancerous, "Yes, that's cancer—cut it out," or "No, that's benign—leave it in." I asked the board if they would keep their findings confidential, and they agreed. I handed the head of the committee the folder with the slides. Eleven out of the twelve wrote down their opinions on paper: "Cancer of an unknown origin." I was dumbstruck! The last of the twelve pathologists sat quietly pondering for a moment, then he said, "I think I know what you're getting at! You think this is cystic fibrosis, don't you?" I nodded my head yes. He asked if the tissue was animal or human. I reminded them all of their promise of secrecy, then I revealed the fact that the tissues were those of an infant monkey.

The sympathetic pathologist pulled a pathology book off of the shelf and flipped to cystic fibrosis. There were only five or six paragraphs under the heading of cystic fibrosis that ended with, "No animal model is known." The pathology committee all agreed that I was going to have a hard row to hoe to get confirmation of the diagnosis, I replied, "There has to be a first someday, and I believe this is it." The helpful pathologist replied by telling me that, "There is a cystic fibrosis expert, Dr. Victor Nasar, in the pediatric department who will be able to confirm your suspicion. If you like, I'll send your slides down to him."

The slides were delivered as promised, and the next day I received the call. "Dr. Wallach, this is Dr. Nasar, I had a good look at those slides that you sent me yesterday." Naturally I asked what he thought. "Oh, no doubt about it! Cystic fibrosis, if I ever saw it!" I responded with, "Are you sure?"

Dr. Nasar came back with, "Absolutely positive." When I asked if he would put that in writing, he came back with, "Absolutely! And seeing as you're just learning about cystic fibrosis, I'll bring over a lot of CF material that I have here—slides, wet tissue, journal articles, that sort of thing so you can have a look—say about noon?" I said, "Noon it is—and please don't forget the confirmation letter."

Dr. Nasar arrived at the appointed hour, and I had to fight to stay calm. As soon as I had his letter in my hand I read it before I even said hello. We sat down at the microscope to look at the rest of my monkey tissue and then Dr. Nasar asked me where I got these tissues. He was obviously curious how a veterinary pathologist had gotten cystic fibrosis tissue for evaluation.

I first asked for confidentiality, which he promised, before I revealed the staggering truth. "Dr. Nasar—you're looking at the first non-human case of cystic fibrosis." Probably, not too many people have heard the expression, "A stunned mullet." The mullet is not a very exciting fish to begin with. One that has been thumped on the head is pretty dull. Dr. Nasar's first reaction was to lean back in his chair with his mouth open; beads of sweat began to break out on his forehead, and it seemed forever before he spoke. "You're kidding me!" Dr. Nasar said with a gasp. I assured him that I was dead serious and that I had done my due diligence. He said, "Here, let me see those slides again!" I had his letter of confirmation and he was under extreme pressure. We looked at the slides again. Even with the revelation that the tissues were those of a monkey, the second look disclosed the same conclusion—cystic fibrosis. Tissue doesn't lie. "There's no doubt about it!" he confirmed, "Nothing else in the world looks like cystic fibrosis! This is cystic fibrosis! I'll stake my career, my life on it!" Then his tone changed, he looked into my eyes and asked, "What animal is it?" Then I told him it was a rhesus monkey. "Man! You've just identified the first non-human case of cystic fibrosis! This is exciting! Where's your phone?"

I asked whom we were calling and he said, "The Cystic Fibrosis Foundation! It's just down the street!" The next day the lab was crawling with CF experts from the Cystic Fibrosis Foundation—they even called the executive director who was fishing in Canada. He cut his vacation short and he was on his way back. They all marveled at the miracle beneath the lenses. They never asked me the ultimate question, so I never gave them the answer. They were all unanimous in their opinion— "the tissues they looked at were in fact classical examples of cystic fibrosis!"

To make sure, the Cystic Fibrosis Foundation sent a set of the monkey tissues to Dr. E. H. Oppenheimer, the world's expert on cystic fibrosis pathology at Johns Hopkins University in Baltimore, Maryland. For good measure a second set was sent to Dr. J. R. Esterly, one of her former pathology Ph.D. students who was now a pathologist at the Chicago Lying—in Hospital. Not a word was mentioned that the origin of the tissue was a rhesus monkey. The only information sent with the tissue sets was that the material was from, "a six-month-old, anemic infant," and a note that said, "We think these tissues are cystic fibrosis, what do you think?"

As sure as God made little green apples, the proclamation from on high was: "Without a doubt—cystic fibrosis!" It was all there in black and white on their department letter head. The world's experts had reviewed the slides and confirmed that the tissues were without a doubt cystic fibrosis. I reread the communications looking for a hint of waffling or weakness, but there was none. The journey had begun. The authorities had agreed and signed their agreement of the diagnosis. History had been made, but, as of yet the discovery was confined to a few people. It was totally a strange situation for me... what should have been the locker-room fanfare and joy was in reality only muffled acknowledgment. This demeanor signaled that we were only at the beginning. I could not move too fast, ruffle feathers, or appear too cocky. Egos were involved!

It was as if I had started at the end instead of the beginning. In reality all I had was a naked fact. I had identified the first non-human case of cystic fibrosis, but it stood in total isolation. I was carrying a piece of dynamite around in my head; I dared not move too fast, drop it, or allow it to pass into the wrong hands, at least until I was ready. That was the key, not until I was ready. There was no accompanying information, no documented history, no source of reference, not anything. Before I moved forward, I would have to fill in all of the blanks.

Why did this particular monkey get cystic fibrosis? That was the million dollar question. Everybody "knew" that cystic fibrosis was genetic and confined to humans. How then did a non-human primate "develop" cystic fibrosis. Where did the monkey come from? How did it get to Yerkes? I didn't have far to go. The monkey had been part of a group of virus-free laboratory raised rhesus monkeys being raised for the NASA space program. Nelly Golarz de Bourne, a behaviorist, was supervising the colony. She was also the wife of Dr. Geoffrey H. Bourne, an anatomist and the director of the Yerkes Primate Center.

There were some fifteen pairs of adult rhesus monkeys kept in small cages. The idea was to have a steady supply of normal, virus-free, captive reared monkeys for the space program. When the babies were six months of age they would be weaned from the mother and raised in a gang-cage with other "teen-age" monkeys. When they reached maturity they would be paired up to produce more captive reared, virus-free, normal monkeys. The ideal was rarely reached in a monkey colony. In addition to having the advantage of being able to demand sexual favors, the males pulled the hair off of the females, gnawed on them, beat them up, and generally abused them. In the wild setting, the female had the opportunity to run away and escape. In the tight cage was another matter.

Dr. Nelly de Bourne noted the hair loss and baldness of the females. She misinterpreted the phenomenon as an essential fatty acid deficiency and decided they were to be given a teaspoon of corn oil each day in addition to their free choice monkey biscuits. Why, she should have asked, if they were all on the same diet, did the males sport a grand hair coat and mane while the females looked ratty and bald? Shouldn't the same deficiency of essential fatty acids affect them all—male and female? There was no questioning her actions here, however. Nelly was the director's wife, and whatever she said was law.

The new directive gave the technicians who fed and cared for the monkeys a major increase in responsibility. Overloaded already, there was no way these technicians were going to go from cage to cage, squeezing each monkey's mouth open to deliver a measured teaspoon of corn oil each day. It sounds simple to do that, but in reality it added hours of work to the day, increased the risk of bites, and created the extra mess of cleaning up the oil the monkeys would sling everywhere and amounted to trying to "force feed" a gang of angry, super-strength teenagers with ADHD and long teeth! They'd rather spit the corn oil in your face than swallow it!

Necessity is the mother of invention. The colony technicians came up with the idea of filling five gallon buckets half full of corn oil, and then filling the bucket to the top with the monkey biscuits and leaving them to soak overnight. The next morning the oil-soaked biscuits were fed to the rhesus monkeys like buttered-popcorn. Several problems were immediately created. The more biscuits a monkey ate the more oil they got. Number two, the extra oil threw the nutrient balance of the commercially prepared ration completely off. In this case, corn oil was notorious for increasing the need for selenium. Even though there was selenium in the pellets, the added oil created a relative deficiency. It never crossed anyone's mind to add the extra selenium. As a result, the pregnant females were selenium deficient, which affected the developing embryos. Likewise, the lactating females were selenium deficient and passed on selenium deficient milk to the infant monkeys. At this point I went back into the colony and examined the rest of them. The hair of the adults and babies had lost the normal gray-green color and the babies were half the normal size and anemic.

I got permission to get a pancreatic and liver biopsy from several of the babies. The classic changes of cystic fibrosis were there, but I said nothing. The time was not yet right. As a matter of standard practice, blood samples were taken from all of the Yerkes monkeys on a monthly basis and frozen for later use should a need arise. I had the blood of the monkey's parents and the infant monkeys tested for signs of a selenium deficiency. Bingo! It was a heady moment, but I still couldn't share it with anyone. Swollen scientific egos at a national and international level were involved and that meant danger if they moved to discredit my research at this early stage.

Nevertheless, it was now a recognized fact that Dr. Joel D. Wallach, veterinary pathologist at the Yerkes Regional Primate Research Center, Emory University of Atlanta, Georgia had discovered the first non-human case of cystic fibrosis. The new darling of the center, I was an overnight celebrity. I presented a feature paper at an international pathology conference held in Atlanta. Emory University put out a news release and the story was featured on the front section of the Sunday edition of the *Atlanta Constitution Journal*. I initiated the process of writing a major scientific paper on the cystic fibrosis monkey.

To top things off, I was given a $1,000 per year wage increase and received letters of congratulations and commendation. NASA was excited that one of their low budget projects had produced a major scientific breakthrough. Mail poured into the center, and there were requests for radio and television interviews. Reporters from journals, magazines, tabloids, radio stations, and television networks called in. The National Institutes of Health began to show serious interest. I was notified that they were going to host an animal model conference at the main NIH campus in Bethesda, Maryland. They wanted me to be one of the featured speakers. I was supposed to present the cystic fibrosis case so others could be on the look out for similar monkeys.

I accepted the invitation and was promptly sent my air tickets, hotel reservations, and a $500 stipend. The NIH also requested a brief abstract for inclusion in the program. I began the task of compiling the abstract that would formerly introduce my cystic fibrosis monkey to the scientific world. Over the years I had done this sort of thing literally hundreds of times. I'd submitted abstracts and had given such presentations to my scientific colleagues, including physicians, veterinarians, and Ph.D.'s, so the task was neither foreign nor formidable. I had done my due diligence. I had made the diagnosis, and I had the diagnosis confirmed by experts in the field. I had backtracked and identified the initiating factors, and I could repeat the process. I could now in fact create an animal model for cystic fibrosis at will. I enclosed appropriate photographs of the monkey tissues for the program. I put the abstract into the envelope, sealed it, addressed it, stamped it, and sent it. I went about my daily business and never gave the matter a second thought.

Shortly thereafter, Dr. McClure returned from his vacation. It was immediately obvious that he was miffed that the cystic fibrosis discovery occurred while he was gone. He would, by his own rules, be the second author on the papers and studies generated by the finding. He had spent fifteen years in the trenches looking through monkey intestines for worms, and the new guy on the block uncovered the biggest discovery ever at Yerkes! McClure was not a happy camper. In the hallway his jaw muscles worked overtime, grinding his teeth whenever I saw him. His office door was closed, a completely new behavior. It now was obvious to me that I was going to have trouble in River City, trouble with a capital "T." Little did I realize how much trouble.

Less than two weeks later, a terse-sounding Dr. Geoffry Bourne summoned me to his office. A week earlier I was making history. Now, inside Dr. Bourne's office, with his face as red as a tomato and veins bulging, he blurted out "You're fired!" Flabbergasted, I asked, "What do you mean I'm fired? I haven't stolen anything. I haven't done anything wrong!" Dr. Bourne responded, "Listen here, Wallach! Everyone knows you can't 'create' cystic fibrosis—it's a genetic disease."

I quickly responded, "Dr. Bourne, I didn't say I could create cystic fibrosis, I said I could create an animal model! All animal models are created by one method or another." He retorted, "Don't you understand, Wallach, they won't allow me to let you say that cystic fibrosis can be 'created'! All of the world's experts have built their careers and their lives on cystic fibrosis being a genetic disease! They won't hear of some young upstart coming along and trying to ram it down their throats that cystic fibrosis could be created! It's out of the question! There's just no way I can keep you, Wallach! You're gone!"

Recovering sufficiently to speak I added, "With all due respect, Dr. Bourne, when I say I can create an animal model for cystic fibrosis, I mean it! I can do it! That's the truth!"

"The truth doesn't matter! No buts, Wallach! You're fired, and that's final."

To add insult to injury, Dr. Bourne called in a pair of armed security guards to have me escorted from the building immediately to prevent me gathering up all my cystic fibrosis material and taking it with me. Bourne didn't want me to take the cystic fibrosis material, but I wasn't going to leave without it! I told the guards, "Look guys I have to get my books, I'll meet you at the door." I went to the lab and put all of my cystic fibrosis records, pertinent references, glass slides, and the 2 x 2 transparencies into the bottom of a box and covered them with my books. The guards checked some of the books at the door, but when they saw my personal stamp on the inside cover they waved me out the door. I left Yerkes forever, with a box full of books and the cystic fibrosis material in my arms. The only ceremony was the armed guard on each side.

That day I swore a silent oath to myself: "They won't win. I won't let them! I simply won't let them." I had the materials I needed. Although the National Institute of Health invitation had been withdrawn, I set to work writing a paper on cystic fibrosis before they wrote it using my own material. I had to beat them to the punch. Throwing all caution to the wind, I decided to bring all my findings into the open in the form of a scientific paper—a monograph. I added a summary of my entire thoughts on cystic fibrosis into the work. I entitled the paper, *The Pathogenesis and Etiology of Cystic Fibrosis*. To be sure, it was bold if not brash to claim I knew the cause of cystic fibrosis. In the face of a calcified scientific community unwilling to hear the truth, this was no time for a weak heart or timidity!

I put together 100 key references and the telling photographs to support the article. I attached the letters that had confirmed the diagnosis and had 100 copies of the package printed and copyrighted. Flying from Atlanta to Bethesda, Maryland a day before the NIH meeting, I got a room and read the cystic fibrosis paper twenty times. I could give it in my sleep. The next morning I took a cab to the NIH campus and arrived at the animal model seminar an hour early. I took up a position at the entrance to the seminar hall where I had been invited to speak. The attendees passing through the great NIH portals were each given a copy of the paper and a smile. It wasn't long before the chairman of the animal model seminar came outside and grabbed me by the arm. "For God's sake, Wallach, what are you doing? We can't have you passing out unsanctioned papers. You'll simply have to leave!"

I responded with, "Well, I guess you have a problem. It's a free country, isn't it?" "Dammit, Wallach, you don't understand! You're disrupting the whole conference!" Demanding to be arrested or allowed to speak, the NIH chairman responded with a, "I will have you arrested, dammit!" Then he disappeared into the meeting. Their problem was that they had printed the title of the cystic fibrosis paper and my name in the early announcements of the animal model meeting and many of the attendees had come specifically to hear my presentation. NIH finally capitulated. "Okay! Wallach, listen here!" I listened. "We're going to give you fifteen minutes to make your presentation. After that, we never want to see your face again! Is that clear, Wallach?"

That was all I needed. I presented the cystic fibrosis paper, showed my slides, and saved five minutes for questions. I left the podium with loud applause ringing in my ears. Revenge was sweet. I learned all too quickly though that this victory would last only a fleeting moment. I had given a stunning presentation and felt vindicated, but I knew that I had trampled on some pretty serious toes. There were bound to be serious repercussions. Naively believing that the truth would prevail, I underestimated the viciousness I would quickly encounter.

NIH was not amused by my behavior. In fact it was the first time in their twenty-five years that the proceedings of an NIH sponsored conference was not published. The proceedings of the 1978 conference are still missing from the written history of the NIH. In their spiteful move to kill publication of my paper, the NIH had unfortunately also doomed the papers of the other presenters! The publication of many world experts papers were derailed for 1978. A lot of scientists were furious at the NIH decision. But the spite didn't end there.

From the moment that I appeared on the NIH steps I was on the "hit list." I didn't realize it at first, but my career in basic research was over. I went to veterinary pathology seminars looking for job announcements; I visited veterinary schools and medical schools applying for jobs as a service pathologist. I wasn't greedy; I just wanted to go back to work. I'd soon find that my work would take on an entirely new direction.

12

20/20

Jobless, I moved from Atlanta back to Missouri. I worked for my father loading trucks just to pay my bills. I applied for the laboratory animal colony director position at the St. Louis University medical school. To my surprise, I landed the job, and began putting my things together, arranging schedules, clarifying responsibilities, and preparing to be employed again. This time I was going to be the director and would make the administrative decisions. To my great shock, just as I was about to begin the position at St. Louis University I received a letter which basically said, "We are sorry, but we have to withdraw our offer of employment. We have just received a letter from Yerkes saying that you are a nut. We are sorry, but we can't have a nut as the director of our animal facility"

Yerkes and NIH had caught up with me again!

I set out again to the veterinary seminars in the hopes of finding a job. I may not be as smart as a lot of people, but no one can accuse me of ever giving up. Persistence paid off. I ran into one of my old veterinary school chums, Dr. John Troxel. John had graduated the University of Missouri veterinary school a year before me, spent some time in the Army doing research, and then opened a small animal practice in Chicago. John was very successful and very experienced in the field veterinary clinical medicine and veterinary research.

I brought John up to date with all of my great days and my more recent termination and the run-in with the NIH. "John, to make a long story short, I'm looking for a job—do you know of anyone who needs a veterinary pathologist?"

"Listen to me, Joel! You're wasting your time! Absolutely wasting your time! They'll never let you back into the system! Believe me! I know! I've seen the mix of ego and bureaucracy in the Army! Take my advice— go retrain and look for something different," replied John.

"But John, this is far too big to let go. Surely someone would be interested in the project?"

"Don't get me wrong, Joel. I'll help you. But right now you don't believe me. So, go try your luck, and when you're totally disillusioned, give me a call. We'll take up the situation from there."

John's statements and assessment of the situation made no sense to me at the time. I still believed that the promise of help for the cystic fibrosis families and children would be so interesting to someone that the curse of the NIH would be neutralized.

In between meetings and seminars, I chopped wood and broke up cast iron bath tubs with a sledgehammer. I had to vent my anger and frustration on something. It was the worst time of my life. Until that point, I was so engrossed in doing my work that it never crossed my mind that politics existed at such a level in science. I finally knew that I had literally been black-balled. The influence of the NIH was everywhere.

It was time to call John Troxel. John of course had been correct from the beginning, but he hadn't tried to force his views on me. John knew it was something I would have to learn for myself. John was not surprised when I called. He only asked, "What took you so long?"

I confessed to John that he was right, "I didn't believe you at the time, but by golly, I do now!"

John came back with, "I understand, Joel. It doesn't make sense that I'm right, but unfortunately, I am. Anyway, that's neither here nor there right now. The important thing is to do something about it. I have a plan up my sleeve that I think will work. Give me a couple of days, and I'll get back to you."

What John Troxel did was to hire the services of the most prestigious public relations firm he could find. They'd been involved in the political campaigns of every senatorial and presidential candidate ever to come out of the state of Illinois. John explained the history and circumstances of my situation and asked them to come up with a plan of action that would bring the matter to the largest possible public audience. In return, John wrote them a check for $20,000.

When I learned how much money John was investing in me, I asked,

"John, $20,000 are you mad? I'll never be able to repay you!" "Don't worry, Joel. I'll get my money's worth. You and I are going to have some fun together," John said with a chuckle. I was dumbfounded. Why would John spend $20,000 just to have some fun?

"Listen, Joel. The money is my problem," John said. "Your job is to get your act together. Have every detail at your fingertips. Be prepared to answer every question, counter every accusation. Know your facts, figures, dates, people, places, and put your story into the best possible format. You do that. I'll do the rest!"

I asked if John thought the plan was going to really accomplish anything. "If it doesn't work 100 percent, it will still do something spectacular, so get your act together and be ready when I call you."

In August of 1978, I found myself in the middle of a media blitz that would have made presidential candidates envious. The cyclone started at the legendary New York Waldorf Astoria Hotel. Every network TV station was there. Every news wire service was represented including UPI and the AP. Medical reporters and writers from every newspaper and magazine had been invited. Media kits with a three page rendition of the basic story of the cystic fibrosis discovery along with a picture of me with one of my monkeys and the original news release from Emory University were handed out to every attendee. I gave a half-hour presentation with slides explaining the value of being able to create an animal model for cystic fibrosis and as a necessary step towards solving the mystery of the terrible disease.

The next day was spent in the 21 Club for lunch with the medical writer for UPI and answering phone calls that were generated by the TV network's airing of the story the night before. The story as we had written it appeared in 1,700 newspapers around the world as a result of the UPI picking it up. The new TV magazine 20/20 contacted me and wanted to arrange a segment for an upcoming program. A lecture circuit was established. I lectured at the invitation of cystic fibrosis support groups. The meetings took place in hospital auditoriums, hotels, and civic centers. I lived with families that had cystic fibrosis children. I ate with the cystic fibrosis patients. I interviewed the parents, looked at their bowel movements, reviewed their hospital and lab records and examined them.

The TV magazine, 20/20, sent a production crew to follow my lecture circuit. They filmed my lectures in VA hospitals, university hospitals, and home living rooms. They interviewed CF families. The 20/20 crew was friendly, but it was obvious they were just going through the motions.

This 20/20 experience was my first with investigative media. I wore my heart on my sleeve and was very open and honest with them. But when the 20-minute story aired, I was surprised to see that 50 percent of the air-time was given to the orthodox view of CF being a genetic disease . . . a view we had completely discredited!

The anti-selenium view on the 20/20 segment was held by the director of the National Poison Control Center in Denver, an MD/Ph.D. toxicologist. It was 1978 and the fact that selenium was an essential nutrient had been known since 1957, 21 years! He actually declared on national television that selenium was toxic and "he wouldn't give selenium to a pregnant woman or healthy baby, let alone a sick child with CF!"

Even though the net presentation of the 20/20 program was neutral, I received thousands of inquiring calls and thousands of inquiring letters. The people themselves wanted to know! The public and CF families were thirsty for information that might help their children. They were all ears. It was obvious that taking the CF story to the public was the right thing to do. The scientific community and the established dogma had actually been a roadblock to progress—certainly nothing new in science.

I lectured in twenty states. I was invited to Zurich, Switzerland and Rome, Italy to lecture to cystic fibrosis families. Cystic fibrosis was the same in Zurich and Rome as it was in the USA. By the end of August, 1978, I had accumulated all of the written material ever published on cystic fibrosis, and without bragging or being arrogant, I knew as much about cystic fibrosis as any medical expert.

The dilemma for proponents of the genetic disease theory of cystic fibrosis was that CF, even CF patients in the same family, rarely exhibited the same form of the disease. In a family with three CF children, one might have pancreatic disease, one would have liver disease, and the third lung disease. Such diversity is hardly the picture of the classic genetic disease. The cystic fibrosis story was the same as the Arctic fox story at the Brookfield zoo.

My experience and training with the Center for the Biology of Natural Systems put me ahead of the knowledge of the day. The established cystic fibrosis experts "knew" that cystic fibrosis was genetic, because that's what they were taught. I was able to come to the table untainted by dogma. As a result, I knew that cystic fibrosis was not a genetic disease, but rather a congenital or perinatal defect caused by a deficiency of the trace mineral selenium in the mother.

I was out of a job. Telephone bills, traveling, airfares, hotels, and restaurants soon consumed my financial reserves. Dead in the water so to speak, I returned to Missouri and worked for my father loading trucks, while I figured out what to do.

Dr. Don Clark, one of my veterinary school classmates, had had a heart attack and asked me to fill in and run his small animal practice for him while he recovered. In addition, he connected me with the Missouri Air National Guard. He had been a jet pilot in the Air Force during the Korean War and had gone through veterinary school on the GI Bill. Now he was supplementing his income as a member of the Air Guard.

The Air National Guard met one weekend each month and required a two week summer commitment. I was inducted as a captain because of my veterinary degree and my Army ROTC background from the University of Missouri. The guard provided extra income and it gave me an escape one weekend each month to continue to work on the book.

The media campaign generated a call from Clinton Miller of the National Health Federation. The NHF was a consumer advocacy group that supported alternative views on health that encouraged the use of vitamins and minerals to prevent and reverse disease. "We're having a convention in Chicago. There will be thousands of people in attendance who will want to hear your message. We'd like you to be a featured speaker. The NHF supports people like you, people who have been downgraded for finding and revealing health truth."

I was very honest and lamented, "I would be very honored, Mr. Miller, except that I'm broke. I couldn't afford the trip." "Don't worry about the money," Clinton chirped, "we'll take care of your expenses and pay you a $500 honorarium."

The NHF convention in Chicago was like nothing I had ever seen. There was an exhibit hall with hundreds of exhibitors. They were a motley crew that included purveyors of water filters, vitamins, minerals, herbs, algae, crystals, books, videos, and beads. There were belly dancers, singers, massage therapists, chiropractors, and iridologists. There were vegetarian and organic food booths of every description: tofu, rice, spices, carrot juice, and blue corn chips. The scene was that of the ancient Persian bazaar. The only thing missing was the sword swallower.

The lectures took place in various ballrooms. Normally there were as many as eight to ten lectures going on at the same time. As a featured speaker I gave my presentation in the main ballroom when there were no other lectures. The room was packed with over a thousand excited people.

My slide presentation lasted for an hour, and I received a standing ovation at the end of my lecture. I felt like the "ugly duckling" had found a home. They wanted to know what I had to say! It was a wonderfully positive experience. There was a refreshing reasonableness about these people. They had a sincere desire to listen and learn. There were no egos, biases, or preconceived notions bogging them down. That NHF lecture turned out to be a milestone and turning point in my career. I had never before addressed a large, receptive public audience before. Previously, audiences had always been comprised of professionals, scientific or medical people, gathered together for some kind of high-level nutrition seminar.

A few days after the NHF convention, I received a call from Dr. Gerhard Schrauzer, head of the chemistry department at the University of California. Dr. Schrauzer was one of my heroes because of his work with Dr. Klaus Schwartz, who determined that the trace mineral selenium was an essential nutrient. Dr. Schrauzer is to selenium what Linus Pauling is to vitamin C. Dr. Schrauzer had read the UPI cystic fibrosis story and called to give me moral support. Schrauzer and others like him had left Germany in 1936 to escape that very kind of manipulation of the truth that I had suffered at the Yerkes Primate Laboratory, being told what to find and what to say by Nazi authorities.

Schrauzer wasn't totally familiar with all of the relationships between cystic fibrosis and selenium deficiency, but he didn't like the way I had been treated. He invited me to address an international conference of Nobel laureates that was scheduled for the following week. Dr. Schrauzer, as program chairman, would guarantee me an adequate hearing despite the last-minute arrangements—and all expenses would be paid!

I went to California and at the University of California, La Jolla campus I put on a 30 minute presentation to the most educated and the most critical audience I had yet encountered. My cystic fibrosis information was well received and I was encouraged to pursue the work "because the truth needed to be exposed to the light of day." Dr. Schrauser went on to say that if I didn't pursue the cystic fibrosis discovery myself, it could be as long as 100 years or more before the concept of a congenital selenium deficiency as the cause of CF surfaced again. I felt that I had been handed a mission and that my observations had been vindicated. After all, if I were totally out of the realm of reasonable certainty, Dr. Schrauzer would have been honest enough to tell me I was wasting my time.

Now, at least I felt I was developing some "20/20" vision with regard to my life's new mission. You wouldn't have known it from the "20/20" television show, though.

13

THE VETERINARIAN BECOMES A PHYSICIAN

Another opportunity arose out of the Chicago NHF conference. As it happened, there were some members of the board of directors of the National College of Naturopathic Medicine from Portland, Oregon in attendance. They had a booth at the expo and were there to recruit students and faculty.

I had never heard of a naturopathic physician or N.D. I didn't know who they were or what they did, so I visited the college's booth, asked questions, and picked up their literature. I was interested because they were fully licensed as primary care physicians in the state of Oregon. Naturopathic physicians could deliver babies, do surgery, write prescriptions, do acupuncture, and primarily differed from the M.D. community because of their strict adherence to the philosophy—"first do no harm."

They were very excited about my background in pathology, nutrition, and teaching so we struck up a conversation. They came to my hour-long nutrition lecture. I used slides that showed a known nutritional deficiency disease in animals and then showed slides of the same disease in humans, making the connection between nutritional deficiency diseases in animals and humans. They took me out to dinner, where the conversation became more animated when they learned I was looking for a job.

I was invited to give a lecture on nutrition to the October annual meeting of the Oregon state association of naturopathic physicians. I was to recount the cystic fibrosis story and cover as much general nutrition as possible in a two-hour presentation. This request was not a problem as I had slides of hundreds of deficiency diseases. Again, expenses were to be paid and an honorarium was given. I didn't know what a naturopathic physician was, but they wanted to listen to what I had to say, so off to Oregon I went.

I was given a tour of the college campus and clinics by the dean of NCNM, board members, and licensed naturopathic physicians. NCNM had been established in 1957 and was the oldest naturopathic medical school still in operation. The classrooms and clinics were housed in the historic postal building. NCNM was a small school in terms of infrastructure, minimally equipped and hardly what I was used to in my associations with the NIH and the great universities across the land. I didn't judge the N.D.s on the limitations of the physical plant of their college, because I knew that a student only gets out of an education what they put into it themselves.

I was shown an architect's rendering for a new campus and had lunch with members of the board and the college faculty. The faculty included Ph.D.s, pharmacologists, M.D.s, cardiologists, N.D.s, and administrative types. The entire group was positive and supportive of my views of nutrition and the ability of supplements to prevent and treat disease. I was treated as somewhat of a celebrity which of course endeared them to me!

An N.D. is a primary care physician and regulated by a state medical board much like M.D.s are. A naturopathic physician can diagnose, treat all diseases, deliver babies, do surgery, get a DEA number, write prescriptions and do other things such as acupuncture, prescribe herbs, and offer nutritional counseling. Naturopathic physicians as primary care physicians were by law required to be paid by insurance companies for their services. In Oregon, the orthodox medical profession looked on naturopathy as a strange old-fashioned offshoot of medicine bordering on quackery. Naturopathic physicians, in turn, looked upon the orthodox medical community as uncaring, arrogant, heavy-handed upstarts, who over-prescribed drugs with harmful side effects, performed unnecessary surgery out of greed, and delivered unnecessary chemotherapy and radiation out of ignorance.

Five states licensed N.D.s as primary care physicians in those days. Today Oregon, Washington, Alaska, Montana, Arizona, Massachusets, Connecticut, Maine, New Hampshire, Vermont, and the District of Columbia license have N.D.s as primary physicians. The naturopathic physician has a reduced scope of practice in many other states because of powerful medical lobbies. Naturopathic physicians were often prevented from delivering babies in states where midwives were allowed to deliver babies. In some states N.D.s were not allowed to puncture the skin of a patient to draw a blood sample when any 18-year-old with three hours of training could be a blood drawer for a hospital or clinic.

The naturopathic audience was an eclectic collection of students at various levels of their studies, academic staff from the college and practicing naturopathic physicians. They were fascinated by the presentation approach of showing slides of the known nutritional deficiency diseases in animals paralleled with the same disease in humans. It was an enraptured audience—they were very interested in nutritional deficiency diseases in humans. They demonstrated their approval with a standing ovation at the end of the presentation. I was in a groove and seemingly among kindred souls; the ugly duckling was starting to look like a swan.

After the presentation I was approached by the chairman of the board of directors of NCNM, the dean of students, and the president. This time the offer was for a job. They wanted me to teach nutrition at the college and create a series of courses that covered nutrition for all four years of the medical curriculum.

I had come to a professional juncture here. Do I totally give up on 20 years of orthodox research and association with the main stream of science and join this maverick band of health care professionals and tarnish my background previously steeped in publication of basic research and credible university affiliations? I remembered what Dr. John Troxal had said, "Joel, they will never let you back in."

I accepted the offer of a teaching position at NCNM—with a single proviso. I wanted to take courses towards completing an N.D. degree at the same time I was teaching. I didn't see any problem. I had done it before at Iowa State University. The task of setting up a series of four sequential nutrition courses of increasing detail and difficulty would be second nature. By no means would it be the first time that I had lectured to a group of highly educated and motivated professional students. My goal and focus was to be able to treat cystic fibrosis patients as soon as possible. My goal was to get the message to the CF community, that I had some cutting edge information to help them and prevent the occurrence of additional CF patients by simple prenatal supplementation of selenium.

After a brief closed meeting, the board approved my request and asked that I be in place ready to teach by January 1979. They projected that taking courses part time I could get my N.D. degree in six to eight years. The projection seemed too long for me as I was already 38. I didn't say anything out loud, but I knew that I would have to speed up the process.

I showed up for work on the 26th of December 1978. The weather was bad. "Black-ice" had ravaged Portland for a week. I let some air out of my tires and arrived safely at the office to find that I was the only one there except for a secretary manning the main office phone, and the school president, Dr. Jim Sensenig. There was no hubub of students yet and in the quiet I went to work. I asked for and got advice and guidance from Jim Sensinig on how to pursue courses with the goal of becoming a licensed N.D. as soon as possible.

By December 31st, I had completed the outline of the courses, ordered the text books and was ready to go, even though classes didn't begin until January 4th.

I remained in the Missouri Air National Guard, but transferred my national guard drill location to the Oregon Air Guard for convenience. I was promoted to the rank of major, and I continued my weekend drills and summer camp schedule. I was eventually promoted to the rank of Lt. Colonial and transferred to the Alaska Air Guard to fill their needs for an environmental health officer to deal with chemical warfare and biological warfare clean up.

Next came the formal application to be a student and application to the curriculum committee for all possible exemptions and advanced standing. Advanced standing allowed me to interact with human patients and begin my residency immediately, including cystic fibrosis patients under the supervision of a licensed N.D. Two weeks later the curriculum committee had approved my advanced standing status. My years of clinical work with animals, my international status as a comparative pathologist, and my publications all contributed to their justifying my advanced student status.

I attacked the massive load of triple projects with the same military approach that had been so successful in getting me through the University of Missouri agricultural school and veterinary school simultaneously. I immediately began to see patients in the college clinic under supervision of staff clinicians and senior students. I visited and toured several private clinics until I found two practicing naturopathic physicians who were willing to take me in and allow me to sit in on their patient visits. One practitioner was a woman, the other a man affording me different gender perspectives.

Within weeks I was delivering babies under supervision, doing office surgery, and connecting IV drips under the watchful eyes of the licensed doctors. During my fourteen years as a veterinarian I had already mastered most of the common clinical and laboratory diagnostic skills. The exciting part was that I was seeing treatment of human disease with nutritional formulas. The doctors I worked for actually asked my opinion and used some of the veterinary nutritional formulas that I suggested.

"Compressing and Condensing" were my watchwords for finishing N.D. school early. Nothing was cut short or left out. I simply had to do the same amount of work as any other student in a shorter period of time. At 38 years of age, I wasn't going to spend eight more years as a student! In order to compress and condense things, I'd commonly be taking classes on one subject while an examiner for another subject would sit beside me with sets of a hundred microscopic slides for normal tissue identification for the histology class, or slides of human diseases for basic pathology courses. I would successfully identify 100 percent even while taking notes on the lecture at hand. Having been a comparative pathologist for over 14 years and having reviewed literally millions of normal and diseased tissue slides from both animals and humans under the microscope over the years made the exercise simple. Using this method, I was able to successfully get equivalent and/or transfer credit for veterinary and graduate classes in physiology, public health, microbiology, parasitology, neuroanatomy, basic surgical technique, medical biochemistry, pharmacology, toxicology, basic courses in clinical laboratory and history of medicine and was allowed to test out of gross anatomy, histology, basic and advanced pathology, and all four courses of nutrition.

In addition to the whirlwind schedule of testing out and advanced clinical study, I had to physically sit in and take courses in the history of naturopathic medicine, medicine, cardiology, pharmacognosy (the understanding of herbs and the extraction of the active principals of herbs for medicinal use), herbal medicine, basic and advanced obstetrics, surgery (which I helped to teach), Chinese medicine, acupuncture, homeopathy, orthopedics, pediatrics, EENT, advanced clinical diagnosis, physical therapy, residency, and internships. The result of this intense program of intellectual warfare was a halving of the projected time frame for graduation—cutting eight years down to three and one half. The naturopathic academic community was in shock. I had passed by the academic level of other instructors who had been on the same track of teaching and studying to be a naturopathic physician who'd started several years ahead of me.

The academic naturopathic community was normally pretty laid-back. Most were ten to fifteen years younger than me, vegetarians, and I don't believe that they were as motivated as I was to just get on with the program. Ten years older, connected to the military, and a habitual hamburger eater, my colleagues saw me as being less "spiritually elevated" than they. Soon they were referring to me as "Conan the Veterinarian!"

I always had clinic duty on weekends because no one else would take it. If weekend duty were assigned to them, many of the other students would just skip out! As a result I probably saw ten times the number of patients as the other residents. Once a month I had my National Guard drill which ended at the same time as the clinic duty started. I would get permission to leave the drill 20 minutes early and stop by McDonald's and get a Quarter Pounder. Arriving at the student conference room in my fatigues, eating a hamburger and reviewing charts simply confirmed their view that I was in fact Conan the Veterinarian.

In 1981, I purchased a small clinic in Canon Beach, Oregon. I paid licensed N.D.s to operate the clinic on my behalf. They also supervised my activities as an advanced standing student. I adapted many of the veterinary nutritional formulas that I had learned in veterinary school to human use. It was no surprise to me that they in fact worked just as well in humans as they did in animals. Perhaps the most popular of these nutritional formulas was and still is the "Dr. Wallach's Pig Arthritis Formula." There are no pigs in the pig arthritis formula. It was called the Pig Arthritis Formula because it was designed to prevent and cure arthritis in pigs.

Seventy-five percent of all Americans over the age of 50 get arthritis of one type or another to some degree. According to the Centers for Disease Control, somewhere between 35 million and 50 million "baby boomers" will get arthritis by the year 2010 and there is not a single medical treatment designed to prevent or cure arthritis! Aspirin doesn't fix arthritis and can cause gastric bleeding and death. Tylenol doesn't fix arthritis and causes 40,000 cases of kidney failure each year, 5,000 of which are so severe you need a kidney transplant. Advil™, Ibuprofin™, and Aleve™ don't fix arthritis and can cause liver disease in five to ten percent of the users. Methotrexate and gold shots don't fix arthritis and they can subdue your bone marrow so they can't manufacture white blood cells, red blood cells, and platelets. Prednisone and cortisone don't fix arthritis either, but they can subdue your immune system so that you're left open to diseases far more horrible than arthritis. These steroids actually speed up the loss of minerals from your bones—something you don't want to have happen if you have osteoporosis or arthritis.

When these over the counter and prescription medicines don't work anymore to relieve pain and inflammation, the only thing left for you medically is joint replacement surgery. These orthopedic procedures rarely work out well, so I never referred my patients to orthopedic surgeons for those procedures. Elizabeth Taylor, for example, had three hip replacement surgeries. Despite having been attended to by the best orthopedic surgeon in Hollywood, she still developed compression fractures. Elizabeth Taylor needed Dr. Wallach's Pig Arthritis Formula.

The advantage my human patients have is that I am a veterinarian as well as a physician and veterinarians have all these nutritional formulas to prevent and cure diseases in animals. We have to since we don't have health insurance for them!

I researched various veterinary nutritional formulas that were designed to prevent and cure arthritis in pigeons, turkeys, dogs, cats, horses, cows, pigs, sheep, lions, tigers, and bears and adapted several of them to human use. Cartilage, ligaments, tendons, connective tissue, and bone itself were regrown regardless of the person's age. I have seen cartilage and bones regrown in thousands of patients. In the 70s and 80s, Dr. Wallach's Pig Arthritis Formula was a mix of 20 to 30 pills and capsules containing gelatin, minerals, trace minerals, amino acids, and vitamins. The pig arthritis formula worked like a charm, but it was inconvenient and expensive to take 20 to 30 pills and capsules three times per day.

Soon, I would have to set up my own shingle and simplify these formulas, but they were adequate for that time and place.

14

They Were Treated Like Dogs, but They Got Better!

Over the years, I ended up with all 28 chapters of the book. "The book" had become "my book" by default! There are a lot of people smarter than me, but there are few who are as persistent or who are willing to work as hard as me. As Carroll Cann, the W. B. Saunders' editor predicted, all of the original book participants except for me had fallen ill, died, or given up in exhaustion.

One thousand pages, two thousand illustrations, hundreds of editorial meetings and eighteen years later, I finished it. In 1983, the tome *The Diseases of Exotic Animals* was finally finished. The book represented 17,500 animal autopsies on over 454 species of animals and several thousand human autopsies for comparison. It effectively reviewed literally millions of microscopic slides and tens of thousands of clinical cases. To sell copies of the book at $140 apiece, W.B. Saunders said I had to add the name of a clinical veterinarian as a co-author of the book and add an obvious clinical subtitle to enhance sales. There are far more clinicians than pathologists in the world. I was to get 90 percent of the royalty and the clinical veterinarian 10 percent.

The book, *The Diseases of Exotic Animals: The Medical and Surgical Management*, is found in every veterinary school and medical school library and in the private library of almost every veterinarian, wildlife expert, and zoologist.

I had hoped that the 23-year collection of nutritional deficienciy truths and their relationship to human disease in the book *The Diseases of Exotic Animals* would bring a revolution in health care. Instead it has become a tome, a reference book that no one can afford to update. It is a classic that any academic professional would be proud to have authored and published, but it didn't stir the medical profession to incorporate nutrition into their treatment programs. The public, of course, is almost entirely unaware of its existence so no health care revolution could be expected from that quarter either. I had done my best, been educated using tax-payer's money to the tune of $7.5 million, used the best science, published peer review and refereed journal articles, published reference books on the subject of nutrition and nutritional deficiencies, but I still felt that I had been unsuccessful in reaching my goal of changing human health in America for the better. I knew that I needed to find another way to be more effective in getting the message disseminated.

I was always very honest with my patients, I told them that I was using veterinary nutritional formulas to treat and reverse their diseases. I proudly hung my veterinary degree on the wall next to the naturopathic medical degree. Most new patients just smiled when they saw the D.V.M., but some were startled and asked, "Doc, I'm here for a physical! Am I in the right place? It looks like you're a horse doctor!" I would fire back, "I won't give you a rabies shot if you don't deserve it!" Then I would put on a full-length obstetrical glove used to examine cows and mares. I would get two predictable reactions: 1) the patient's eyes would get as big as saucers and 2) the patient, especially the ones in gowns with the split up the back, would back stroke out of the examining room with all due haste.

The nurse would hunt them down and would often times find them cringing behind the water cooler exclaiming, "It's not my turn!" Once they got used to my sense of humor, patients would tell their friends and relatives, "If your not happy with what your doctor is doing for you, go see Doc Wallach. He'll treat you like a dog, but you'll get better!"

I delivered babies, sewed up chain-saw wounds, put casts on fractures, treated earaches, ringing in the ears, Bell's palsy, spinal stenosis, trigeminal nerve neuralgia, anemia, colic, diarrhea, constipation, obesity, allergies, ADD, ADHD, depression, bed-wetting, athlete's foot, hemorrhoids, varicose veins, arteriosclerosis, heart disease, cancer, arthritis, menopause, osteoporosis, bone spurs, low back problems, loose teeth, diabetes, hypoglycemia, chronic fatigue syndrome, and high blood pressure. My goal, of course, was to prevent all of these diseases and help people live to be 100 years old, but few people came to my office for advice on how to prevent disease. Most of my patients were people who had suffered for many years from chronic disease, followed their multiple doctors' and specialists' advice and were frustrated because they were not making the progress that they had hoped for.

Ben Franklin said that, "an ounce of prevention is worth a pound of cure," so this chapter is designed to pave the way for my discussion of preventative programs as well as therapies for existing diseases. I often hear our patients say, "I just can't take all of these supplements and medications!" To which I reply, "The inconvenience of taking supplements is a small exchange, cheap insurance if you will, in return for the prevention of a major disease such as heart disease, diabetes, arthritis, or cancer."

We go to a great deal of expense and effort to prevent major automobile wear by changing oil, filters, and transmission fluid. Why not treat our bodies as well as you do your "Beamer"? Preventive maintenance of our bodies can cost as little as $1 to $5 per day depending on whether you want a $10,000 or $50,000 "insurance" policy (smoking and drinking cost considerably more!!!).

A daily baseline supplemental program of vitamins, minerals, and trace minerals are essential to preventive health goals. It is impossible to obtain enough nutrition from our food to reach the maximum genetic potential of 120 to 140 health-filled years. Therefore, I recommend taking supplements at preventive levels in divided doses t.i.d. (three times per day) to keep blood levels elevated for at least 12 hours per day. All recommended supplemental levels of nutrients for specific diseases are to be taken in addition to the base prevention amounts.

This basic supplement information was issued to my patients by means of single sheet handouts. Over the years the information I collected for the handouts and the questions and feed back I got from patients from the hand outs were the basis for the *Let's Play Doctor* book that Dr. Ma Lan and I wrote. We used a format for *Let's Play Doctor* that was similar to that used for The Merck Manual. People found *Let's Play Doctor* so useful as a home health reference that it became a best seller with over 300,000 copies sold.

I continued to lecture for the NHF and other alternative health groups, including the Cancer Control Society, Whole Life Expo, and New Life Expo. I even put on my own freestanding lectures by putting ads in various newspapers and began appearing as a guest on talk radio shows. All of these activities built a loyal following of all kinds of patients with chronic health problems that had been intractable to standard medical treatment. Cystic fibrosis families found me through word of mouth and media contacts.

I was particularly interested in my weight loss patients because of the challenge. I really paid great attention to their complaints and comments. As a result, I learned that the overweight person has similar cravings and binge eating habits as pregnant women. They craved salt, fried foods, sugar, spicy foods and even non-food items such as clay, hair, finger nails or they chewed on paper. It didn't take long to determine that the common thread between the "munchies" displayed by pregnant women and the obese patient was a deficiency of minerals. They both demonstrated the behavior known as pica or cribbing. Binge eaters, "chocoholics," and anyone else who "can't eat just one" and suffer from being overweight are always, 100 percent of the time, mineral deficient. As a result my weight loss programs always contained complete mineral supplement programs. Hair analyses were often done to personalize the mineral supplementation program.

The results were wonderful. Patients lost weight and they kept it off. Patients were able to eliminate their binge eating habits and lost their cravings. It didn't take long for the news of my success with weight loss patients to spread. The start of office hours had to be pushed back to 5:30 a.m. Two nurses were hired just to weigh everybody in, take their blood pressure, and refill their supplements and their weight loss medications.

One of the more interesting "cancer" patients was a 60-year-old man from Idaho who had been diagnosed with testicular cancer by a medical doctor. He drove all the way to Portland to see the horse doctor who treated people. On examination, his scrotum was as large as a grapefruit and rubbery, like a water balloon. I got the old pocket flashlight out and turned off the lights in the examining room. I placed the flashlight to one side of his scrotum and turned on the switch. The light revealed a hydroceole of the scrotum, which was filled with about a pint of clear fluid.

Using a topical anesthesia on the scrotum, I drained off the fluid using a 50-milliliter syringe and a switch-valve. The man stayed overnight in a nearby motel and returned the next morning. Examination revealed a normal scrotum and testicles with no return of the fluid. Quite obviously he had not had "cancer." If a chiropractor or naturopathic physician had made the mistaken cancer diagnosis, there would have been a huge outcry for the elimination of such quacks for the safety of the public. Since a medical doctor made the "mistake," it was just "one of those things." Since no harm had come to the patient, the patient couldn't sue and get any compensation!

These basic patients with every day, common complaints were the bread and butter of my practice. I used as much veterinary nutrition as I could to improve their health and reverse their problems. The patients and I had a lot of fun together. I gave them useful information and I certainly learned a lot from them. All of this medical activity was entered into to support my interest in treating CF children and families with cystic fibrosis and muscular dystrophy. The word spread and they came, cystic fibrosis and muscular dystrophy patients of all ages.

As a result of my speaking schedule and media campaign, I saw an average of fifty patients per day, an outrageous load for a naturopathic physician. My day started with weight loss patients at 6:00 a.m., new patients appeared at 9:00 a.m., and patients that required special procedures were seen after lunch until 3:00 pm. I realized quickly that my schedule was going to be overloaded, and I would have to generate some passive income if I were going to be able to have time off and escape the rigors of the around the clock demands of a heavy patient load.

Most N.D.s averaged about six to eight patients per day compared with my fifty. As a result, my colleagues believed that I had some mafia, gangland, or illicit drug connection. The fact that I drove a new Cadillac and lived in a large Victorian house while they drove ten year old Volkswagens and lived in basement apartments added fuel to their envious fantasies.

About a year after graduation I entered into a three-way partnership with another N.D. and an M.D. We purchased a twenty-five year old osteopathic practice and took over the 3,000 patient files. The M.D. was the primary instructor of medical diagnosis and surgery at NCNM. He and I shared an office and he was sympathetic to our naturopathic nutritional approach to preventing and treating disease. He was a vegetarian, practiced yoga and meditation, so he was looked upon as a non-threatening partner. Our new association and joint practice grew. We each took an equal sized draw each month and all seemed to be well.

The association gave me some extra time to develop a source of passive income. I looked at developing an insurance business. I considered buying a McDonald's franchise. I priced Oregon beef farms. I took an insurance management course and passed the test for the state of Oregon insurance license. I took the management course from McDonald's. All of these types of business ventures were capital and labor intensive, so they were ruled out for the time being. The management and sales training turned out to be very useful though.

I was eventually invited to a business seminar in downtown Portland by another naturopathic physician. I was told only that a marketing expert was going to give a free seminar on how to build a passive income type of business. In the pursuit of identifying some source of passive income, I decided to accept the invitation and go.

I arrived at the appointed hour to find about 500 well dressed men and women already seated. There was a high level of excitement. Everyone had a tape recorder and a pad and paper for notes. They were obviously very professional and highly respectful of the promised speaker.

The speaker, Jack Daugherty, was introduced as a former potato-shed foreman from Idaho! I thought to myself, "What could I learn from a potato-shed foreman—I am a doctor!"

What I learned was, that if I could identify my goals and if I focused on my goals, success was inevitable. I learned that if I could help others get what they wanted, I could get what I wanted. He said, "All you have to do is plan to work and work your plan." It seemed obvious, but nobody had ever quite verbalized the thought quite as simply as Jack did.

Then Jack started drawing sponsors, circles, "legs," downlines, and dollar signs. He talked about making an extra five-thousand dollars per month with just a few hours per day required. Jack talked about network marketing, and Amway, whatever that was. I immediately knew that I could do this network marketing thing, whatever it was—as long as it was legal, and I would have to check that out. Maybe this network marketing was the method of training and communication that I needed to get the nutritional information out to the general public! I needed an army of motivated people who would be rewarded for their efforts. I would help them to get what they wanted, and in return, I would get what I wanted—the prevention and elimination of most disease through nutritional supplementation!

My sponsor was a naturopathic physician. Her sponsor was a naturopathic physician and his sponsor was a pig farmer! I was 42 years old and had never been approached by anyone before to investigate network marketing. I must have been considered a terrible prospect.

They gave me tapes, books, catalogues, price lists, and a starter pack that included laundry soap, dish washing soap, window cleaner, shampoo, and a box that contained a month's supply of Nutralite multivitamins. The whole pile cost me about $200, but I couldn't figure out how to make money selling the stuff. Did I need a store? Did I need to hire sales people? The margin of profit was so low, I would have to sell thousands of boxes of product per month to make it work.

I asked more questions. My up-line leader, Bill Heard the pig farmer, said he would come to my house to explain everything if I would get several couples to come over to hear about the opportunity. As promised, I had five couples who were neighbors and friends. Interestingly enough, I couldn't get a single naturopathic physician to participate. The N.D.s expressed concern that network marketing had a bad reputation. They were afraid to participate because their association with network marketing might tarnish their professional image that they had worked so hard to gain. Obviously they didn't see network marketing as a tool to disperse nutritional information like I did.

Bill appeared about a half-hour early dressed like a bank president and set up a white marker board. I was amazed. I had expected bib-overalls and smelly boots. Bill didn't look or act like any pig farmer I had ever met. He lectured with a good-natured and humorous style for about an hour on his personal experience that brought him to network marketing, America, "The Dream," financial opportunity, financial freedom, lifestyle, the process of duplication, helping others, and a company by the name of Amway. It was 1982 and I had never heard of Amway, but I knew I could do it.

Two determined young men who had failed many times at trying to start up a business partnership had founded Amway. They had finally, through shear force of will, formed a company that sold a liquid organic cleaner—LOC. Their success was finding a product that was useful and which came in a one-month supply which people needed to reorder. Seven years later they acquired the Nutralite supplement company and entered into network marketing. Today, Amway has a million U.S. distributors and is an $8 billion a year business.

There are many individual marketing groups in Amway. The one that I had hooked up with was called "World Wide Dream Builders." Each marketing group had its own flavor and style. World Wide Dream Builders stressed wholesome family values and directed its business energies towards recruitment and education. Recruitment was accomplished primarily by putting on home meetings, seminars, "drawing circles" and "showing the plan." There was also cold contacting, the three foot rule, mailings, and plastering parking lots with flyers.

The education came in the form of seminars, "tools" such as books, audio and video tapes. The whole idea was to train a volunteer sales force, each of whom had the same opportunity for an enhanced lifestyle, financial success, and financial freedom as their goal.

To succeed though, everyone has to learn different things. Because I was a teacher and practitioner of nutrition, I did not have to spend a lot of time understanding nutrition or the education process, but I did have to learn how to qualify a prospect, how to test close, and how to close the sale and "get the check." In the early days I must have read every Zig Ziglar book ten times. Then there were positive motivational books, including Og Mandino and Robert Schuller. One couldn't communicate with prospects if they were down in the dumps. I learned that you had to get ten "no's" before you got to the "yes." The quicker one got the "no's" out of the way, the quicker you got to the "yes," so even the "no's" brought joy!

I sponsored my business partners into Amway and began to incorporate Amway's Nutrilite nutritional supplements into the office pharmacy. In turn, my Amway upline and downline referred patients to us and our practice grew in fame and income. Amway patients paid when they received the service and they transmitted the nutrition information they were given "upline" and "downline." Each day at 3:00 p.m. I would leave the office and ply the neighboring office buildings looking for business builders, looking for customers, setting up appointments for home meetings, and above all, "showing the plan."

On the way to one of the NHF seminars in Long Beach, California we had a great adventure. One of the things we did at the seminars was have a microscope at our booth to view blood samples of attendees. We would give them some health insights based on what was seen in a smear of blood. Part of the process for the blood test included cleaning the finger skin with ether to remove skin oils. We packed the ether in a tight metal can and double sealed the can with paraffin. The can was placed in plastic bags and sealed. The sealed package was placed in my brief case along with other papers and forms and we were off to Long Beach.

About an hour into the flight, I smelled ether. In those days people were still smoking on airplanes so I knew there was a potential problem. I pushed the call button to attract a flight attendant. When she arrived I suggested to her that she put the No Smoking light on because we had some leaking ether. The attendant blanched, turned on the No-Smoking light and screamed down the isle that there were ether fumes loose on the plane. When we arrived at the John Wayne Airport in Orange County, we went to the baggage claim to pick up our belongings and the microscope. While waiting I noticed about six seedy looking guys wearing fatigue jackets with peace signs painted on them. These guys had surrounded us and they were slowly tightening the circle.

I thought they were muggers, so I alerted my partner. We stood back to back and we readied ourselves to repel muggers. As they got closer, one man flashed a badge and a gun. He identified himself as an under-cover DEA agent. He and his gang wanted to search our bags for cocaine. The ether incident on the plane had been called forward and they thought we were free-basing cocaine. They brought the dogs up to sniff our bags, they searched us, and in the end turned us loose to go on our way. The only "stuff" that we had with us was a bottle of vitamin C tablets.

In 1985, I was returning from one of my Alaska Air Guard summer camps. Instead of going home I decided to stop by the clinic to see how things were going. I entered the clinic to find that during my absence, our M.D. partner had formed a new clinic corporation, hired our nurses away from the partnership, took all of the patient records, and had evicted the third partner and myself. He wanted us to continue to pay for the original lease, but we would have to start up a new practice on our own!

He had decided that in the great scheme of things he was worth more than we to the clinic operation, so he decided to take it over. Even though this M.D. was a vegetarian, even though he did meditation and Yoga and was an alternative doctor, he was still an M.D. An M.D is an M.D. and almost all believe they are immortal and god-like.

When I arrived, the clinic pharmacy was locked with a nurse inside to guard the inventory. The patients who filled the waiting room were totally unaware of what had happened or what was about to happen.

My first instinct was to break the pharmacy door down, which is what I did. I backed up ten feet, ran at the door and threw a football shoulder into it. Wood splintered everywhere, the nurse inside the pharmacy ran out of the rear door screaming. The other nurse ran down the hall and called the police. When they arrived I assured the police that the door was mine, and if I wanted to break it I could, would, and did.

I went to an attorney to file suit against the M.D. partner. After 30 days we had a settlement hearing with a judge who looked at our partner-ship agreement and said it was valid and that somebody would have to buy out the other partners. Until that was worked out, I had no clinic practice.

Amway joined up with MCI at about this time. Ma Bell was dismem-bered and it was a free for all as the small long distance companies tried to get a share of the "Dial 1" long distance business. MCI didn't have the time or the capital to hire and train thousands of sales representatives and some clever MCI executive came up with the idea to enlist Amway distributors to sign up new MCI customers. Amway distributors got two dollars for signing up a household and ten dollars for signing up a business with MCI. A residual income of one and one half per cent of the new customer's long distance phone bill was paid as long as they kept that number.

I had time on my hands while everyone decided what to do about the clinic partnership so I looked into the new MCI opportunity. I called a few neighbors and knocked on a few doors. The average home long distance phone bill at that time was only about $25. I folded my tent and prepared to give up the MCI business . . . I thought.

The holidays were approaching and there were lots of parties. I was a guest at one of these galas and out of habit I asked a few of the other guests if they had a long distance phone bill of any size. All but one said they didn't.

Surprisingly, the largest bill belonged to a trucker. He wore a denim vest with no sleeves and jeans, had leather wristbands with metal spikes attached and tattoos all over his bare arms. When I asked about his phone bill, he lit up like a Christmas tree—"Man do I have a phone bill, it's $800 per month!"

Now I perked up and asked if all truckers had such large phone bills.

He said, "Heck yes, mine is a small phone bill compared to most. Trucker's phone bills can run up to thousands of dollars per month."

My next question was to ask where truckers hung out. "Truck stops," he said. I asked where the biggest truck stop was. "The 76 Auto Truck Plaza at the junction of I-10 and I-5 at the north side of L.A."

I honed my skills at signing up truckers into the MCI "Dial 1" program at the local Jubitz truck stop in Portland. I had a month before the legal process ran its course for my suit against the M.D., so I decided to head down to L.A. and sign up some truckers into the Amway-MCI system.

My first job was to get a motel room on the truck stop property. I got a monthly rate that included a microwave and a refrigerator. I started signing up truckers. I signed up an average of 100 per day for 30 days. The best part was that several truck stop owners liked the idea, so they signed up their college-aged kids to ply the truck stops and sign up truckers after I left. Many truckers signed up other truckers as they crossed the country, so the organization grew.

While waiting for the legal process to be completed, the spiritually elevated M.D. just packed up all his belongings and left town in the middle of the night. I sold my share of the practice to the naturopathic partner, packed up, and moved to Houston, Texas to buy a yacht with some of my Amway earnings and get a life. The oil crisis had hit Texas and the bottom was falling out of oil prices. A barrel of oil had been $35. Now it was $8 per barrel and banks were repossessing Texas yachts at a rapid rate. It was one of my Amway dreams to live on a yacht and it was the right time to make it happen.

15

THE AGE BEATERS

My first boat was a 25-foot sloop, a single masted sail boat that was docked in a marina in Clear Lake, Texas adjacent to Galveston Bay. I learned how to sail, I fished, and I started courting a very pretty, very tall, cheerful, and athletic Chinese medical doctor named Ma Lan. We had a lot in common with our interest in helping people with their health, the outdoors, sailing. Yet we had a lot of differences because she was raised in mainland China in a communist political and business system. An internationally known microsurgeon who had taught at Harvard Medical School, she knew little of capitalism, marketing, nutrition, and nutritional supplements.

Our dates consisted of fishing and eating our catch. We cooked, listened to music and talked about the Amway business, nutrition and science and medicine. Ma Lan taught me how to use a throw net to catch shrimp and fish, and I taught her how to use a spinning rod to catch redfish and catfish.

After six months of courting and fishing we were married on Valentine's Day, 1987, and our lives have been a joint venture, adventure, and a continuing educational experience ever since. More about Ma Lan and our courtship later. Suffice it to say that we grew in our need for space so we graduated to a 40 foot sloop christened *The Elixir*. It slept eight and had every amenity and navigational device that could be attached to a civilian boat. We had to learn how to seriously sail, operate the satellite navigational and radar systems, and maintain the engine and electronics. Every American dreams of living on a yacht. It's a lifestyle that every American equates to luxury, early retirement, success, and financial independence. It was in fact the lifestyle that I had taped to my refrigerator door for one of my Amway goals.

The concept of network marketing had made early retirement and financial success happen for me. The concept of network marketing and the residual income it generated worked, and I was only 48-years-old!

I ran my Amway business from the deck of *The Elixir* under the sun of Galveston Bay by telephone and had lots of time to spend with my new bride. I believed that I was living the lifestyle of kings. In this newfound leisure I had lots of time to think and plan how to best help patients maximize their health and their longevity. I thought if I could focus on longevity and add 20 to 50 years to everyone's life, I would be doing the righteous thing. I would have accomplished my goal.

How old could a person really live if they did everything right? All species have a "genetic potential" or upper limit for longevity. For mice it's 700 days. For dogs—23 years; horses—32 years; elephant—45 years; chimpanzee—52 years. Man? 168 years. Unfortunately Americans don't do a very good job when it comes to longevity. An American's average lifespan is 75.5 years, about half of our genetic potential for longevity of 120 to 140 years.

In 1990, the World Health Organization examined the top 32 industrialized nations for health and longevity. The United States ranked 17th in longevity. Sixteen other countries actually live longer than we do. We ranked 19th in healthfulness, which means that 18 other countries live longer than we do before they develop heart disease, diabetes, and cancer.

We as Americans have the highest priced and most technologically advanced health care system in the world, yet this highly regarded health care system, the envy of the world, has failed to make us the healthiest and the longest lived nation in the world. The American healthcare system has failed because it has failed to educate the public on how to prevent and cure diseases with nutrition. The information necessary to make Americans the healthiest and the longest lived people on earth through supplementation of vitamins, minerals, and trace minerals already exists in the veterinary and medical literature, therefore, one must conclude that American health and longevity is not a doctor's primary goal.

Whether or not an individual of a particular species reaches their genetic potential for longevity depends on their being able to negotiate successfully through two basic concepts.

Concept number one: avoid stepping on the land mines or eliminate unnecessary and wasteful death from predators and road accidents. Don't smoke, don't abuse alcohol, don't do drugs, avoid agricultural chemicals and industrial wastes in food, air and water. If at all possible, avoid going to the doctor. Given half a chance they will kill you.

American Mormons and the American Seventh Day Adventists live to 82 years on the average—six and one half years longer than the average American. What is their secret? It turns out that it's not what they do, it's what they don't do. Mormons and Seventh Day Adventists live to be 82 years of age on the average because they avoid caffeine (i.e. coffee, soft drinks, tea, iced tea, etc.), alcohol, smoking, and fried foods (i.e. pork, catfish, shrimp, lard shortening, etc).

Concept number two: Now that you have avoided the land mines, do all those positive things necessary to make it to 140 years of age, including consuming all 90 essential nutrients in optimal amounts each day to warranty that you will properly develop, maintain, and repair your body.

Assuming that you avoid the "land mines" of life, longevity depends on how faithfully one consumes optimal amounts of the 90 essential nutrients—the raw material necessary for health and longevity—each and every day. Supplementation is the only way that you can guarantee you will consume the optimal amounts of all 90 essential nutrients and assure yourself that you are going to make it healthfully to 100 or more.

Remember, plants can't manufacture minerals like they do vitamins. And nothing works in the body without mineral cofactors—nothing! Vitamins, DNA, RNA, chromosomes, enzymes, hormones, energy, not even oxygen works without mineral cofactors. Minerals are in fact the limiting factor for health and longevity—they are in fact the long sought out "fountain of youth."

Unfortunately Americans have been taught by our health care system that they can just eat well, eat the four food groups, and get everything they need to lead a long healthy life. The equivalent scenario would be that you take a bag full of dirt from Texas, throw it into the oil pan of your car, and exclaim, "I don't have to put oil in my car because I just put dirt from Texas in there and there is oil in Texas dirt." Even the village idiot wouldn't do that to a twenty-year-old Volkswagen! Yet every American has been trained and directed by the credibility of the American medical system to throw away half of their health and longevity potential just by eating well—"You can get everything you need from your four food groups."

The sentence, "You can get everything you need from your four food groups," has killed more Americans than all the foreign enemies in the 220 years we've been a nation. Blind faith in doctors by our parents and grandparents has resulted in a national disaster. The credibility we have given doctors has resulted in Americans being miserable in the last 12 years of their lives and has resulted in Americans giving up 50 percent of their longevity potential.

Americans made doctors demigods, similar to political figures, athletes, and movie stars. The T.V. series *Dr. Marcus Welby, M.D., Dr. Ben Casey, Dr. Kildare* and *E.R.* have drilled into American's heads that doctors are our health advocates and that doctors will throw themselves on the pyre to save their patients. No one points out that doctors have mortgages, Mercedes payments, college tuition payments for their kids which all must be dealt with. The American patient is the source of their money, their lifestyle, and their credibility, yet we have been cheated because American health and longevity are not the doctor's priority— their own lifestyle is their priority. Doctors of course will vigorously deny this observation; however, the proof is in the pudding. Americans only live to be 75.5 on the average and we rank 17th in longevity and 19th in healthfulness. So what's hidden in the pudding we've been eating? Obviously not the minerals we need!

Nutrients are called essential when we need them to prevent disease and death and our bodies can't manufacture them. We must consume essential nutrients every day as food or supplements. On the average we get 10 deficiency diseases for each essential nutrient that's missing from our diets for several weeks, several months, or several years depending on the nutrient. That's a whopping potentially 900 diseases that are preventable by supplementing with all 90 essential nutrients.

The nice thing is, that if you have any of these 900 deficiency diseases (except 100 congenital defects that are not reversible by supplementation) you have every honest expectation to get some recognizable benefit if you supplement properly, maybe even get a 100 percent better.

An analogy of our "genetic potential" for longevity is the engine of a Mercedes, which is a wonder of German automotive engineering. The engine is designed to run 300,000 miles before it needs a major overhaul or needs to be replaced. Yet if you, the owner/driver, don't maintain the Mercedes engine by supplying the essential air filters, oil filters, fuel filters, coolants, lubricants and motor oil, that wondrous engine designed to run 300,000 miles won't run 50 miles! Without filters, oil, and coolant, even a Mercedes won't make it to the engineered potential ("genetic potential") of 300,000 miles (in humans 120 -140 years).

The association between maximizing one's longevity and the intake of optimal amounts of essential nutrients by supplementation is well documented in the laboratory for many species and in isolated Third World cultures in remote far-flung areas of the Earth. While the people of the long-lived Third World cultures do not have Ph.D.s in biochemistry or nutrition, western medicine, doctors, or health insurance, they have by serendipity set up their homelands in an idyllic biochemical Garden of Eden, and as a result many live to 120 to 140 years and some extraordinary individuals live to be 150 to 160. While these long lived cultures and their idyllic homelands are superficially quite different, it is their similarities, their common threads or common denominators, that give the net result of healthful longevity that we can learn and benefit from.

All of the long lived cultures were persecuted peoples for religious, racial, or monetary reasons and they fled the kings' armies looking for refuge in desolate high mountain valleys ranging from 8,500 to 14,000 feet in elevation. By chance, the long lived cultures have set up their homelands in regions that have 60 to 72 minerals in the parent rocks and soil that they chose to live in. They picked places to live that were arid and had less than two inches of precipitation per year. They had to pick places that had dependable permanent sources of water. By chance, the long-lived cultures on earth picked glaciers as their permanent sources of water.

Glaciers move up and down the mountains in synchrony with the seasons, growing in winter and shrinking in summer. Glaciers literally weigh millions of tons. As they move up and down the mountain's slopes, they grind up tens of thousands of tons of rock into rock "flour" each year. This rock flour containing 60 to 72 minerals comes out from under the glacier suspended in the water by turbulence and small particle size. This rock flour suspension is known as "glacial milk."

Each of the long-lived cultures has built canals or aqueducts to carry the "glacial milk" to their valleys. Not only do these age-beaters drink the "glacial milk," they irrigate with the mineral-laden glacial milk or have fields on flood plains that get replenished with mineral-laden silt every spring when it floods. Their grains, vegetables, fruits, and nuts convert the inorganic elemental minerals in the fields to plant derived colloidal minerals. It is the plant derived colloidal minerals in their grains, vegetables, fruits, and nuts that are their common threads giving the age-beaters their health and longevity. It is the plant derived colloidal minerals that are in fact the Fountain of Youth!

The search for health and longevity is as old as man himself. We have expended resources, money, energy, and have in fact died in droves looking for the Fountain of Youth. Literally the Fountain of Youth has been under our feet since the beginning of time. The answer is almost anticlimactic; it's minerals.

History is a revolt against death. While the search for life comes to us in what appear to be merely odd legends or stupefying prescriptions for strange behavior, some in fact reveal a scientifically justified quest to find and preserve the minerals which are the stuff of life in the midst of the oddity.

The oldest known story relating to the active human search for the secrets of longevity is the 5,000-year-old saga of Gilgamesh. The Sumerian King from Uruk, along with his good friend and general of his armies, Enkidu, decided they would live forever. Enkidu died suddenly in the mid-years of his life, causing King Gilgamesh to panic. The king decided to place his entire fortune and energies into a do or die search for eternal youth and immortality.

Gilgamesh climbed to the tops of the highest mountains, searched in the dense forest, and deep into the depths of rivers and oceans in his legendary and fanatical search for youth and longevity. Gilgamesh was regarded as a gerontological myth until the discovery of 12 clay tablets that archeologists determined were 5,000 years old. Pieced together after their discovery in the ancient city of Sumar, the tablets confirmed that Gilgamesh was in fact a king, adventurer and hero of his times who led a great quest for the "key to immortality." He called for a "revolt against death itself!"

As the legend goes, Gilgamesh eventually and heroically found a wise old man in the high mountains, who spoke of a fragrant flower that "looked like a buckthorn and prickled like a rose." The wise prophet shared with Gilgamesh that the plant could be found at the floor of the world's deepest sea. By coming into possession of this plant and tasting it, one could regain his youth.

Gilgamesh located the plant, however, before he could eat sufficient quantities to rejuvenate himself, it was, according to the legend, stolen from him by a serpent seeking to regenerate a new skin.

Hyperborean legends of longevity tell of the Island of Blest, where according to the ancient Greeks Strabo and Pindar and Pliny, the Roman lived as "Blessed Humans" with very healthy and exceedingly long lives. "Hyperborean" translates to "beyond the North Wind"—a wondrous legendary place of health, joy, and pleasures of the unknown and a place of great difficulty to reach. Many cultures still have deep beliefs in the ability to attain immortality by "masters" and still embrace this "Golden Age" (Hindus, Iranians, Celtics, and Chinese).

The Chinese Taoists developed a whole way of life to ensure immortality through training and self-discipline directed at conservation of what limited resources one was given at birth.

The word "Tao" means "The Way," the way to immortality. Through the accomplishment or mastery of the Taoist techniques one would become a "hsien" or an immortal or man-god. If you could master the knowledge of primal substances (alchemy and knowledge of minerals and metals) and quintessence of life and sex and become a hsien, you could control physical reality and be a master magician, course through the air as a bird, control the weather, take different animal shapes as you wish, become invisible, become immortal, and thus be ageless.

The three basic truths of Taoism are naturalism, empiricism, and special skills.

According to the Tao, everyone begins their life at birth with a fixed or given amount of Qi or Life Force, which you must conserve as a major factor in attaining immortality. Conservation of Qi requires progressing towards a state of "effortless action," thus gaining optimal benefit in life, health, and longevity with a minimal expenditure of energy or Qi, kind of like a professional couch potato.

The Taoist techniques include respiratory, dietary (alchemy, minerals and metals), gymnastic, sexual, and meditative exercises. Meditation is applied as a basic for mastering all the Taoist techniques. To become a hsien you must reduce your rate of breathing, "on exhalation swallow the breath for nourishment, and while the breath is internal, direct it on a specific course through the body and cause it to ascend to the brain, the main organ to maintain and rejuvenate because it controls all others."

The Taoist dietary practices include avoidance of grains, meat, wine, and most vegetables. Strict Taoists subsist on roots and fruit. The master hsien are able to live on "breath for meat and saliva for drink." The dietary, sexual, and breathing techniques are meant to prolong life long enough to allow one sufficient time for making the elixir of immortality. Kung Fu was designed to be the gymnastics of the hsien or Toaist masters. Its function is to eliminate obstructions from within the body which are expelled through the external circulation of breath and sexual essences.

In Tao, during sex one reaches sexual fervor to the point of orgasm, but does not ejaculate. Instead one meditates. While this seems strange, it is in fact quite consistent with what we know about minerals and health. Men lose 420 mcg of zinc per ejaculation. The ability to enjoy the ecstasy of sex without ejaculation is a zinc conserving practice.

The 20th century Taoists include the practice of Chinese Chi Gong, Yoga, mind-body duality, and the body, mind, spirit practitioners who use crystals, pendulums, and dowsing rods.

Roger Bacon in his *Opus Magnus* wrote:

> The body of Adam did not possess elements in full equality....
> but since the elements in him approached equality, there was
> very little waste in him; and hence he was fit for immortality,
> which he could have secured if he had eaten always from the
> tree of life. For this fruit is thought to have elements
> approaching equality.

Bacon felt he could extend life by 100 years if he could "reduce the elements in some form of food or drink to an equality or nearly so and have taught the means to this end." For talking and writing about a balanced diet and essential elements that could promote health and extend life, Bacon was put in jail for his heretical remarks!

Paracelsus (1493–1541) came to his end in a bar room brawl in the White Horse Inn in Salzburg, Germany. Paracelsus straddled the end of the Middle Ages and the beginning of the Renaissance. A university professor, a legendary physician, a social outcast, and an insatiable traveler, he brought Chinese alchemy to western cultures as a form of ritualized chemistry. Paracelsus described alchemy as "the ultimate matter of anything, that state in which the substance has reached its highest grade of exaltation and perfection." It was this state that Paracelsus felt could provide health and extended life or immortality.

The German physician Christopher Hufeland (1796) published the book, *The Art of Prolonging Human Life* (later the title was changed to *Makrobiotik*) which featured hygiene to maintain health and the dietary and health practices of makrobiotik to attain longevity.

Benjamin Franklin (1780) wrote a letter to Joseph Priestly. In it, he stated:

> Agriculture may diminish its labor and double its produce.
> All diseases may by some means be prevented or cured,
> not excepting even that of old age, and our lives
> lengthened at pleasure even beyond the antediluvian
> standard.

Dr. Alexis Carrel (1912) grew fibroblasts (connective tissue cells) from chicken hearts in flasks fed with extracts of blended chicken embryo and the cells kept multiplying and growing for 34 years (two years beyond Carrel's own death). Carrel's colleagues got bored with the experiment and threw the fibroblasts out. The experiment resulted in the theory that cells are inherently immortal if fed a perfect diet and kept in a perfect environment. Carrel was not just your average physician. He had won the Nobel Prize in Medicine for developing the end to end anastomosis (joining of transected ends) of blood vessels with fine suture.

Unfortunately for the Carrel and the immortality of the cell theory, a Dr. Leonard Hayflick came along and used artificial growth media with major mineral deficiencies for human fibroblast propagation. In his experiment (faulted from the beginning), human fibroblasts could only divide 50 times before dying out and showing accumulations of ceroid lipofucsin, the pigment of aging that indicates lipid peroxidation and a selenium deficiency. Hayflick attributed Carrel's success in unending propagation of healthy chicken fibroblasts to the contamination of the growth media by embryonic fibroblasts from the chick embryo media— rather than admitting that poor and limited nutrition prematurely ended the life of his human fibroblasts. The 50-replication limit of fibroblasts is known as the "Hayflick limit."

James Hilton made "Shangri-La" famous through his 1934 Pulitzer Prize winning novel, *Lost Horizon*, where people lived healthful, loving, productive, and long lives. The novel was made into a classic movie of the same name in 1937 and remade in the 1960s as a color film entitled, *Shangri-La.* In the original novel and the original movie, the people of Shangri-La attributed their youthfulness, health, and longevity to a Spartan diet, peaceful attitude, a work ethic devoted to gardening and farming, and a rich Christian faith and lifestyle. The remake of the film version portrayed an eastern type meditation as the basis of their health and longevity, which contributed to the passion for eastern meditation by the "hippy" movement of the 1960s and 1970s.

The modern day "Cryologists" have such faith in the technology of medical science as a route to immortality that they pay huge sums of money up to $45,000 for a head and $120,000 for a whole body to have themselves quick frozen in liquid nitrogen, "Cryonic Suspension," after they die to be stored until a cure is found for their terminal malady.

The Immortalists of the Flame Foundation (also known as "CBJ") believe that "if you become cellularly alive, you will not be influenced by the mass program of death." The Immortalists, like Gilgamesh, are having a revolt against death. "CBJ" is derived from the first initials of it's three founders, Charles Paul Brown, Bernadene Sittser, and James Russell Strole. All three are ordained Christian ministers who no longer preach the word of God—they now "preach against death."

The Immortalists claim an active membership of over 4,000 rabid followers and in 1994 celebrated their 26th anniversary as an organization. The CBJ faithful believe "we die because we think we must." To "neutralize" the "death program" a strong and equal but opposite action or belief is required. "People [must be] reinforcing the idea that you don't have to die; to live as an Immortalist people need to close off their 'exits,' things like a belief in heaven or hell or reincarnation or even holding onto a family burial plot."

There are all kinds of food preservatives, drugs, and pharmaceuticals (i.e.-BHT, GH3, Deprinel, DHEA, etc.) that are touted as the answer to longevity, yet there are no living centenarians who have tried these chemical shortcuts to support the theories with truly extended years. There are all kinds of proponents of exercise as a major progenitor of health and longevity, yet neither human history nor human experience bears out the exercise theory.

The great distance runners, Jim Fixx and Dr. George Sheehan, believed that exercise was the elixir of health and the foundation for longevity. To that end they ran and jogged almost every day of their adult lives. Neither took vitamin or mineral supplements.

Jim Fixx, who started the whole running craze with his best seller, *Jog Your Way to Health*, died at age 52 following multiple cardiomyopathy heart attacks—a simple selenium deficiency. Fixx was convinced that if he took supplements the water would be muddied and people wouldn't know if it was the exercise or the supplements that got him to age 100.

Fixx asked sports medicine doctors, trainers, nutritionists, and coaches if he needed to take nutritional supplements. They all assured Fixx that he could get everything he needed nutritionally by simply "eating the four food groups." In actuality, when one exercises and fails to take supplements, exercise becomes a negative because athletes sweat out their essential minerals!

Then there was Dr. George Sheehan, medical editor *for Runners World Magazine* and a "runner's runner." His only concern with diet and nutritional supplements was that, "they didn't interfere with running." Dr. Sheehan died of widely disseminated prostate cancer at the age of

76. All that running and all that pain and sweat without supplementation bought him six months longer than the classic American "couch potato" who averages 75.5 years. According to the medical school at the University of Arizona, JAMA Dec. 25, 1996, selenium supplemented at 250 mcg/day will reduce ones risk of developing prostate cancer by 69 percent.

Jesse Owens, who won four gold medals in track and field in the 1936 Berlin Olympics, died at the age of 66. None of the "Flying Finns," the track team from Finland and legendary for dominating three Olympics in a row during the 20s and 30s, reached the age of 70. Athletes sweat out more minerals in five years than couch potatoes sweat out in 50 years. If you sweat out all of your copper and don't replace it by supplementation you are at high risk of dying of a ruptured aneurysm. If you sweat out all of your selenium and don't replace it by supplementation you're at high risk of developing a cardiomyopathy heart attack or cancer. If you sweat out all of your chromium and vanadium and don't replace it by supplementation you're at high risk of developing adult onset or type 2 diabetes. If you sweat out all of your calcium, magnesium, and sulfur and don't replace them by supplementation, you are at high risk of developing arthritis, osteoporosis, and kidney stones.

The United States government has hired and isolated 350 longevity scientists in an abandoned military facility in Arkansas to study aging and how to slow aging down on tens of thousands of mice and rats on calorie restricted/nutrient dense diets. Clive McKay's caloric "undernutrition" (60 percent reduction of calories from free choice) in the mid 1930s doubled the 50 percent survival rate and doubled the known life span of laboratory rats. Undernutrition (low caloric intake) without malnutrition (diet contained the same amount of vitamins, minerals, and trace minerals as the free choice diet) experiments show great benefit even when the low calorie/ high mineral diet is begun in mid-adulthood. Low calorie, nutrient dense diets (high levels of vitamins, minerals, and trace minerals) are not for children as there is a relatively high mortality on the front end of this program. Children will flourish and do well on optimal calorie/ nutrient dense programs.

Biblical patriarchs are notable for having had great longevity, including Methuselah at age 969 years and Noah at 950 years. As time moved ahead chronologically in the Bible, from the Creation, the recorded longevity for the patriarchs declined. Did this decline in longevity reflect a gradual loss of minerals and trace minerals from the soil or a covering of inert sand dropped on mineral-rich soil by the Great

Flood of Noah's time?

Anthropologists have theorized the maximum lifespan of ancient man based on physical traits and cultural skills and assets:

"Missing link"—43 years maximum lifespan
Australopithecus—47 years maximum lifespan
Homo erectus—72 years maximum lifespan
Homo sapiens—120 to 140 years maximum lifespan

The maximum survival rate or longevity for fish has been extended by 300 percent in the UCLA laboratory of Roy Walford. He accomplished this increase in longevity by maximizing the level of vitamins, minerals, and trace minerals fed to the fish as well as by lowering the water temperature by just a few degrees.

Before the "Industrial Revolution," man as a species survived the "Age of Pestilence and Famine"—from before written history to the 1700's wars, famine, and epidemics of infectious disease combined to kill 30 to 50 percent of the human populations of the various continents. As more calories and protein became available, more cultures increased their average age of survival. The wealthy (including royalty, merchants, priests, and doctors) always did well as they acquired mineral rich food in a wide variety and excess quantities from far flung corners of their spheres of influence. The organized searches for new land, treasure, herbs, and spices to support a king's adventures always included a search for the "Fountain of Youth." Ponce de Leon was in fact a clerk on one of Columbus' ships that journeyed to the New World with a Royal Charge to find the "Fountain of Youth" if it existed in the New World.

Despite "heroic" efforts by the 20th century "health care" professions, the maximum life span of 120 to 140 for human beings hasn't changed for urban man since the days of ancient Rome. The 50 percent survival rate has increased 300 percent from 25 to 75.5.

Humans must come to grips with the fact that if we are to reach our true genetic potential for health and longevity we must become independent of our minerally depleted soil and food and the poisoned environment. We must not bet our lives on modern medicine or the random distribution of essential minerals being or not being in our food or we will surely fail in our quest for health and longevity.

As an ag student, I knew in 1958 that minerals were necessary to prevent debilitating and life threatening diseases in animals. As a comparative pathologist, I have known since 1962 that the same concept of disease and death prevention with supplements would work in people, too. In 1965, I began to communicate these observations to the medical community through lectures, scientific articles, and books, all to no avail. In 1978, I began to lecture to the general public on the concept of disease prevention and longevity using mineral supplements—the average person initially reacted by saying, "That's interesting, but I need to ask my doctor."

In 1993, the baby boomers found out they were not immortal and they do not want to wind up like their parents—sick, miserable, and financially broke from the yoke of medical and health care bills. By 1998, more than 30 million Americans have heard the tape *Dead Doctors Don't Lie* and are ready to do what ever is safe, economical, and effective to eliminate disease and add years to their life—even take vitamins, minerals, and trace minerals as supplements.

In examining our options for reaching our maximum genetic potential for longevity we have two control groups to evaluate for an optimal and rational approach in humans:

1. Those who as a group do not take supplements. In fact, this group pooh-poohs the use of supplements and fully believes one can get all of the essential nutrients they need from the "Four Food Groups." This homogenous, non-supplementing control group is made up almost exclusively of medical doctors, whose average lifespan ranges from 58 to 69 depending on whose research one looks at.

2. Those who, as a group, do not take supplements yet live to be well over a hundred years of age. This control group includes several ancient cultures which have common denominators that are in fact the long sought after "Fountain of Youth."

While there is some controversy as to whether these people actually do live to be 160, we know for a fact that humans can live to be 122 years and 162 days because the Guinness Book of World Records says so. None can argue that these long lived centenarians from Third World countries do a much better job than we do in reaching their genetic potential for longevity. We will set aside for a time the cynical comments of the naysayers and examine the positives that are obvious.

There are eight well-known cultures whose peoples routinely live to their maximum genetic potential of 120 to 140 years of age. These cultures were written up in the January 1973 special issue of the *National Geographic Magazine*. The fact that all eight cultures are Third World countries is significant. The longest average longevity held by an industrialized nation are the Japanese who live on the average to 79.1. On the other hand, the Himalayan Tibetans from the northwest of China, the Hunzakut from the Karakarum Mountains of eastern Pakistan, the Russian Georgians from the Caucasus Mountains in western Russia (and their sister cultures of Armenia, Azerbaijian, Abkhazia, and Turkey), the Vilcabamba from the Andes of Ecuador, and the Titicacas of the Andes of Peru are all famous for their high percentage of centenarians.

The common denominators of the eight long-lived cultures include:

1. The communities are found at elevations ranging from 8,500 feet to 14,000 feet in sheltered mountain valleys.
2. The annual precipitation is less than two inches.
3. Their water source for drinking and irrigation comes from glacial melt and is known universally as "Glacial Milk" because the highly mineralized water is an opaque white or gray in color and because of the presence of an enormous amount of suspended rock flour.
4. There is no heavy industry or modern agriculture to pollute their air, water, or food.
5. Only natural fertilizer including animal manure, plant debris, and "Glacial Milk" is applied to their fields.
6. Western allopathic medicine was not historically available to these cultures, so they are able to avoid stepping on "land mines."

Himalayan Health

The Tibetans were the inspiration for the Pulitzer Prize winning book by James Hilton, *Lost Horizon*. Tibet's oldest people are found on Chang Tang or the northern plateau, elevation 15,000 feet, which consists of salt lakes fed by glaciers from the eastern slopes of the Himalayan Mountains. This mountain culture has about 500,000 people who are devout Buddhists. The Tibetans are a mix of nomadic herdsmen, merchants of salt, farmers, and great cavalrymen on camel or horse. Tibet makes up almost 10 percent of China's land mass and was founded in the 7th century by King Songtsan Gambo. The Chinese government took over Tibet in 1950 by sending a large army to establish a military governor. Since 1965, the region has been administered by a military governor and known as the Tibetan Autonomous Region (T.A.R.) of China.

The herdsmen there build their corrals, huts, and roads out of salt bricks carefully cut from dried salt lakes on the top of the plateau. They hunt Marco Polo sheep, antelope, gazelle, wild asses, and yak. The yak, which translates to "wealth," provides meat, sausage, milk, cheese, yogurt, butter, wool, skins, and animal power for plowing, carrying freight, and for riding. The staple diet consists of "Tsampa." This smelly, hand-mixed paste is a concoction of lightly toasted barley flour, yak butter, salt and black tea. Tsampa is served with turnips, cabbage, potatoes, trout, egg omelets, and beans. Tibetans routinely drink 30 to 40 medium sized cups of black or green tea daily to prevent dehydration, because of the dry air encountered in the high elevations. Each cup of tea is flavored with a chunk of rock salt the size of a Concord grape and two pats of yak or goat butter.

The Tibetan capital city of Lhasa (translates to "Place of the Gods") was the inspiration for James Hilton's legendary city of Shangri-La. The city is found at an elevation of 12,000 feet where temperatures can fluctuate as much as 80 to 100 degrees each day. The center of old Lhasa is the holiest shrine in Tibet—The Jokhang built in 650 A.D. The Jokhang is the "Mecca" to the Tibetan Buddhists. Many of the faithful would trek through the mountains for years to come and pray at this holy site.

In the mountains west of Lhasa is Drepung, a gigantic monastery that houses 10,000 monks and 25,000 serfs and assistants working 185 estates and tending over 200 pastures. The Potala, "High Heavenly Realm," is the sprawling mountain top palace of the Dalai Lama (translates to "Ocean of Wisdom" and represents the living prophet of the Buddhist faith and the inspiration for the ancient prophet in James Hilton's, *Lost Horizon*) built into the mountain 700 feet above Lhasa. The Potala is famous for its 1,000 rooms, 10,000 altars, 200,000 statues of Buddha and eight gold gilded tombs of past Dalai Lamas. South of Lhasa are tens of thousands of acres of terraces fed and watered by mineral rich "Glacial Milk" that originates in the Himalayan glaciers and supplies an endless source of minerals to replenish the fields.

Li-Ching-Yun reportedly lived to the age of 256; he outlived 23 wives! Li of Kaihsien, in the province of Szechwan, China was born in 1677 and died in 1933 at the age of 256 years. Li was the inspiration for the 200 year old leader of Hilton's Shangri-La. Professor Wu-Chung-Chien, the Dean of the Department of Education, of Minkuo University, claims to have found records showing that Li was in fact born in 1677 (the Chinese have the most accurate of all census records in the history of man), and that on his 150th birthday in 1827, Li was congratulated by the Chinese Imperial Government. Fifty years later, in 1877, Li was sent another official congratulations on his 200th birthday. Fifty years later, at the age of 250 years, Li lectured to a thousand medical students in Beijing on the art of living a long and healthy life. His advice: "Keep a quiet heart, sit like a tortoise, sleep like a dog."

The May 6, 1933 edition of *The London Times* noted: "Telegrams in Brief—A telegram from Chungking in the province of Szechwan, China, states that Li-Ching-Yun, reputed to be the oldest man in China and presumably in the world, has died at KiahSien, at the alleged age of 256 (Reuters)."

And from the Associated Press on April 21, 1998: "Nepal's oldest man, Bir Narayan Chaudhuri, a regular smoker who never set foot in a hospital died Monday April 20, 1998, at the age of 141. Chaudhuri lived in Khanar, a village 125 miles east of the Nepalese capital of Katmandu, and had been a cattle rancher [presumably not a vegetarian]. 'Villagers recall tales about Chaudhuri leading the first land survey team in 1888,' said Narayan Wagle, a reporter who first wrote about Chaudhuri two years earlier. Chaudhuri, a regular smoker, subsisted on a diet of vegetables, pork, beef and rice."

Georgian Longevity

The Russian Georgians as well as the Abkhazians, Azerbaijianis, and Armenians are found at the timber line of the Caucasus Mountains which have peaks of 12,434 to 13,274 feet above sea level. They live in simple stone houses without electricity. Their blood pressure is typically 104/72 at age 100. Women continue to have children after the age of 52. They typically drink an eight-ounce glass of vodka with breakfast and have a large glass of wine with lunch and dinner. Almost all of the old people are from rural backgrounds or occupations such as farmers, shepherds and /or hunters.

This group of centenarians from the Caucasus Mountains is found between the coasts of the Black Sea and the Caspian Sea and mountain villages at or above 4,500 feet. The region supports over 500,000 people, 4,550 to 5,000 of whom are over 100 years of age. The oldest known person from the Caucasus region in 1973 was Shirali Mislimov. At 167 he still worked in the village tea plantation in the small Azerbijiani village of Barzavu on the Iranian border. His wife was 107 when he turned 168 in May of 1973. He died a few days prior to his 169th birthday. They feel that youth is up to 80 years of age, 80 to 100 is middle age and 100 to 160 years of age are the seniors. Many married couples are married for over 100 years.

In studying over 15,000 people over the age of 100, it was learned that only the married individuals attained advanced age and still had an active sex life after the age of 100. Mejid Agayev celebrated his 140th birthday in February 12, 1975. Agayev was the oldest living citizen in the Azerbijiani village of Tikyaband that bragged of having 54 people over the age of 100 years. Work relegated to centenarians included weeding fields, feeding livestock, shepherding, picking tea, washing laundry, house work, and baby sitting. Women over 100 years of age usually had between four and 11 children during their child bearing years.

The staple diet of the Caucasus region includes chicken, mutton, beef, goat milk, cheese, yogurt, butter, bread, tomatoes, cucumbers, green onions, garlic, fruit, pita bread, boiled corn meal mush (abusta), red pepper, tea, wine, and salt. Their total caloric intake per day ranges between 1,800 and 1,900. Their fields have been irrigated with glacial milk for over 2,500 years.

Ecuadoran Centenarians

Ecuador's star-shaped "Sacred Valley of Longevity" (Vilcabamba) is actually five valleys that converge and sit between two Andean Mountains at 12,434 feet above sea level. The western skyline of Vilcabamba is dominated by the summit of Mandango, the tallest mountain whose glaciers supply the mineral rich glacial milk which is used to irrigate the terraced fields. The glacial milk originating from the high peaks of Podocarpus National Park pours into the Rio Yambala which converges with the Chamba River which is also used for irrigation.

In 1971, a census revealed nine people over 100 years of age for every 819 or an astounding one centenarian per 100 people! Miguel Carpio at age 123 was the oldest living Vilcabamban found at the census—he still smoked, drank wine, and "chased women." The staple diet of the Vilcabamba Indians includes corn, beans, goat meat, chicken, eggs, milk, cheese, and a soup known as "repe" which is made from bananas, beans, white cheese, salt, and lard. The average total calorie intake of the Vilcabamba Puruvian Centenarians ranges from 1,200 to 1,800 calories per day.

As legend holds, the first Incas came to Earth on an island in Lake Titicaca, to start what was to become the most advanced civilization of pre-Columbian America. Titicaca is found in the Andean highlands of Peru at 12,506 feet above sea level. The main city of Titicaca is Puno (population 32,000). The people of the Altiplano (high plains) are divided into the pure Indians and the "mestizos" who are a mix of Indian and Spanish. The treeless hills that form the Altiplano surrounding Lake Titicaca are covered with "pata pata," or the stone terraces built by the Incas to provide level farming areas, and as catchments for the mineral-rich glacial milk from the great Andean Mountain, Mt. Cardillera Real with which they irrigate their crops.

The original Indians of the Lake Titicaca region are the Aymara. The Quechua, who still speak the language of the Incas, were descendants of Inca slaves after the Inca occupation in the 12th century.

Glacial milk fed Lake Titicaca which is over 3,200 square miles in surface area, 122 miles long and 47 miles wide. When viewed from a plane, the outline of the lake looks like a jaguar ready to pounce on a rabbit, thus the name Titicaca translates to "Rock of the Puma (or jaguar)." The Rio Desaquadero originates from the effluent of Lake Titicaca.

Quinoa, an indigenous grain of Titicaca, begins to ripen in late April or May. It is used as Europeans use wheat, barley, rye, and oats. At 15,400 feet barley never ripens to seed heads, so the Indians use it for cattle feed. The Titicaca shepherds live and work at the 17,000 foot level.

Macedonian Vigor

The story of the Hunza began 2,300 years ago with Alexander the Great. Alexander's father, King Philip, was murdered by an errant officer, leaving Alexander with a troubled Macedonia. He was besieged on all sides with restless and dangerous enemies. The barbarians that had been conquered by Phillip's armies were anxious to be governed by their own princes. Alexander quickly became a mighty general, conquering foes on every side. Ultimately he was forced to battle the Persian empire. A strange twist of fate conspired to create another long-lived people.

In the midst of fighting for his life and empire against Darius of Persia, Alexander learned that three of his trusted generals had Persian wives. Also, these generals had most likely given council to Darius regarding a dearly won (and nearly lost) battle. Alexander sent members of his personal bodyguard to execute the three generals and their wives. The generals in turn, learned of the execution orders. Forewarned, they were able to fight their way free and with their wives fled northeast following the Indus River. Eventually they crossed through the pass of

Babusar and across the 3,000 foot deep Hunza River Gorge via a suspen-ded bridge made of braided goat hair. The three generals and their wives formed the nucleus of a warrior tribe that initially flourished by preying on and raiding the trade routes and caravans that flowed from China to India and back again.

The Hunzas were not always known as Hunzas. Up until the turn of the 20th century, the valley was known as the Kanjut and the people known as the Kanjuts. When the Indian Girkis tried to invade Kanjut, they gave the valley and the people in it the name Hunza, because all of the people in the valley were allied and united as arrows in a quiver. In the Burushaski language (a mix of ancient Macedonian and Persian) the name Hunza translates to "arrow."

The indigenous plant life of the Hunza Valley was rather limited. Ninety-nine percent of the original valley was bare rock. Cultivated plants included barley, millet, wheat, buckwheat, potatoes, turnips, carrots, beans, peas, pumpkins, tomatoes, melons, onions, garlic, cabbage, spinach, cauliflower, apricots, mulberries, walnuts, apples, plums, peaches, cherries, and pears. Pomegranate trees are scattered throughout the valley. The Hunza consume milk, buttermilk, yogurt, and butter (which they put in their tea and use as a cooking shortening). Hunza children are breast-fed until two to four years of age.

A large variety of indigenous wildlife including ibex or "Markhors," Marco Polo sheep, geese, ducks, pheasants, and partridge provided the early Hunza with meat. The Hunza do not cook the majority of their food because of a lack of fuel. Even the animal manure is added back to their fields. The Hunza salt supply is mined from hills near the Shimshal and Muztagh Rivers and used in their tea and for cooking in its raw brown state. The salt's brown color comes from various trace minerals included in the salt deposit when the ancient seas dried up.

There are 14 Hunza practices that contribute to their longevity:

1. Basic diet is grains (whole grain and sprouted), vegetables (raw or steamed), fruits (fruits are dried and reconstituted in water or diced and served in gelatin from goat and mutton tendon and cartilage). Meat is consumed at two to four pounds per person per week. Mutton, goat, yak, beef, poultry, brain, kidney, and liver are eaten as available. Dairy, including whole milk, butter-milk, yogurt, cheese, and butter, are staples. A grape wine known as Pani is consumed daily. Contrary to popular belief the Hunza's are not vegetarians.

2. Their farm soils are maintained by organic agricultural practices, "That which is taken from the soil is returned to the soil." Composting, plant debris, and animal manure is turned back into the soil.

3. All Hunzas work 12 hours each day, seven days each week—to them there is no Sabbath (work doesn't appear to kill anyone).

4. Fat sources include whole milk, butter, ghee, apricot oil, and animal fats.

5. Total absence of additives, preservatives, or chemicals in their air, food, and water.

6. Daily consumption of salt by adding chunks of rock salt to their tea and in cooking vegetables and meat.

7. No agricultural sprays or chemicals of any kind.

8. All children are breast fed for two (girls) to four (boys) years. Traditionally there have been no vaccines or antibiotics. There are few if any birth defects recorded except for two hermaphrodites or "mukhanas" in the 2,300 years of recorded Hunza history.

9. All grains, vegetables, and fruits are dried for storage by use of the sun.

10. Native herbs are used for medicine, seasoning, and food. There are no western style hospitals or doctors in Hunza. Part of their longevity success is due to the avoidance of injury and death found in industrial nations at the hands of high tech health practitioners.

11. Glacial milk is the exclusive water source used for drinking and irrigation purposes. The fields are flooded with glacial milk and when the water soaks into the soil, a thick layer of mineral silt or "rock flour" is left on top of the soil. The silt is plowed into the soil before planting. The crops convert the metallic rock flour into colloidal minerals for their own metabolism. The farmers then eat the colloidal mineral rich crops. As a result of regular consumption of the essential minerals, the people are relatively disease free and live well past a hundred.

12. Apricot oil is used for cooking along with ghee (clarified butter) and yak, beef, mutton, or goat fat (tallow).

13. Whole grains are used exclusively—no processed or white flours.

14. The Hunza eats 1,800 to 2,000 calories each day.

The Hunza remained unvanquished in battle until 1891, when the British Empire conquered and pacified the Hunzas by installing an Islamic ruler known as the Mir.

The annual precipitation in Hunza is less than two inches. The surrounding mountains, the Karakorum Range, is only 300 miles long, the mountains are bare of plants, naked and almost metallic grey in color. Mount Rakaposhi, 25,550 foot high, overlooks the 8,500 foot high Hunza Valley along with more than 60 summits higher than 22,000 feet. Mount Rakaposhi is one of the most difficult mountains on Earth to climb. It took 23 attempts to conquer its summit. The first 22 attempts failed, but in 1958 a British expedition finally succeeded in scaling the nearly sheer face. Maps refer to this Karakorum Range at the junction of many countries such as the Pamirs—the Afghanistan Pamir; the Russian Pamir; the Chinese Pamir, etc. Pamir translated from Persian means "Roof of the World." Tibet is often called the "Roof of the World," however, Lhasa is at an elevation of only 13,000 feet and is surrounded by summits only 18,000 feet high or less.

A few miles above the junction of the pearl gray waters of the Hunza River is a village called Secundersbad. It is here that the Hunza Valley begins. The Hunza Valley follows the Hunza River up to its sources beyond Misgar, almost on the Chinese border where it originates from glacial torrents spewing from under the 5,000 square mile Ultar Glacier. The Hunza Valley is barely 200 miles long. There were no naturally fertile valleys in Hunza as compared with the Willamette Valley in Oregon. The Hunza Valley was originally bare rock, the soil only being carried basket by basket up the 3,000 foot gorge walls and placed in hand crafted stone terraces. This soil is continuously replaced by hand from mineral laden silt dredged by hand from the bed of the Hunza River 3,000 feet below.

Then there was the problem of water in the barren "safe haven" of Hunza. Fortunately one of the original rebel Macedonian generals was a military engineer. He was able to locate a year round source of water roaring from under the Ultar Glacier 50 miles away. The Ultar Glacier originates on the 25,550 foot high Mount Rakaposhi. He was able to design and construct a gravity-propelled aqueduct which carried water for drinking and irrigation. The aqueduct was a wonder of engineering as it was made from grooved logs attached to each other to form a 50 mile long trough which was hung from sheer cliffs by steel nails hammered into the rock walls.

The water originating from under the millions of tons of ice grinding on the parent rock of Mount Rakaposhi was so rich with minerals that it was bluish white, hence the inhabitants coined the term glacial milk. Generation after generation, crop after crop and year after year for more than 2,300 years the Hunza people have drunk and irrigated their terraced fields with glacial milk, unwittingly assuring their people of an optimal intake of the more than 60 minerals in the glacial milk of the Ultar Glacier!

Except for the polar glaciers, the Karakorum Range has the largest collection of glaciers in the world. Millions of tons of glacial ice (in some places hundreds or thousands of feet thick) grind four inches of living mountain rock into a fine "rock flour" each year. That rock flour is then carried in suspension to the land below. No rock, no mineral, and no metal is resistant enough to be exempt from the grinding forces of these millions of tons of ice. The glacial milk emerges from under the glaciers in great white water "nullahs." Thousands of glacial nullahs merge and join the Hunza River, very quickly the Hunza River joins the Gilget River; the two rivers, now merged, join the Indus River. The Hunza and the Gilget Rivers are purely glacial rivers, almost entirely made up of glacial milk, whereas the Indus River is a conglomerate of hundreds of smaller brooks, streams, and rivers that drain the great Indian and Pakistan watersheds.

There are sister mountain ranges paralleling the Karakorums. The Hindukush (translates to "the Hindu Killers") and the Himalayas have most of the world's tallest peaks. Yet their glacial milks are not as complete or as dense with minerals as the glacial milk from the Ultar Glacier that feeds the Hunza Valley. Glacial milk is a mixed liquid, a solution of ionically dissolved elements and a suspension of the finely ground rock dust or "rock flour" ground from the living parent rock of the mountain by glacial friction. The suspended minerals in the glacial milk are referred to as metallic colloidal minerals.

If one boils away a quart of glacial milk, the resultant deposit of minerals averages two inches in the bottom of the quart jug. By contrast if one boils away a quart of Evian or Perrier water, you will only get enough mineral to cover the head of a pin—a huge difference. The average particle size of the colloidal minerals are 7,000 times smaller than a human red blood cell, so small they can only be viewed with an electron microscope. The individual elements in glacial milk are not found in their separate pure atomic form, but rather as aggregations or mini-alloys forming suspended solute particles. The presence of these aggregate particles (ranging in size from one hundred thousandth to one ten millionth of a centimeter in diameter) are only detected by chemical analysis or the electron microscope. The raw rock inorganic colloids cannot pass through semipermeable membranes and therefore produce little or no osmotic pressure, depression of the freezing point of water (unlike a salt solution), or elevation of the boiling point. These molecular mini-alloys or aggregates carry a uniform negative electrical charge.

Plants, including wild forms and crops such as grains, vegetables, fruits, and nuts, take up these inorganic metallic colloids and convert them into intracellular (within the cell) organically bound plant colloids. These organic plant colloids are the form of minerals found in and used by all living cells of plants, animals, and humans. It is the eating of the plants rich in organic colloidal minerals that is the secret of health and longevity of the eight long-lived cultures known as the "Agebeaters."

In May, 1994 Margaret Skeets, of Radford, Virginia turned 115 before she died. *The Guinness Book of Records* identified Margaret Skeets as the oldest documented living American, age 115 at that time. They said there were other Americans older than she, but they didn't have the paper work to back up their claim.

Susie Brunson died at age 123 in December of 1994. Her family based their claim that she was the oldest American when she died on her birth date December 25, 1870 which was recorded in the family Bible.

In August of 1996, Christianson Mortenson from San Raefel, California turned 114 years old.

In July of 1995, Dorah Ramothibe, from South Africa, turned 114.

Francisco Barasneujavo Choperina, from a small mountain town just outside of Bogata, Columbia turned 125, in October of 1995. He attributed his longevity to drinking a gallon of goat's milk every day.

Jean Calment of France died at the age of 122 years and 162 days old in August of 1997, and according to the *Guinness World Book of Records* was the oldest documented woman at that time.

Hamudi El Abdullah of Syria turned 133, just before he died in July of 1993.

Masumi Dousti of Iran died at age 161 January 1995, according to the Rocky Mountain News Wire Service in Denver. A lot of credibility has to be given to this obituary because she was survived by six living children ranging in age from 120 to 128 years of age.

Sherali Mislimov according to the *National Geographic Magazine* at age 167 years was the oldest documented human in January of 1973. Five months later Mislimov celebrated his 168th birthday in May of 1973—his wife was 107 years of age.

People do live to be 120 to 140 years of age. They do it all of the time.

Some extraordinary individuals will live to be 150 and 160. The only question is how can we get there from here without moving near a glacier?

16

THE KILLING FIELDS

The life of retirement, success, and leisure actually became boring. One could only scrub the decks on *The Elixir* so often. Hanging out at bars didn't interest me, so I began to visit the Jones Medical Library at the Texas Medical Center in Houston to keep up on medical and nutritional research. At the same time I called my friend Clinton Miller from the NHF to seek an association with a Mexican alternative hospital, one where nutritional treatments were a major health approach. It was during one visit to the Jones Medical Library that I came across that very tall, very beautiful, very happy and very intelligent Chinese lady named Ma Lan. Let me tell you more about our courtship now.

Ma Lan and I sat across the library reading table from each other. It was hard to avoid looking at her because she is very tall for a Chinese lady. She towers over almost all 600,000,000 Chinese women at a height just short of six feet. Ma Lan played basketball in China for seven years. I still don't know if I made her uncomfortable by looking at her or if she really wanted to know how to pronounce a word from a journal article in English. As a result, out of curiosity, I asked Ma Lan to join me for lunch. After three overtures, Ma Lan accepted the invitation to join me, and we talked about each other's academic background, our mutual interest in sports, and our love of fishing. Ma Lan's favorite food is fish.

It was immediately obvious that Ma Lan was a gentle, soft-spoken person, yet there was an inner strength that radiated from her. Ma Lan's first weeks in Boston would be enough to send most people packing and headed back to their homeland, but gentle Ma Lan is also tough, so she persisted. Walking back to her dormitory on a snowy January night, only three weeks after arriving in Boston, she had a heavy long coat on and her purse hanging off of her right shoulder. She was hunkered down against the chilling wind. Three teen-aged boys with Saturday night specials accosted her and grabbed her purse. A scuffle ensued and to make a long story short, Ma Lan used her martial arts skills to send the three gun-toting teens running. She kept her purse intact, by the way.

Ma Lan was in medical school during the Chinese Cultural Revolution. She was arrested along with all academics and put in the countryside in a forced labor program in the rice fields. She, along with the other captives, was restricted to a simple diet of corn meal, pork fat, and salt for three years. Many millions died, but Ma Lan kept herself alive by adding river grass and mud to her meals. The ancient practice of flooding the rice fields with muddy river water returns a certain amount of silt, clay, and organic material back into the fields each year, thus enriching the soil and providing minerals that can be incorporated into their crops. Chinese culture has been historically intertwined with herbs and acupuncture for over 5,000 years, but supplementing with vitamins and minerals was a new concept to Ma Lan.

Having come to the United States as an exchange scholar with Harvard to teach microsurgery to graduate medical doctors, she had also done microsurgery research at Harvard Medical School. Ma Lan had written and published several papers on her successful use of laser and suture methods of joining the cut ends of small arteries the diameter of human hair.

Microsurgery is a tedious and exacting procedure conducted under the magnification of a microscope. Ma Lan had become an expert in microsurgery because of both natural talent and attention to detail. Her skills were refined in the crucible of her seven year tenure as a general surgeon at the Canton Air Force Hospital. During the Vietnam War, Ma Lan was recalled from the labor camps and her expertise was enhanced through numerous military wound repairs. She was quickly noted for her ability to repair damaged tissues and restore the disrupted blood supply. While most micro-surgeons reported a respectable success rate of 65 percent by joining together the major arteries and veins, Ma Lan boasted a 95 percent success rate because of her ability to repair small arteries and veins the diameter of human hair, in addition to repairing the larger vessels. This provided a much more complete blood supply and almost guaranteed success. She was now doing microsurgery research and teaching at the St. Joseph Hospital, part of the Texas Medical Center complex in Houston.

Fishing was our recreation. Ma Lan would cook our catch in traditional Chinese fashion in the galley of *The Elixir*. The fish and shrimp were fresh, the taste was great, and Ma Lan ate the fish bones! Ma Lan gave me the steamed or baked fish fillets. I was very surprised when she simmered the bones of fish, chicken, pork, and beef in a vinegar solution. The vinegar would leach the calcium, magnesium, manganese, boron, copper, sulfur, and other minerals out of the bones into the soup. As a culture the Chinese do not eat dairy products. It's just not part of their cuisine, yet they require calcium like all other humans. If you go to a Chinese restaurant, there are no cheese dishes. I often wondered where the Chinese people got their calcium. They get their calcium from animal bones.

After six months of sailing, fishing, learning to eat animal bones, and courting, Ma Lan and I were married. As a surgeon, Ma Lan wasn't trained to regard nutrition as important. She had no concept of the importance of nutritional deficiencies as a cause of everyday diseases. As a result she wasn't historically interested in nutrition or nutritional deficiencies or the Amway business. But as a friend and wife she was very supportive and helpful. Ma Lan would have library searches done for me on Keshan Disease, selenium deficiency, and cystic fibrosis. She would proudly present me with abstracts on any current nutritional journal article, and we would discuss them. In this way Ma Lan began to understand my interest in nutritional deficiencies and their profound affect on human health.

We made several failed attempts to sponsor some of Ma Lan's academic friends and associates into Amway, but they were more interested in science and basic research than they were in transmitting health information to the general public and residual income. After all they had "good jobs." About this same time, I received a grant of $5,000 from the Association of Eclectic Physicians, an international research support group chartered in 1823. The grant was to support a study of Keshan disease, a selenium deficiency disease in Chinese children. To do this study, Ma Lan and I went to China for three weeks. Ma Lan made all of the local arrangements in China for hotels as well as the contacts with the appropriate government agencies so we could establish joint studies with the Chinese pathologist and clinicians who were experts in the field of Keshan disease. The idea was to study tissue from large numbers of children dying of a confirmed selenium deficiency disease known as Keshan disease.

During the Japanese occupation of Manchuria prior to World War II, Keshan disease killed 13 out of every 1,000 Chinese preschool children. It is characterized by a sudden acute onset of cardiomyopathy, a kind of muscular dystrophy of the heart muscle. Keshan disease was originally thought to be caused by viruses and the young Japanese soldiers were so afraid of Keshan disease that they chose to go to the stockade for refusing to occupy Manchurian towns, rather than risk dying. During the 1950s, the Russians theorized that Keshan disease was caused by aflatoxins produced by *Aspergillus flavus*, a fungus contamination of stored corn. They sent a team of scientists to help modernize the Chinese grain storage system as a result. The grain storage system was improved, but the rate of deaths in Keshan Province children remained at 13 per 1,000.

The World Health Organization was called into Keshan Province by the Chinese government in the 1970s to help find the cause of Keshan disease. The WHO team noticed that calves, lambs, and pigs died of the same cardiomyopathy heart disease that the Chinese children died from. They also noted that the children of railroad workers living in Keshan Province seemed to be strangely immune to Keshan disease. It was discovered that the general population of Keshan province was a minority culture moved there by the Chinese government to populate formerly uninhabited land, much like American Indians being placed on reservations. They were ordered to grow corn as the grain of choice. The poor peasants ate only the corn they grew locally. The railroad workers had food imported into Keshan province on the trains. There was something missing from the food grown in Keshan Province.

An analysis of the soil showed that the soil of Keshan Province was almost totally devoid of the trace mineral selenium. The Chinese peasants ate only the corn grown on the selenium deficient soil and lost 13 out of every 1,000 children to Keshan disease. The railroad workers ate food imported into the province on the rail line and lost none of their children to Keshan disease—the mystery was solved!

Cystic fibrosis was thought by the medical profession to be a genetic disease transmitted by a simple Mendelian gene that is found in one out of every four white Americans with a European background. According to that theory, CF was only supposed to occur in children from a middle-European background. A simple computer search of the pediatric literature showed that cystic fibrosis had been diagnosed in black Africans, Eskimos, East Indians, American Indians, African Americans, Japanese, and Chinese. Even a sexually hyperactive missionary carrying a cystic fibrosis gene couldn't spread the disease that fast and that universally. My theory was that, if there were CF changes in the Chinese children with the known selenium deficiency disease, Keshan disease, I could make an irrefutable connection between CF and selenium deficiency.

The trip to China was highly successful. More successful than I had hoped or dreamed. Ma Lan and I visited the three Chinese medical schools that were considered to be the holders of all knowledge on Keshan disease. We examined the microscopic tissue slides and preserved organs of 1,700 Keshan victims. As we'd hypothesized, the microscopic changes of cystic fibrosis occurred in significant numbers. A landmark paper resulted from our Chinese study comparing the microscopic changes of Keshan disease to cystic fibrosis that was published in a peer review scientific journal, *Bio-organic Chemistry* in July of 1991. All of the reviewers noted in their comments that the study was unimpeachable.

The results of the Chinese study prompted the awards committee of the Association of Eclectic Physicians to bestow upon me the Wooster Beach Gold Medal. In 1990, they formally forwarded a nomination to the Nobel Committee in Stockholm, Sweden and nominated me for the 1991 Nobel Prize in Medicine for establishing the basic understanding of the relationship between the genesis of cystic fibrosis and a maternal deficiency of the trace mineral selenium. There was little doubt now that cystic fibrosis was and is the result of a congenital selenium deficiency.

I was honored and humbled by the nomination. The fact that peers and colleagues held my work in such high regard was the pinnacle of my scientific career. The nomination for the Nobel Prize in Medicine, however, only created a jealous rage from many medical doctors and fellow doctors of alternative medicine in later years. After all, who was Wallach, and how could such a maverick deserve such a hallowed and coveted nomination?

Upon my return from China, Clinton Miller, my long time friend from the National Health Federation, was able to get me a staff appointment with one of the more well-known alternative hospitals in Mexico. The hospital, Hospital Santa Monica, located in Rosarito Beach, Baja, Mexico was owned and operated by Kurt Donsbach. Donsbach was a highly successful alternative health chiropractor who built a nutritional empire by publishing a dozen small booklets on various popular nutrients and common diseases. Selling 11 million of these popular booklets allowed Donsbach to start a small "degree by mail" institution that he called "Donsbach University," the equivalent of "Hamburger University" established by McDonalds to train store managers.

The Donsbach University program was designed to train health food store owners and managers how to recommend vitamins and minerals for various diseases. The correspondence courses were designed to teach the student how to use a computer program that was designed to suggest individual nutrients or products for specific diseases. Donsbach was one of the most financially successful of the alternative health practitioners of his time. As a result, he became the lightening rod for every attack by every unhappy medical group or government agency looking for a scapegoat. It was the logical response to these attacks that drove Donsbach to establish an alternative hospital in Mexico.

Ma Lan and I went to Mexico and began to learn what might be considered the cutting edge of alternative medicine as practiced by the hospital's naturopaths, chiropractors, acupuncturists, herbalists, and maverick M.D.s. The orthodox medical profession viciously attacked the philosophy of alternative medicine as quackery, yet people came to Mexico by the tens of thousands for this "unorthodox" treatment. Terminally and chronically ill patients, including cancer patients, diabetics, arthritics, stroke patients, and Alzheimer's patients poured into Mexico. They fled the U.S. by the tens of thousands. What were they fleeing from? After all the United States had the most expensive and the most technologically advanced medical system in the world we're told!

I was sent out on the road by Donsbach to lecture at health expositions and health seminars and inform the public of the available alternative health services at Hospital Santa Monica in Mexico. I talked with the American public, I interacted, I listened. They were fleeing from the orthodox medical doctors with their "Cut, Burn, and Poison" treatments that rarely cured anything! These people were simply acknowledging the fact that our medical treatments had failed the American public in many ways. First of all, the orthodox medical approach was expensive; second, it didn't cure anything; and third, medical treatment itself could be dangerous and life threatening!

In a January 1993 news release, Ralph Nader and Sydney Wolfe declared that "doctors kill 150,000 to 300,000 Americans each year in hospitals alone, as a result of medical negligence." Everybody in the alternative health field knew this horrible statistic, but it was the first time that anyone with any credibility in the main stream had verbalized the widely known fact. I made an overhead transparency of this news release and began to use Ralph Nader's data in my "Dead Doctors Don't Lie" presentation. The United States had lost 56,000 military personnel in Vietnam over a ten-year period, for an average of 5,600 per year. Millions of people poured out into the streets to protest these lost lives. We had political anarchy for the last three years of the Vietnam war because of these deaths. And because of those deaths, God forgive us, we shot and killed American students at Kent State in Ohio, who were just exercising their First Amendment rights to free assembly and free speech. Yet no group was out marching in the streets with placards protesting the killings by the medical profession.

In July, 1994, another Ralph Nader survey pointed out that 70 percent of doctors who treat Medicare patients flunked the exam on how to treat seniors safely and effectively. What would happen to American Airlines if 70 percent of their pilots flunked the exam on how to fly? What would happen to American Airlines if they killed 150,000 to 300,000 passengers per year? Everyone would "go Greyhound!" Medical doctors reacted violently to the Ralph Nader statistics that I routinely quoted in my "Dead Doctors Don't Lie" tape. They wrote articles in their own defense and went on talk radio to try to reduce the amount of damage to their image as all-knowing saviors of the American public. Doctors admitted killing 80,000 Americans each year, but it was too late. The genie was out of the bottle and the spin-doctors couldn't put Humpty Dumpty, M.D. back together again!

Harvard Medical School, in a heroic attempt to soften the negative effects that "Dead Doctors Don't Lie" was having on the image of American doctors, created what they thought was the ideal study to determine just how many people were really killed each year by the American medical community. After putting together a scientifically correct study, Harvard turned the study over to the Rand Corporation of Boston to actually conduct and collate the results of the study to avoid any possible accusations of Harvard tampering with the results. On November 5,1996, the Rand Corporation and Harvard Medical School jointly published the survey that appeared in every newspaper in America. The article's aptly entitled, "Examining the Casualty Count," showed that doctors kill 180,000 Americans each year in hospitals alone as a result of medical negligence. It further demonstrated that 1.3 million people are injured each year from medical negligence. That's 1.5 million casualties a year inflicted upon the American public by one trade!

In March of 1998, the Centers for Disease Control stated that two million infections occur each year in hospitals alone as a result of medical negligence. Doctors simply don't wash their hands between patients or after they use the toilet. Add two million infections per year to 1.5

million casualties, and you get 3.5 million casualties per year in hospitals alone as a result of medical negligence. Why are we so concerned about biological warfare or germ attacks from Iraq when we have these "attacks" going on? If Iraq, Iran, or Libya were to inflict 3.5 million casualties upon the American people, the American government would immediately and without hesitation declare war! Tomahawk missiles would fly, stealth bombers would launch, and the Marines would sail.

According to Ralph Nader, Sydney Wolfe, the Centers for Disease Control, Harvard Medical School, and the Rand Corporation, doctors inflict 3.5 million casualties on the American public each year. Despite the casualty rate, they are still revered by 90 percent of their victims and 98 percent of the survivors of their victims.

Many people cringe when I attack the medical profession and ask sarcastically, "How would you describe the ideal doctor?" That's an easy question to answer. First a doctor should do no harm to patients. How many people do herbalists, acupuncturists, chiropractors, naturopathic physicians, homeopathic physicians, and nutritional consultants kill each year? Compare the true-benefit-to-damage-ratio and the alternative health care givers would win every time. Money should not be the driving force in the doctor's soul. Don't get me wrong, I believe in free enterprise and reward for effort, but the money stream comes effortlessly with good service.

Mother Teresa was given the Lincoln Continental limousine used by Pope Paul VI during his visit to India. Mother Teresa raffled off the limo and used the money to build a hospital for lepers. Could you see many medical doctors doing that? When Mother Teresa was awarded the Nobel Peace Prize for her work with the poor of the world, she declined the traditional award banquet and used the banquet money for a Christmas dinner for the world's poor. I couldn't imagine in my wildest dreams a doctor giving up the recognition of winning the Nobel Prize in the world press in exchange for a Christmas dinner for his poor patients.

Lest you think I'm critical of every medical doctor, let me tell you about a few that should be revered. One of the last modern clinicians to win a Nobel Prize was Dr. Albert Schwietzer. He could be described as the Mother Teresa of medicine. He was a religious missionary as well as a physician. He brought love, respect, hygiene, medicine, and gentle care to the people of Lamberine, Gaboon in Africa who would otherwise have been forgotten and abandoned by the modern western medical profession. These poor patients paid with firewood, chickens, and bread, and they didn't have insurance!

Then there was Dr. Fienstein, a white doctor in black Harlem who should have won the Nobel Prize in Medicine. He died in 1996 at his dinner table after seeing his last patient of the day at age 97. It was not his durability that should have gotten him the Nobel Prize, but the fact that for 70 years he took roasted chickens, pies, bread, and service (house cleaning and laundry) in exchange for his services.

Drs. Schweitzer and Fienstein probably made mistakes in diagnosis and choices of treatment. They were only human. The thing that separates them from other doctors is that they loved their patients more than they loved their own comforts. They first "did no harm." They respected their patients, and they didn't milk the community they served like the Sheriff of Nottingham.

Back at Hospital Santa Monica, I saw many excellent doctors at work—the kinds that should be rewarded. It was there that I began refining my nutritional formulas. The original formulation of the Pig Arthritis Formula was relatively expensive, costing as much as $500 to $1,000 per month. The large number of pills and capsules caused a great deal of gastrointestinal problems that the patients affectionately called "B and F Disease," an abbreviation for belching and farting! The ninety pills and capsules per day were also an inconvenience. People got bored with the need to carry a shopping bag full of bottles or a box full of pills with them wherever they went. As a result of the high cost and the problem of managing so many pills every day, people began taking Dr. Wallach's Pig Arthritis Formula until they began to get results. Then they went off of the program for several months till symptoms returned, back on again until they felt relief in a vicious cycle. Even though the formula would regrow cartilage and bone, long term compliance was difficult to maintain.

At Hospital Santa Monica, I learned that there was a liquid multiple trace mineral supplement available for the patients known as Mineral Toddy. Mineral Toddy was produced by Rockland U.S.A. from a unique prehistoric plant deposit that had never been compressed into oil or coal. It had never been fossilized or petrified. The value of this tea colored liquid was that it contained 77 minerals in the plant derived colloidal form. Because they were plant derived colloidal minerals instead of from ground up rocks, they were up to 98 percent bio-available. The plant derived colloidal minerals were offered in the hospital cafeteria as part of the patient's supplement program.

The plant derived colloidal minerals were very astringent. Taken "straight," they'd "shrink wrap your lips over your teeth" if you drank them without juice. The fascinating thing about the patients was they all voluntarily put one or more ounces of the liquid minerals in their juice at every meal. Because the plant derived colloidal minerals were liquid, they were easy to add to vegetable and fruit juices that were already part of the alternative cancer programs.

I recognized immediately that the liquid plant derived colloidal minerals would solve an enormous number of problems for those who needed to supplement with vitamins, minerals, and trace minerals. Because there were more than 70 minerals in the product, one didn't need to have 30 different bottles with various individual minerals in them. This one formula saved the patient a lot of money and inconvenience. As an added benefit, the plant derived colloidal minerals prevented "B and F Disease."

I got excited about this new-found nutritional tool, and I gathered every piece of information that I could find on plant derived colloidal minerals. I had never heard of colloidal minerals until this moment in my professional career so I began to educate myself. I gathered every book and every article that had ever been written on colloidal minerals and within three months I was familiar with just about everything historically and currently known about colloids and plant derived colloidal minerals.

I had been trained at the cost of $7.5 million by the NIH to understand and gain expertise in a variety of scientific subjects and specialties using a library search technique. I used the information search technique during my research work with The Center for the Biology of Natural Systems and the St. Louis Zoo. I used the same technique to gather information for the book, *Diseases of Exotic Animals*, and now I applied the same technique to learn everything I could about plant derived colloidal minerals.

The plant derived colloidal minerals were not a "cure all" snake oil type of product. There were problems that would have to be overcome. The Toddy colloidal minerals taken by themselves were so astringent they would make you squirm just a little bit! Those foolish enough to attempt to drink the colloidal minerals straight would never take them again. The colloidal minerals were all present in trace amounts. They required an additional source of the major minerals and electrolytes such as calcium, magnesium, manganese, zinc, and potassium to even come close to the published RDAs. I revamped "Dr. Wallach's Pig Arthritis Formula" to take advantage of the liquid multiple minerals in the Toddy. This allowed the reduction of the number of pills in the formula from 30 three times per day to six capsules of the collagen, glucosamine sulphate, and chandroitin sulfate twice per day. The patient response was immediately positive to this new approach to a time tested, animal tested, and veterinarian approved formula.

The Toddy's plant derived colloidal minerals were put in five ounces of calcium enriched Minute Maid orange juice. The calcium enriched orange juice totally masked the astringent properties of the Rockland Toddy minerals so that even children would drink the mixture which provided a significant amount of additional calcium. The second ingredient in the revamped Pig Arthritis Formula was 100 percent Kosher beef gelatin. I originally used Knox gelatin in the pig arthritis formula, but when I learned that Knox contained pork, chicken, and beef gelatin depending on market availability, I switched to the Willamette Valley brand which was always 100 percent Kosher beef gelatin.

Gelatin is primarily collagen, but it also provides small amounts of chondritin sulfate and glucosamine sulfate. These three substances are the basic building blocks of cartilage, ligaments, tendons, connective tissue, and bone matrix.

Bone matrix is the gelatinous foundation of bone. Bone matrix makes up as much as 25 to 40 percent of the total bone weight, depending upon the age of the individual—40 percent in kids and 25 percent in adults. Without the gelatinous bone matrix, most new supplemental calcium could not be retained in bones and most of what is absorbed is just urinated out of the body.

A simple high school biology experiment illustrates the need for bone matrix. Take the bone from a chicken drumstick and place it in a quart of vinegar for a month. At the end of the thirty days you can tie the bone into a knot because the minerals have been leached out of the bone by the vinegar. All that remains is the rubbery gelatinous matrix.

The third ingredient in the Pig Arthritis Formula was one ounce of the Rockland Mineral Toddy, the plant derived liquid colloidal trace mineral supplement. These colloidal minerals were up to 98 percent absorbable and contained up to 77 plant derived colloidal minerals, including trace amounts of all of the known 60 essential minerals.

The fourth ingredient was Total Toddy, a liquid multiple nutrient supplement that had Mineral Toddy as its base, plus sixteen vitamins and eighteen amino acids.

The total mix came to seven and one half ounces of liquid in an orange juice base. It tasted good and was easy to take. It was also very economical. An added plus was that the B and F disease was eliminated!

Patients loved the new, almost totally liquid approach to the Pig Arthritis Formula. They told their friends, they told their relatives, and they told their colleagues. People began to look for our booth at trade shows and health seminars and the movement spread like wildfire.

17

THE KLUNK-A-KLUNK BUSINESS

In October 1989, the fortunes of Ma Lan's and my employer, Kurt Donsbach, began to fail. He was a good nutritionist but a bad business-man. Donsbach University had been shut down. His mail-order nutritional business had been delivered a nearly mortal blow by a small multilevel business known as Nutrition Express. Donsbach owed a considerable amount of money to some of his staff and consultants. Two became the owners of what was to become Nutrition Express. In a settlement agreement, Donsbach gave the Nutrition Express group the rights to use his nutritional formulas privately labeled under their name. Donsbach, though, didn't understand the power of network marketing. As a result of the ballistic growth of Nutrition Express using his formulas, that small company all but obliterated his antique style mail-order business that depended solely on his personal effort for its sales.

In a last ditch effort to salvage something of his teetering alternative health empire, Donsbach assembled all of his business leadership into his office and asked for suggestions. Some suggested a road bus cam-paign almost like an evangelistic tent rally. Some suggested advertising campaigns. Others suggested mailings and phone boiler rooms to re-energize old customers. I suggested that since he had a well-known product that was respected by many people, that he should take his products into the network marketing arena. After all, in network market-ing, people were paid only when they made a sale. Overhead was cut by as much as 75 percent!

Donsbach hated network marketing because of the Nutrition Express experience. Instead of embracing the idea, he cut my suggestion off with a terse and snide response, "If you think network marketing is all that great, get a license and start your own company. I have a warehouse full of product I can't sell. I'll sell it to you at my cost!" Everyone in the room laughed. In fact, they belly laughed and roared till tears ran down their face. Most of them had worked for Donsbach for ten or more years and they knew that "Donsbach knew best."

At the meeting's end, I marched out of the office and drove to the San Diego town hall. I bought a business license and formally registered our new business. Wellness Lifestyle MLM was born. Sitting down at the computer, I assembled a catalogue of prices and products. I pounded out a business manual and a compensation plan for Wellness Lifestyle MLM. I knew the Amway compensation plan backward and forward, so instead of reinventing the wheel I just used the Amway compensation plan in its entirety. Ma Lan and I collected aluminum cans on weekends to help capitalize our business. We literally worked seven days each week and almost twenty-four hours each, taking occasional catnaps.

The products we sold included Donsbach's mail-order nutritional products and the Rockland Mineral Toddy—the liquid plant derived colloidal minerals that had been used so successfully in Hospital Santa Monica. My wife, Ma Lan, and I rented a four hundred square foot warehouse on the second floor of a small strip mall, right above a Mexican car insurance company. It was about a mile from Donsbach's corporate offices and warehouse.

Each morning for two years, Ma Lan and I had crossed over from our little house in Mexico into the United States at the San Ysidro border crossing and returned back into Mexico every night. Getting into Mexico at night was easy. It took only seconds. Americans bring their dollars so they always waved us through. The morning lines back into the United States were long and slow because the border guards checked the identity papers and work permits of each Mexican citizen passing into California. San Ysidro border crossing was noisy, hot, and dusty, and it sometimes took up to an hour to get back into the United States.

We bought a small two-bedroom beach house from a little old American couple in Playa Santa Monica. It was within two hundred yards of Hospital Santa Monica and was private and convenient. It allowed us to walk to work everyday. If there was an emergency at night we could get to the hospital within minutes.

Fortunately, the warehouse afforded us the choice of staying on the

American side of the border and saving the time of crossing back and forth. The warehouse had a phone, an answering machine, a 1.5 cubic foot icebox, a microwave oven, shelves, a couch, shipping tables, and a two-wheeled cart—all purchased at local garage sales. We contracted for an incoming 800 number. We were now a national business.

Ma Lan and I bought a 1978 Chrysler K-car station wagon for $1,700 to haul products into our warehouse. Then we'd haul the packaged orders out to the UPS shipping center. The cases of products were brought up the stairs to our second floor warehouse on the two wheeled cart. The cart made a klunk-a-klunk sound as it was hauled bumpity-bump up the stairs.

Orders were taken off of the answer machine each evening, then processed and packaged for shipping. We ate supper on the shipping tables and slept on the couch. Sleeping on the warehouse couch saved us three hours each day by cutting out the trek to and from Mexico. The next morning we ate breakfast on the shipping table. Then the boxed orders were taken down the steps on the two-wheeled cart—klunk-a-klunk! The boxes were then driven to the UPS center for shipment before we reported to work in Donsbach's office.

Ten percent of the monthly profit was to be paid to Donsbach, the major supplier of our products. In exchange, I was allowed to introduce the network concept to the patients in Hospital Santa Monica. Only ten percent of the patients attended the optional weekly marketing meeting. For most, their attendance at the meeting was initially just curiosity or an event to kill time. But when they found out that they could save up to 30 percent on their supplement costs, they got excited and spread the word to other patients and their relatives.

I was invited to give a series of lectures in eastern Montana by one cancer patient and her sister. She was so excited about the results that she had experienced in the hospital that she wanted her friends to hear about the anti-cancer nutrition program and the network marketing opportunity. I toured through the little towns in Montana giving the "Dead Doctors Don't Lie" seminar. Miles City, Glendive, Circle, Jordan, Sydney, Lewistown, Fort Peck, and Billings were all included in the schedule. The audience ranged from 50 to 200 people and the "Dead Doctors Don't Lie" message instantly clicked with the ranchers and farmers. They gave their livestock minerals to prevent and cure diseases and save on veterinary bills, but they didn't take the minerals themselves.

I slept in feed rooms, trailers, living rooms, and cars. We would drive all night to get to the next town in order to do an early morning live in-studio radio program. Pennsylvania was next on the list. A cheese maker invited me to give lectures to the Amish community. The Amish are wonderful, hospitable farm families. I learned a lot from them, ate at their dinner tables, stayed in their homes, and went to their seminars in their horse drawn buggies.

The Amish are your basic 19th century farmers. They recycle animal manure and compost. They use horses to pull and operate their farm implements. They burn wood and coal to heat their homes. They use oil and kerosene lamps to light their homes. They are born in their homes and they die in their homes. They use herbalists, acupuncturists, chiropractors, naturopathic physicians, and midwives. And they take care of their elderly in their homes.

The Amish tend to have six, eight, or ten children per family. I observed that those families that did not supplement with vitamins and minerals had younger children with congenital birth defects such as cleft palates, cleft lips, spina bifida, hydrocephalis, Down's syndrome, PKU, autism, hyperactivity, ADD, clubbed feet, hernias, muscular dystrophy, and heart defects.

The Amish also breastfeed their babies. If they didn't supplement the mother, she would become more and more depleted of minerals with each succeeding child. As a result of this pattern, the younger children tended to have the birth defects and middle aged mothers tended to have a variety of degenerative diseases including lupus, arthritis, osteoporosis, high blood pressure, diabetes, and heart disease. The high rate of congenital birth defects in the Amish community resulted in the common myth about the Amish that "they marry their cousins, practice incest, and inbreed." These myths about the Amish are sad, cruel, and quite false. These people are very humble, religious, honest, family orientated, and industrious.

The Amish don't have health insurance by choice, so they tend to do as much for themselves as they can when it comes to health care. I showed them pictures of birth defects in animals and people that were caused by vitamin, mineral, and trace mineral deficiencies. They very quickly saw the value of taking vitamin, mineral, and trace mineral supplements because they historically gave minerals to their animals but not themselves.

Back home, we had moved our forty foot sloop, *The Elixir*, from Kemah, Texas to the "J" street marina in Chula Vista, California. We had used it as our primary U.S. residence, but it was obvious with the growing volume of our business we needed more space. Ma Lan never liked to tell people we lived on a boat, so when I told her we needed to find a house she got very excited. In China "boat people" are looked at as ghetto or slum dwellers. When we went to China, Ma Lan admonished me not to tell her parents that we lived on a boat, because they would be mortified that their surgeon daughter was living like "boat people." I told her that we lived on a yacht not a boat, the dream of every American, and that living on a yacht was a luxury lifestyle—all to no avail. Ma Lan wanted a real American house. We had no credit of any kind, so our criteria was that we looked only at houses that were for sale by the owner and where the owner was willing to carry the note.

We looked through the classified ads every day. There were lots of houses for sale by the owner. It was 1989 and the real estate collapse had gripped California for over a year. It was a buyer's market. If the owner wanted to be cashed out with a bank loan, we didn't even waste the time to go look. If they were desperate enough to carry the note, we took the drive and looked at the house. We found a perfect 3,500 square foot two story, three bedroom house that had an office and a three car garage. The owner was a real estate salesman who had been strapped with two house mortgages for over a year. He was ready to sell. We wrote the contract on the back of an envelope and walked out with the keys to the house. We had gotten into the house with the payments of a thirty-year mortgage, but with a large balloon cashout that was due in five years. We now had a race. We had to get our klunk-a-klunk business up and running so that in five years we could meet the balloon payment, or Ma Lan's new house would go back to the owner.

Once inside the car I gave Ma Lan the keys to the house and asked her how she liked her first American house. Ma Lan was dumbfounded. "It is ours?" she asked. "How did you do that so quickly?" Everything was perfect for a win/win situation. He needed to get rid of a house. Being a real estate agent, he was not emotionally attached to the house. As an incentive for us to buy the house, the real estate agent threw in about $15,000 worth of furniture and wall hangings and dropped $100,000 off of the asking price. We didn't have a house that we needed to sell so we could move quickly. We needed a house and had the respectability of two doctors plus enough cash flow to make monthly payments.

We began to fill our new three-car garage with an inventory of supplements and books. We bought a floor model demonstration computer for a significant discount. We started appearing at trade shows and health exposition booths in earnest. We handed out "Dead Doctors Don't Lie" audio-tapes and educated people on the need for minerals and trace minerals.

I was even invited to Ada, Michigan by a man who was a warehouse manager for Amway. The meeting was held in his living room like one of my old Amway house meetings. Six couples attended and signed up as wholesale buyers. Wellness Lifestyle MLM was off and running in Ada, Michigan. I went to the East Coast of Florida to put on meetings for several other people. We were cash poor, so my travels down the East Coast of Florida were by Greyhound Bus. The bus station culture is a world in and of itself. I watched people eat, made mental notes of their health problems, and made notes on deficiency diseases just like I had done in my college days.

Each Florida town meeting drew fifty to 200 people. Most of the people were seniors and they were very interested in the "Pig Stuff."

When I was on the road, I would strip the orders off of the answering machine after my seminars, put them in a very clean and orderly format and fax them to Ma Lan. In turn, Ma Lan would run the credit cards and fulfill the orders. We had a plan and we worked it!

Once I was invited by a hair-dresser to give presentations in Hyannis, Massachusetts. It was the first time I had visited any of the New England states. The people were fun and were very interested in nutrition. A viable group was built, and I visited Hyannis three times per year to give seminars to the growing marketing group.

The commissions for the some 300 plus distributors in our klunk-a-klunk business were calculated by hand each month. We didn't have the money to get a computer program to keep track of the down line genealogy, so folders were established for each downline group. For awhile this would be all right because the Amway business structure required that you keep track of all your downline business yourself. Individual distributors had to calculate their downline commissions by hand and pay them until they reached $25,000 in monthly sales volume for three months in a row. Fortunately for us, no one was at that level yet. I would deal with that problem when we got there.

The monthly commission checks were faithfully sent out by the 15th of the following month. Every time we sent out a check we enclosed an order form and a price list. As a result the distributors got excited and ordered more and more of the Wellness Lifestyle MLM supplements. The business grew and we were very, very busy.

By April 1990, our little klunk-a-klunk business was in a major growth curve. Two of us were soon handling more orders than the 100 employees in the larger Donsbach mail order business. Informed of our growth by his warehouse manager, Donsbach now demanded 50 percent of the profit. It was outright theft and an outrage, but we had no choice except to comply with his demand since 80 percent of our sales were of his products!

Unknown to Ma Lan and I, Donsbach, our major supplier, had purchased the nutritional division of Rockland USA, the small Oklahoma based network marketing company that sold Mineral Toddy, even though he was notorious for his hatred of network marketing! Mineral Toddy was the liquid colloidal minerals that I had used for patients in Hospital Santa Monica. Elmer Heinrich, the owner of Rockland USA, had put together a contract with Joe Namath to sell water filters and had contacted Donsbach (the formulator of the Rockland products) and asked if he wanted to buy the nutritional business. Donsbach couldn't resist. He had seen how well Ma Lan and I were doing in such a short period of time with Wellness Lifestyle MLM and decided to get into the network marketing business using the uniqueness of the plant derived colloidal minerals as his vehicle.

Donsbach now demanded that our little Wellness Lifestyle MLM business and its 800 distributors be turned over to his new company which boasted less than 400 active distributors; he called it Eagle International. Again, I had no choice but to bow to his demand to combine forces and bring our klunk-a-klunk business and our 800 distributors into Eagle International as a marketing group of the larger new company if I wanted to be able to continue selling these products. In exchange for my cooperation, I was promised the position of president for the new company. At the last minute, though, another network marketer from a failed Canadian company that had sold bee pollen was brought in to be the president of Eagle International. I was given the position of vice president of marketing. I had no authority, but it was a great title.

18

On the Road Again

In short order, the bottling line equipment, storage tanks, filing cabinets, and computers from Rockland USA arrived in San Ysidro, California. A week later several 6,000 gallon tankers filled with the pure plant colloidal minerals arrived and disgorged their champagne-colored contents into the storage tanks. We were in the mineral business.

The original Rockland—now Eagle International—bottling line was a low capacity hand operated piece of equipment that was labor intensive. The large boxes filled with the empty bottles were dumped into a hopper at the start of the line. The same person would set the bottles upright by hand onto the conveyor belt. The conveyor belt delivered the bottles to the actual filling point, the eight bottles to be filled were stopped in position by a steel pin set in place by a second technician. The fill button was then pushed and a set of eight hydraulically driven fill nozzles lowered into place and delivered a quart of the pure colloidal minerals into each bottle.

The next step was to pull the steel pin that held the bottles in place and allow the eight filled bottles to move down the line where a third person placed a cap on each one by hand. A hand drill with a rubber fixture attached to the bit was used to tighten each cap one at a time. Some times they were so tight you had to blast them off! Other times they were so loose that half of the minerals would leak from the bottle during shipping.

The next step was for the individual tightening the caps to slip a clear plastic sleeve over the neck and cap of the bottle. The bottles then moved by the conveyor through a heat tunnel that shrank the plastic sleeve around the cap and the neck of the bottle as a security seal.

At the end of the line a fourth individual pulled the filled and sealed bottles of Toddy from the line, packed four to each case and taped each case shut. When everyone felt good and the equipment in the bottling line was working perfectly we could fill 120 cases in four hours. This sounded good in the beginning, but we soon realized that two pallets of 120 cases each per day was going to be a severe production limit.

The various ingredients for the multiples such as Total Toddy were put into a 300 gallon mixer and two pallets of 120 cases each, a total of 240 gallons, were produced with each full batch.

Murphy's Law set in and whatever could go wrong did go wrong. Hoses sprung leaks. Bottles of Total Toddy sometimes literally blew up like Molotov cocktails. Raw materials didn't arrive on schedule. The staff called in sick. Customers' checks bounced. UPS lost orders. But we had the sense we were doing good work and moving forward with our new business. Ma Lan and I worked hard day and night seven days a week to build Eagle, Donsbach's new network marketing company. When I wasn't on the road lecturing and training, I helped to bottle minerals and fill orders. Ma Lan worked in the warehouse, bottling minerals and moving pallets with a forklift. A Harvard microsurgery instructor doing manual labor in a warehouse—I love this country!

I hit the road again, giving lectures, educating, manning booths at expositions, sending out mailings, and conducting conference calls. Everyone was excited. Teamwork took form, and we were in business again. Ma Lan and I bought a floor model booth display out of our own pocket for half the listed price so we could be more professional in our trade show presentations. We had special signs and displays constructed for the booth.

Our first outing for the booth display was a San Diego Whole Life Expo. I had given lectures for the Whole Life Expo before, but it had always been for Hospital Santa Monica. Now it was for our own business. Familiar attendees came by the booth and they were very interested in our new colloidal mineral products, but they didn't like the taste or the astringent quality of the pure minerals. Again we heard the complaint: "They shrink wrap your lips over your teeth!" Many visitors to our booth just wanted literature to show to their doctor before they made their purchase decision. I could tell that introducing a new concept in mineral supplementation to the general public was going to be a heavy duty educational process!

My lecture schedule increased from 100 presentations per year to 300 per year. Plane schedules, hotel reservations, and product movement increased to a dizzying level. The three man Eagle International phone crew couldn't keep up. To relieve the pressure, Ma Lan and I continued to take orders and ship to the smaller customers and distributors from our three car garage. The San Ysidro warehouse from our klunk-a-klunk business was dropped at the end of the one-year contract and all of our business was now done from our home office and our three car garage. Ma Lan hired two college students to help with the nightly packing and shipping. Calls and letters from the public began to pour in. They were still fleeing the medical profession and they wanted some information and tools to help themselves! We had found a need and were attempting to fill that need.

Over the years, my lectures at health expositions had been taped and sold by the taping companies. They gave me a master, which I duplicated and gave away. The message was the same from the very beginning. I was a veterinarian and physician, and I was able to treat human disease with veterinary nutritional formulas. You can't get the minerals and trace minerals that you need from food because plants can't make minerals and there are few, if any, nutritional minerals in the fields where our food is grown. You have to supplement with vitamins, minerals, and trace minerals if you want to be healthy and if you want to reverse some diseases and if you want to live to be 100 or more.

It was also important for the audience to know that doctors and their medical advice were potentially dangerous. They needed to realize that doctors are not the holders of all knowledge about health and longevity, and that doctors were ignorant in the field of nutrition. I began to incorporate news stories of doctors who had done terrible things to patients and of doctors who had died early in life from nutritional diseases. So began the 90's version of the "Dead Doctors Don't Lie" presentation.

There was no company money to build tools, such as books, videos, or audio-tapes. I began to write handouts to answer these questions. The handouts only fueled the thirst for information so I decided that Ma Lan and I should write a self-help book directed to the general public to answer their unending questions—*Let's Play Doctor* was born!

Donsbach told me that the book *Let's Play Doctor* would never be accepted by the general public—after all, "Who was Wallach?" He thought that there were already dozens of great self-help books written by famous alternative health experts on the market already. I believed that Ma Lan and I had a different approach than the other alternative health doctors, so we steamed ahead with the book anyway.

Let's Play Doctor differed from the other self help books on the market because it was written to allow the reader to answer their own questions. The other self-help books on the market were simply the dietary or herbal views and spiritual philosophies of the author. The funds that resulted from the sales of the book *Let's Play Doctor* were used to pay for mailings to our personal downline. Eagle didn't initially mail information to the downline, so we mailed useful tidbits of health information and order forms along with a price list. Our Wellness MLM down line grew to the point that it was 85 percent of the total Eagle sales each month.

To conserve money, Donsbach terminated Ma Lan from her position in September of 1990 in Hospital Santa Monica and from her job with Eagle International. Initially this created a financial crisis. Ma Lan, however, had always wanted to work for the University of California. My long-time friend, Dr. Gerhard Schrauzer, was a professor of chemistry at the UCSD campus so we looked at these events as a forced opportunity. Schrauzer arranged for Ma Lan to volunteer as a research associate for six months until she could find a full time paying position.

We worked the network marketing business harder and made up the difference in lost income with increased commissions. And we still collected aluminum cans on weekends to help out. In six months Ma Lan's dream of working for the University of California came true. She was hired by the pharmacology department to do microsurgery research. Again Ma Lan persevered and the temporary disaster worked out for the best. And, in addition to her new position at the University of California, Ma Lan still helped fulfill our orders for our personal marketing business.

Donsbach and his business manager Peter Holliday went to Europe in March of 1991 to establish business activities in England and Poland. Before leaving, Donsbach terminated me from my position as vice president of Eagle to try to save additional money. While in Europe, Donsbach terminated Peter Holliday, believing that he would stay in England with his wife Jacque's wealthy family.

Donsbach's alternative health empire was now in chaos. Unknown to me, Kurt Donsbach, the original purchaser of the Toddy colloidal mineral business, had failed to make his monthly payments to Elmer Heinrich at Rockland USA. At the end of April 1991, the Eagle International colloidal mineral business was foreclosed on and taken back from Donsbach by Elmer Heinrich. Heinrich was heavily involved with his water filter division of Rockland USA by this time and was in the process of landing a contract with Joe Namath to market the water filters in discount stores. He didn't want to deal with having to run the mineral business again. Hauling the storage tanks and bottling equipment back to Tulsa, Oklahoma seemed like just too much trouble. So he decided almost overnight to resell Eagle International.

Elmer met with Peter Holliday and me in the "J" Street Marina sandwich shop where Ma Lan and I kept our boat. We had a long discussion and Elmer decided to sell Peter and I the Eagle business. Peter with his MBA, banking experience, and commitment to alternative heath due to his wife's alternative cancer treatments at Hospital Santa Monica was to be the CEO, set up the office, and take care of building the inventory. I, as president, was to use my Amway network marketing experience to build a network of distributors through seminar training and education. Because Peter and Jacque initially had more money than Ma Lan and I did, they wound up with 51 percent of the new company. Ma Lan and I had 44 percent. Elmer's son Rocky had five percent. And there was a first right of refusal stock buy-out clause if either of us died or we wanted to sell and there was an annuity bought for Peter and I so that the surviving partners could buy the dead partners' stock. I felt comfortable with the arrangement.

So on May 1, 1991, Ma Lan and I became the second largest stockholders of Eagle International. Satisfyingly, I became the president of a "previously owned" network marketing business that had recently tried to fire me!

19

DEAD DOCTORS DON'T LIE

I had been lecturing on health and nutrition since 1964. Initially my presentations were given to academic audiences made up of fellow pathology researchers, professors, and medical and veterinary clinicians at the various nutrition seminars that were sponsored by universities, the National Institutes of Health, zoological societies, and pharmaceutical companies.

The early lectures were officially recorded and made available to the attendees as audio cassettes and printed proceedings. The original cassettes ranged from one half-hour to an hour. They were designed to be succinct, educational, and scientifically correct. These academic lectures were not in a format that would have been interesting to the average American and hardly had enough time devoted in them to educate the public on the concept of mineral deficiencies.

I began to lecture to the general public in earnest in 1978 when I repeatedly told the cystic fibrosis story to small but interested CF parents' support groups. Through experience, trial, and error I learned that to be successful in communicating with the general public, a lecture had to be a blend of truth, real science, education, and entertainment. To keep the audience with your line of thought they had to be made one with the presenter. Science by itself was too boring for the average person. Education could be too structured for the poorly motivated. And without a story that was illustrative and entertaining, the cause was lost even on the devoted listeners.

I tested different techniques for holding an audience's attention for 30, 60, 90, and 120 minutes. The presentation had to be entertaining without being corny. If it were too corny the science would be discounted. It had to have a focus, a direction. A presentation had to take away the most common objections to a new concept, answer questions, and deal with an issue that was of great personal interest to the average person in the audience.

If I failed in my responsibility to take away all of the objections during the presentation, there would be too many questions at the product sales table and only a few could be served. If I was successful in taking away the objections, a high percentage of the attendees would purchase books and products. It was easy to tweak the presentation based on the response of the audience.

I literally made thousands of tapes over the years and learned how to get laughs and nods of agreement and understanding from the audience. I learned how to bring them to tears and how to drive home an important point. The more hard hitting the example, the fewer examples were needed to take away the objection or make the point. If weak examples were used to make a point with the audience, one needed six to ten or more of them to get the same end effect as two blockbusters. In an effort to keep the length of the presentation within the two-hour limit, I opted to use small numbers of high impact facts and examples.

One of the toughest objections to deal with after a seminar or a phone conference was, "That's all very interesting Dr. Wallach, but I'm on two prescription medications so I think I had better ask my doctor before I make my purchase." I decided I had to deal head on with the blind adoration and respect that the general public heaped upon doctors. I started the hobby of collecting articles that reported on crimes that had been perpetuated by doctors. I even collected the obituaries of young doctors to build a case against the medical profession's seemingly spotless image.

Statistics showing that a few doctors sexually abused their patients, that some actually murdered their spouses, patients, or partners, some were arsonists, and that some had embezzled money from Medicare brought laughs from the audience but didn't put a dent in the numbers of people who still wanted to "check with their doctor." Someone's M.D. may be an ax murderer, but their personal doctor is still considered a "medical god." For many, the medical profession's credibility in the area of health knowledge had not been tarnished. The obituary collection was inserted into my presentation as obituaries of young doctors showed up in the newspapers. It was immediately obvious from the audience reaction that I had hit a chord. Obituaries of doctors who had died of obvious complications of nutritional deficiencies was the tool I had been looking for to illustrate the point that the medical community was not the group to ask for health and nutritional advice.

Obituaries of young 38 to 48-year-old doctors who had died of ruptured aneurysms (copper deficiencies) and cardiomyopathy heart attacks (selenium deficiencies) were very common and created quite a response in the live audience. Oncologists that died of cancer, sports medicine doctors that died of heart attacks while jogging, endocrinologists who died of diabetes, and orthopedic surgeons who died of complications of a hip fracture were of particular interest to the audience.

General Sheridan in his ten years of Indian Wars in the American Great Plains rallied his soldiers to a passionate and murderous genocidal fever with the motto that "The only good Indian is a dead Indian."

The book "Uncle Tom's Cabin" and it's evil character, Simon Lagree, was used to bring the industrial north to a passion sufficient to support the federal government's expenditures and press the Civil War to a successful conclusion.

I wanted to rally the attendees of my nutrition seminars to the same level of passion to take control of their own health. I wanted every patient to be informed and demand second and third opinions from alternative health doctors. It was time for nutritional supplementation to be a serious tool in preventing and curing human disease just as it was for the animal industry.

It was during the question and answer period after a formal seminar in Coconut Grove, Florida that my search for a battle cry was answered. An irate attendee by the name of Richard Dennis asked, "I came here for nutritional information. Just what is the purpose of the doctor obituaries at a nutrition seminar?" I blurted out a form of the hip quip: *Dead doctors don't lie!* Thus, the "Dead Doctors Don't Lie" title was born.

The Health Options Exposition had its first health seminar in Denver, Colorado in 1991. We only had tables to display our colloidal mineral product. The crowd was small but I ran into Robert Snook, who would become one of our bigger distributors. He asked if he could video my presentation. I said, "By all means." Later, Robert told me that other alternative health lecturers had refused to let him record their lectures and that my willingness to let him tape my lecture gave him great confidence that I was honest and factual.

Robert was an engineer for Wonder Bread. A detail oriented person, he was dependable and a self-starter. I went to Colorado every three months, and Robert and I built a large Eagle business. Part of his large downline was built in Iowa, Missouri, Kansas, Montana, and Nebraska. Robert became a dedicated bloodhound when it came to finding great newspaper articles revealing the felonious activities of doctors, doctor's obituaries, and positive articles on vitamins and minerals. Robert's persistent efforts resulted in him developing a downline of over 50,000 distributors. Now that's duplication!

I myself spent a considerable amount of time in the medical library at UCSD looking for studies on doctor's health and longevity. There I found an obituary study in the June 15, 1895 issue of the *Journal of the American Medical Association* that showed that American doctors lived to an average of 54.6. I reran the same type of obituary study 97 years later using the same obituary technique from JAMA January 20, 1993 using a random collection of 44 doctors obituaries and found that American doctor's longevity had increased from 54.6 in 1895 to 57.6 in 1993. I rounded the number up to 58 years of age to give doctors the benefit of the doubt and included the statistic in my tape "Dead Doctors Don't Lie." This little statistic would later send doctors into a tizzy.

Doctors were not as healthy and didn't live as long as the average American "couch potato." They only lived to an average of 58 years of age while the average American lived to be 75.5. My simple reasoning went, "If doctors knew what they were talking about when it came to health and longevity, they should be healthier and live longer than the average American. Doctors should in fact set the standards for health and longevity. Doctors, because of their education and access to nutritional supplements, should come closer to the human genetic potential for health and longevity than anyone." Doctors had failed to perform. Scrutiny of their health and longevity statistics showed very clearly that they had racked up a big fat "F."

The reason doctors as a group don't live to 75.5 were quite clear. The fact was that as a group they didn't understand clinical nutrition or take vitamin and mineral supplements. This early age of death for medical doctors and their ignorance of nutrition hit a nerve in the ranks of embarrassed and flustered doctors. It also hit a motivating cord for a large segment of the American people who had had numerous negative experiences with doctors. Americans of all ages, following their doctors advice to have annual physicals, give up red meat and chicken skin, had become vegetarians, ate whole grains, exercised, given up smoking, salt, saturated fat and cholesterol for 50 years and had not gained any significant health benefit! They might as well have remained beer bellied, cigarette smoking, meat and salt eating "bubbas." Where had they gone wrong?

Seniors who had battled for the institution of Medicare, dutifully followed their doctor's advice and had been through the mill of the medical system. After 10 doctors, 25 medications and perhaps even damaged in some way by medical malpractice seniors were still miserable in the last 12 years of their life and died at the same average of 75.5. Baby Boomers didn't want to wind up like their parents and grandparents, miserable, debilitated and broke as a result of outrageous medical bills.

I had at last identified a common thread to excite all Americans about nutrition and coined a universal war cry that transcended age, race, religion, politics, economics, gender and education. The demigod doctor's apparent and perceived immortality had been proven to be a lie. The emperor wasn't wearing any clothes, the emperor was naked! **Dead Doctors Don't Lie!**

Doctors went crazy over my tape. They were shocked, angry, and resentful and they refused to believe that doctors didn't live as long as the average American. "Wallach has to be lying!" Doctors wrote editorials, pontificated on radio talk shows, and wrote letters to their patients. I had struck the mother of all raw nerves! In response, doctors ran their own longevity studies in an attempt to prove that doctors did live longer than the average citizen. "Wallach's study of 44 doctors was too small to be valid!" They screamed and they ranted. Doctors contacted insurance companies and ran actuarial studies on 250,000 doctor deaths. They found out in their studies that doctors lived to be 62 or 69 depending on whose interpretation one used. Whatever interpretation one uses, that lifespan is still far short of the 75.5 that the average American couch potato will reach. The concept of "Dead Doctors Don't Lie" had survived the full weight of the most vicious counter attack of the medical profession!

In addition to the failure of their statistical counter attack, their irritation and public clamor only added more curiosity for the general public.

Even though their own studies showed that doctors didn't live as long as couch potatoes, doctors failed to step up to the plate and admit that they had failed to set an example for health and longevity for the American public. Typical of the arrogant doctors, they tried to "spin doctor" their own study and crowed, "You see Wallach lied, doctors don't die at 58, they die at 62!" They were so intent on proving me wrong that they ignored the fact that their own studies showed that doctors don't live as long as the average American couch potato.

The next question I had to ask was, "What do doctors die from?" Everybody defended doctors. They died early because of the "stressful responsibilities they have." They died early "because of the long hours they worked!" The excuses were pretty lame. There were many professions that required more hours and had more stress attached to them than did the medical profession. They still couldn't fess up. Doctors as a group are too arrogant to admit they could have been so wrong.

Doctors commit suicide a lot. They get cancer and don't want to go through the rigors of chemotherapy and radiation. Doctors get caught stealing drugs from hospitals and don't want to go to jail and wind up in a cell with two big horny guys with AIDS. Doctors kill themselves with overdoses of recreational drugs. Doctors kill themselves while driving under the influence of drugs and alcohol. They buy airplanes and kill themselves flying into mountains because they're too egotistical to take flying lessons.

Doctors kill each other in murder plots and love triangles. I actually gave a brief series of lectures entitled "Dial M.D. for Murder," but many people felt the lecture was too grim. Doctors kill each other in surgery just like they kill everyone else. Dr. Ian Monroe, the 73-year-old editor of *Lancet,* the most prestigious British medical journal, died of "complications of surgery." That's a politically correct way of saying that the surgeon screwed up and killed him!

Whatever is left after eliminating all of the above causes of death is due to natural causes, which are in fact nutritional deficiency diseases 100 percent of the time. Doctors die of diabetes, a deficiency of chromium and vanadium. Doctors die of ruptured aneurysms, a deficiency of copper. Doctors die from asthma, a deficiency of magnesium, manganese, and essential fatty acids. Doctors die from cardiomyopathy heart disease, a selenium deficiency. Doctors die of cancer, an indirect deficiency of selenium. Dead Doctors Don't Lie!

In June 1994, we professionally video taped a two hour lecture that I gave in Kansas City, Missouri in front of an audience of 900 people. The video was made available in it's unedited form. The sound track of the video was edited down to 90 minutes and it became the legendary "Dead Doctors Don't Lie" audio tape.

The June 1994 version of "Dead Doctors Don't Lie" tape was copied by the thousands by Eagle distributors. I allowed them to do it and encouraged them to do it because it was good for the company even if they weren't in my downline. For the first time, I had a 90 minute audio cassette tape that perfectly duplicated my message. We gave vitamins, minerals and trace minerals to farm animals to prevent and cure disease but not humans because the medical profession had the "malignant dumb" belief that "you can get everything you need from the four food groups." That little sentence has killed more Americans than all of our foreign enemies put together in the 200 plus years that we have been a nation. You can't get everything you need from the four food groups because plants can't make minerals like they can vitamins! Plants can't make minerals!

An enterprising Eagle distributor from Missouri scheduled me as a guest for the Jan Michaelson talk radio show on WHO AM1040 in Des Moines, Iowa just before a seminar. The station WHO is 50,000 watts and covered four states through the air waves. I was supposed to be the guest for one hour, but Jan liked the "Dead Doctors Don't Lie" concept so well that he kept me on for a full three hours! The call-in lines literally buzzed. As soon as one line was cleared, it immediately filled up again. The farmers of Iowa, Nebraska, Kansas, and Missouri knew exactly what I was talking about in 30 seconds. They gave their animals minerals. They ate out of the same fields as their livestock but didn't take any minerals themselves! Farmers were suffering and dying from diseases that we had eliminated in the animal industry. What a concept!

The seminar was to be held in the Des Moines Botanical Gardens that held a seated capacity of 450. To our surprise 1200 excited people showed up to hear the message! Excitement was high and people were sitting on the lawn outside the building trying to figure out a way to get into the packed facility. The state police shut off the highway exits, thinking that an overturned 18-wheeler had blocked the exit ramps. Radio was to the "Dead Doctors Don't Lie" seminar what air power was to World War II and Operation Desert Storm. "On The Air Strikes" became a standard tool to invite the public to our seminars.

We were able to squeeze an additional 150 people on the floor, in the center isles and the rows along the wall for a total of 600 people. I gave a short version of the "Dead Doctors Don't Lie" presentation and then gave a second seminar immediately afterward to a second 300 people. The balance of the crowd drove two hours north to Vinning, Iowa, the next town that we had scheduled a meeting for. The same distributor got me on the Mike Murphy morning show on KCMO in Kansas City, Missouri. The response was the same. We had overflow crowds in Kansas City, Missouri, Overland Park, Kansas and St. Joseph, Missouri.

The overwhelming positive response was the same everywhere we went—"Dead Doctors Don't Lie" was a hit.

The reason we don't get nutritional information from doctors is because doctors get thirty seconds of clinical nutrition information from four years of medical school. "Dead Doctors Don't Lie" was handed out, mailed out, and placed in every order that was shipped. The ultimate health and nutrition message was being duplicated and spread.

The average size of the audience for the "Dead Doctors Don't Lie" message grew from 50 per seminar to 300 to 500 per seminar.

The new Eagle company was grossing $17,000 per month when we took it over in May of 1991. That's not great but it was cash flow. At the end of the first year we were grossing $50,000 per month.

The reason for Eagle's relatively slow growth rate for a network marketing company was that Peter Holliday, the managing and controlling stock holder, paid commissions only on occasion, not monthly as is the tradition with network marketing companies. If Eagle needed money, Peter just appeared to "borrow" it from distributors that month by not paying commissions! In addition to not getting paid by Eagle, distributors suffered from devastating back orders of up to three months for Total Toddy, the only liquid colloidal multiple product on the market. Peter didn't seem to get the idea of duplication and geometric growth. He rarely filled the warehouse. And when he did the back orders were filled first, so the full warehouse was empty in three days. Peter's management policies were effectively a sea anchor on Eagle's growth.

Despite administrative setbacks, the Eagle distributors were loyal to the message. You can't get what you need from the four food groups. You have to supplement with all 90 essential nutrients. They used the products and they passed on the message—Dead Doctors Don't Lie!

The administrative, cash flow, and shipping problems of Eagle grew as the size of the company grew. Distributors constantly asked, "What would happen if Eagle went under and went bankrupt?" I said, "Don't worry, we would have product within thirty days if that happened." I knew that the collapse could happen any moment. Professional network marketing people avoided Eagle like the plague because it was well known that Peter didn't pay commissions on time and that most people took product in lieu of money.

In December of 1994, Rockland refused to ship any more tankers of Toddy colloidal minerals to Eagle because Peter had run a bill of $75,000 dollars. "Pay up the bill or there would be no more minerals." Instead of doing the righteous thing and setting up a payment schedule, Peter went to a competitor and nemesis of Elmer Heinrich and Rockland USA called T.J. Clark.

By comparison to the Rockland operation, the Clark mining operation was very primitive. The Clark family had a bitter dispute when the father died and the three brothers split off into competing companies. The Clark minerals were not pure plant derived colloidal minerals. They were according to Bob Musac, the Clark marketing man, "a secret blend," that only T.J. Clark knew. According to Dr. Gerhard Schrauzer, an analysis of the blend showed that the mineral content of the T.J.Clark product varied significantly in consistency from batch to batch.

About this time an algae growth appeared in the minerals causing large numbers of bottles to be returned. We lost distributors faster than we could recruit them. I probably should have started my own company at that time, but I was loyal to the distributors who had stuck with Eagle and with me. I knew that I would disrupt their business and their lives if I made the move at that time, so Ma Lan and I just buckled down and worked harder; after all, we had the buy-sell agreement in place.

Holliday hired Steve Scott, the famous distance runner who had broken the four minute mile 147 times, as a spokesperson for a sports drink Peter wanted to create. His idea was to develop a sports nutrition line to go head to head with Power Bar, Gatorade, Powerade, and other fluid replacement drinks. Peter literally spent millions of dollars for ineffective advertising without consulting me. When I asked why he didn't ask me about these things he said he could out-vote me anytime, so why waste the effort? Jealousy over Ma Lan's and my ever increasing commissions was apparently beginning to rear its ugly head.

In April of 1995, I got a call from a man in California by the name of Bob Schmidt, who wanted to use the "Dead Doctors Don't Lie" tape to market minerals. When I inquired if he was an Eagle International distributor he said he wasn't, "But the message was so important, that he would really like to use the tape in a generic way." I thanked him for his positive feedback on the content of the tape, and declined to give permission because he wasn't an Eagle International distributor.

In August of 1995, I got a call from San Diego Audio, one of my tape duplicators, who stated that the "Dead Doctors Don't Lie" tape was getting very popular and that, "One individual distributor had ordered 70,000 copies!"

The duplicator gave me the toll free number that had been placed on the cassette label and sent me a copy of the tape. The duplicator was concerned because the distributor was not an Eagle distributor and had added the name of their company and product into the tape where I had talked about Eagle and the Toddy minerals.

I called the number and got an order operator for a distributor of a new network marketing business called New Vision. I asked for the telephone number of the main company in Phoenix, Arizona. I called the company and asked to speak to the president. In short order B.K. Boreyko comes on the line and introduces himself as the New Vision President.

I said, "B.K., we've got a problem! One of your distributors has inserted the name of your company and products on my taped message without my permission!" I went on to say, "I fully expect to be paid a royalty for the tapes and I am prepared to sue you if necessary."

After a moment, B.K. asked what I wanted. I said, "B.K., I want whatever the standard industry royalty is for intellectual material. I'm going to be in Seattle for a health expo in a couple of weeks, and it would be a good time to settle this matter." Before we ended the call, B.K. threw out an offer, "How about ten cents a tape and fifteen cents per bottle of minerals sold?" This of course was a righteous offer. But in good faith to my Eagle International downline I couldn't accept the offer of a royalty on their mineral sales because it would be a conflict of interest. I countered by saying, "How about twenty five cents per tape?"

B.K. said, "We'll see you at the expo."

Before the Seattle expo I met with John Valenti, the 23-year-old New Vision distributor who was using my tapes as a recruiting tool. We had lunch and I took him for a tour of the Eagle facilities and introduced him to the Eagle administrative staff.

John asked if there was anything that could be done about the 90 day to six month delay in commission payments. He also asked about having to take product in lieu of commissions. The twenty-one day shipping delay was also a major concern as was the need to have distributors ship product. John said, "There was no way that professional MLM business builders would accept these growth strangling constrictions!"

John pointed out that historically, tape mailings in network marketing netted about five to ten distributors per thousand tapes mailed out. The "Dead Doctors Don't Lie" tape produced 35 to 50 new distributors per thousand tapes depending on the skill of the person getting the call. John said, "The 'Dead Doctors Don't Lie' tape will revolutionize network marketing!" The Eagle staff was rude and discounted young John and the value of the "Dead Doctors Don't Lie" tape. They said with a laugh, "Why should we change things for you? Everybody else has accepted these rules and guidelines! Besides we don't like the 'Dead Doctors Don't Lie' tape, it's too controversial." Without saying another word, John got up and left the meeting shaking his head.

In the parking lot, John quipped, "Doc, I can recruit a lot of people into the mineral business using your 'Dead Doctors Don't Lie' tape, but I can't do business the way that Eagle operates. Sorry."

I said, "John, I understand where you're coming from, however, please don't use the 'Dead Doctors Don't Lie' tape until we have a contract." We shook hands and parted company.

The Eagle monthly sales were stalled at about $150,000 per month after four years. We were still working hard, but not smart. Peter's attempt to develop a popular sports drink before the 1996 Olympics in Atlanta had cost Eagle millions of dollars with no return. Peter, it seems, was convinced that Eagle was going to collapse within a year.

The weekend of the Seattle health expo arrived and I went to Seattle having forgotten about the suggested meeting with the New Vision people. I arrived a day early to set up the booth and locate the product that was to be shipped in advance. The books and tapes that I had shipped were at the hotel, but in typical Eagle fashion the product was not at the hotel. The airfare, cab, hotel room, and food all had come out of my pocket. If I didn't have product to sell I would lose money big time. I called and learned that the product had never been shipped even though the order was submitted two weeks earlier. I demanded that the product be put on an air freight flight with direct delivery to my booth in the exposition hall.

After my Saturday morning lecture the booth was swamped with eager people interested in plant derived colloidal minerals. I sold them books and tapes and took orders for the minerals. John Valenti popped up in the crowd and actually helped me with the sales rush. The New Vision crew headed by B.K. Boreyko arrived and I picked a new Eagle sign-up out of the crowd and had them watch the booth in exchange for a couple of sign-ups while we retired to the restaurant to talk. There were several possible scenarios, but I had to exclude any direct association with their colloidal mineral sales even though it meant giving up millions of dollars in royalties each year. When it comes to loyalty, Eagle distributors knew that the Wallachs were so loyal that they could bet their mothers' eyes on our support and trustworthiness.

I knew that if I didn't get a contract with New Vision, their distributors would pirate the "Dead Doctors Don't Lie" tape anyway and it would cost me millions of dollars just to police the illegal use of the tape. So the lesser of the evils was to hammer out the contract, let New Vision use the "Dead Doctors Don't Lie" tape, and collect a royalty. A second factor in my decision to allow New Vision to use the tape was a letter from Peter asking me to stop using the controversial "Dead Doctors Don't Lie" tape. Peter was never encouraging and didn't understand the rough and tumble world of network marketing. He never left the confines of his office to go on the road. Peter arrived at the office at 7:30 a.m. and left for the club and martinis at 3:00 p.m.

The contract with Benson Promotions would accomplish several things: First, New Vision agreed to pay me a royalty of twenty five cents per tape which was retroactive to include the 70,000 tapes they had already sent out. They wrote out a check for the full amount of $17,500 on the spot and handed it to me with a smile, "We know there are going to be many more checks!" Second, New Vision would police the illegal pirating of the "Dead Doctors Don't Lie" cassette themselves. And finally, there was no way to predict how many "Dead Doctors Don't Lie" tapes New Vision would sell, but at least I would get something for their using my tape and I had some control.

Within a month I was getting calls from angry Eagle distributors complaining that they had gotten one of my "Dead Doctors Don't Lie" tapes in the mail from a New Vision Distributor. I never told them that I had given up millions of dollars of personal income to protect their sales. The calls and complaints began to roll in by the hundreds! New Vision, under the guidance of John Valenti, had begun to mail out tens of thousands of the "Dead Doctors Don't Lie" tapes.

In effect, New Vision was "chumming the water" with the "Dead Doctors Don't Lie" tapes. I pointed out to our Eagle distributors that New Vision would get 35 to 50 new recruits per thousand tapes they sent out, the other 970 were potentially ours if we just went out and got them! About the same time, Terry Porter, a man from Idaho, appeared at one of my seminars. Terry Porter owned a small advertising business in Meridian, Idaho and saw an opportunity in the colloidal mineral business.

Terry, a former college basketball player, is six foot five and weighs about 245 pounds. He smiled a lot, had salt and pepper gray hair, and walked with a limp in his right leg. I learned that Terry had broken his neck some years earlier sliding down a snow mountain on an inner tube. He had a Christopher Reeves type fracture and had spent three years as a quadriplegic in intensive physical therapy with a traction "halo" bolted to his head. Terry was told he had a life expectancy of seven years. During the three years of physical therapy, Terry's hair had turned snow white. Terry's son had been given the Toddy colloidal minerals by a chiropractor friend. The chiropractor said the colloidal minerals had helped his diabetic patients get off of their insulin and was very excited about the business opportunity.

Despite his son's urging, Terry initially refused to take the colloidal minerals, but Darwin's mother Verdon did. Darwin's mother had bursitis in the shoulder so severe she had to sleep in a chair because rolling over in bed caused her to wake up with excruciating pain. After three weeks all of Verdon's pain went away. After the seeming miracle of Verdon's shoulder healing, Terry decided to give the colloidal minerals a try. Terry took the minerals once per day, just to avoid the wrath of his wife. At the seven-month mark, Verdon was cutting Terry's hair and remarked that the color was coming back into his hair! Terry started to take the full "Pig Arthritis Formula" twice a day, which resulted in a fifty-percent return of his hair color over a six month period. He had more muscle strength, was not tired, and slept like a rock.

Now he was ready to take the message to the world.

20

AIR STRIKES AND ROAD KILLS

I had stopped using the concept of financial freedom as a marketing and recruiting tool in 1993. Peter was so bad about paying commissions in a timely fashion while having our key products perpetually on "back order" that distributors wanted to hang me when I came back into their town. So I preached the DDDL concept and the health wonders of plant derived colloidal minerals. The "Pig Stuff," as happy users referred to it, worked so well that consumers stayed with our program because the Pig Arthritis Formula worked, not because they wanted to build a business or make a lot of money.

I had taken on four regular weekly radio talk show programs to keep activity going in well-established downlines. One hourly radio program was KSCO AM1080, in Santa Cruz, California. This program covered San Jose, Santa Cruz, Monterey, Carmel, Scotts Valley, and Watsonville in north-central California. A large nucleus of faithful users of plant derived colloidal minerals developed in the south bay area including Michael Zwerling, the owner of the KSCO station. His interest blossomed into a passion to spread the DDDL concept using his contacts with other station owners. We began to spread the alternative health concept and the benefits of the "Pig Stuff" via the airwaves. A second hourly program was aired on Saturday mornings from Palm Springs, California. This station, KPSL AM1010 covered Palm Springs, Palm Desert, Desert Hot Springs, 1000 Palms, 29 Palms, Indian Wells, and Yucca Valley. This show was rebroadcast every Sunday evening to double the exposure.

All of the radio programs produced numerous health turn-arounds that could only be described as "health miracles." One of the most remarkable is the Inge Reagen story. Inge, from Desert Hot Springs, had been flat on her back with a total disability for 12 years with osteoporosis, osteoarthritis, bone spurs, ankylosing spondylitis, fibromyalgia, and high blood pressure. Inge had nine doctors including three orthopedic surgeons, three rheumatologists, an internist, an endocrinologist, and a podiatrist. To pay all these doctors and follow their "prescriptions," Inge had spent the life insurance proceeds received after her husband died AND refinanced her house. She spent $250,000 to install wheel chair ramps, elevators, and special plumbing to accommodate her wheel chair. Her son Rudy would pick her up out of bed every morning, strap her in the wheel chair, feed her, and then head out to work. Every evening he would return from work and reverse the process. This went on 365 days per year for twelve years.

Inge had cervical vertebrae fused. She'd had several finger joints replaced. The surgeons wouldn't replace her hips, knees, and shoulders because her bones were too crumbly. One physician described her bones by saying they were "just like saltine crackers!" She kept complaining about hip and knee pain so the surgeons suggested that her legs be amputated and that would solve her pain problem. Despite being on several drugs for pain, depression, and to counter the side effects of the original drugs, Inge was alert enough to say, "Let's think about this first."

The surgeons referred Inge to a psychiatrist whose job it was to convince Inge to get the amputations. About this time Inge heard one of my interviews on KPSL and decided to try the Pig Arthritis Formula. In six weeks she was able to slip out of the wheel chair into a walker. After several more weeks she was able to slip out of the walker and use a cane. A few weeks more and Inge was able to function at 100 percent without pain or restricted motion. Inge has since become one of our greatest supporters of the DDDL concept. Inge is now known as "The Angel of Palm Springs" because she has introduced literally thousands of people to Dr. Wallach's Pig Arthritis Formula.

The third regular radio show was Talk America Radio Network emanating out of Boston every Saturday morning. This show was syndicated and was heard on as many as 52 AM talk radio stations in the United States as well as short wave radio world wide. A fourth station came on line, KCEO AM 1000, that covered San Diego and Orange Counties for two hours every Sunday afternoon.

The idea of course was to answer health questions for our customers and distributors and to let the recipients of the DDDL cassette know that we wanted them to join us! The air time was paid for by Ma Lan and me out of our own pocket, but the sale of the books and tapes covered the cost. Any distributors that were picked up were a long-term source of residual income.

Terry Porter contacted me and said he wanted to build an Eagle downline using all of his advertising expertise. We cut one-hour radio and 30 minute TV infomercials. We did more and more live radio interviews. The DDDL seminar attendance grew to 300 to 500 per night. Because of Terry's ability to get crowds and field a crew to man tables, I assigned ten days per month to Terry. The other twenty days were to be divided amongst all the other distributors.

I literally used all the tape royalties generated by DDDL sales to air the radio and TV infomercials. I also used the royalties to help my leaders build their own downlines while I was giving live seminars for the Porters. When the distributor couldn't afford the cost of infomercials Ma Lan and I paid for them as a reward for their loyalty. The DDDL seminar crowds grew to 800 to 1200 per night. There was electricity in the air!

In a short time I was actually able to help more people with their health challenges through the DDDL concept and the Pig Arthritis Formula than I had been able to help in my private practice on my busiest day! I had stumbled onto a way to help literally thousands of people with arthritis, osteoporosis, heart disease, diabetes, etc. by teaching them how to help themselves!

By this time, 18 audio duplicating companies had become licensed to reproduce and sell the DDDL tapes. Forty different nutritional companies used my tape, even ones that sold bee pollen, herbs, and blue-green algae. The message was universal. You can't get everything you need from your four food groups because grain, vegetables, fruits, and nuts can't manufacture minerals. The 40 companies that used the tapes signed up 30 to 50 distributors per thousand tapes. Using "air strikes" and seminars (we called them "road kills") we had the opportunity to recruit the remaining 950 people.

Even though the tapes were being used by the "competition," it was my sincere belief that Eagle distributors would be able to recruit more than their share of new distributors as a result of New Vision's DDDL tape mailing program. That was quickly proven true. The old adage, "A rising tide raises all ships," is quite true. This success aside, at the Eagle annual meeting in June of 1995, Peter gave me legal notice that he had an offer for his stock of $6 million and that according to our contract I had 30 days to match the offer. I matched the offer in 24 hours; after all, this was the moment I had planned for in order to buy Peter's stock. But Peter then rejected all offers saying, "If my shares are worth $6 million now, they'll be worth $20 million in a year or two." Peter's goal was to sell his stock or to take the company public with an IPO.

The "Dead Doctors Don't Lie" tape and the concept that there are not enough minerals in our food took flight. The DDDL cassette sales soared into the millions. The Eagle monthly sales grew to $1 million by January of 1996. The commission checks for just about all the Eagle distributors who were actively working the program (not just buying the product for personal consumption) went up. Everyone was excited and got down to building their business in earnest. The Eagle had landed! Eagle was gaining a life of its own, and I could actually see starting to cut back on my road schedule and enjoying life at home by the end of 1997.

In June of 1996, Eagle had its fifth annual meeting in Atlanta, Georgia just prior to the opening of the Olympic Games. At a private breakfast meeting between Peter and I the day before the annual meeting, Peter again promised that if he had any offer to buy his stock he would honor our stock agreement contract and offer his controlling shares of stock to me at the offered price. Peter also told me at this time that he was getting an accountant from a large stock exchange company to "massage" the books and get them ready for a public sale of Eagle stock. I would have preferred that Peter just sell me his stock. Because he owned 51 percent of the stock and could out-vote me at any time, I constantly mentioned my preferences in the matter. The meeting between Peter and me was amicable and all seemed well.

Every year since the start of Eagle, Ma Lan and I gave out achievement awards to our downline out of our own pocket since Eagle under Peter's stewardship had never done any of these things. 1996 was no different. Ma Lan and I had earned a cruise for meeting sales levels of the marketing plan, and we planned to leave on the island cruise immediately after the annual meeting. Ma Lan was also to receive a new 1996 $38,000 Cadillac during the awards ceremony for her sales volume. She was photographed getting into her new car with a big grin. She'd worked hard for many years and was the first Eagle distributor to earn the car award. What a country! To make the victory even sweeter, Ma Lan's car award would soon be followed by new car awards to eight of her downline distributors. This was a testimony to her leadership and hard work and the power of the DDDL tape. A rising tide raises all ships.

Peter gave his usual state of the company address at the annual meeting and talked about the plans for foreign subsidiaries in Europe and New Zealand. Peter had been talking about foreign holdings for Eagle in New Zealand for about three years so the same old lecture was naptime for most of the long time distributors. The popularity of the DDDL tape and the books *Let's Play Doctor* and *Rare Earths* opened up a new way to pass on and duplicate the message that Americans had to supplement with vitamins and minerals if they wanted to live healthfully to be 100 years of age. Radio programs became an integral part of our method of passing on the message and inviting the public to our free seminars. One full time person was required just to schedule my seminars, arrange tickets, and schedule radio and television in cooperation with other Eagle distributors.

We outgrew our three-car garage so we bought a small 6-acre "ranch" just down the street with barns and two houses. We immediately built a four-car garage as a staging and shipping area for easy UPS pick up. We had grown from a 400 square foot second floor warehouse in our original klunk-a-klunk business to a six-acre complex.

In order to protect our downline from the fits and starts of Peter's management style, we accumulated over $500,000 in inventory. In addition, we shipped product in 24 hours—unlike the Eagle company. And if people wanted cash for their Eagle checks we would get them to sign their checks over to us and give them the cash. We turned their checks back to Eagle and increased our inventory.

United Parcel Service gave Ma Lan and me a full set of shipping computers so we could generate our own bar codes and track our own packages. We hired a shipping manager from UPS to be our office manager. She brought with her four people who had been with UPS part time for three or more years. Our little shipping department was as big as Eagle's and our personnel were professionally trained and more experienced. We even procured our own computer and software to monitor and track orders that we were turning in to Eagle. Eagle was legendary for screwing up orders, and since we were turning in up to $25,000 worth of orders per day it was important to monitor them. The computer was also to be a safety valve in place and ready to go in case Eagle went under and we were forced to start our own company.

In August of 1996, I unofficially learned that Peter had ignored our stock buy-sell agreement and sold his controlling shares of Eagle stock to John Wilson, an accountant, without giving the stockholders a chance to match the offer. Peter had sold his shares to John at 70 cents per share while everyone else had paid $12. I wasn't too surprised though. John Wilson was the accountant who was preparing the Eagle books for the public sale. My antennae and red flags went up immediately. Accountants inspecting company records prior to a stock offering are supposed to be neutral and not benefit from anything they find in the audit. Did John find some hanky-panky that precipitated the sale?

The first thing that came to my mind was that Peter may have gotten his hand caught in the cookie jar by turning in excess expenses to get a few extra thousand dollars per month. Peter didn't have a downline to generate commissions and according to the company records, he was only getting a $5,000 salary each month. John Wilson could have found such a bookkeeping problem with Peter's records and forced him to sell. I started looking around and asking questions about the sale of Peter's stock to John Wilson.

As a result of my inquiries, John Wilson appeared at several of my seminars in Seattle and introduced himself as the new president and CEO of Eagle. I offered to buy as much Eagle stock as necessary to become an equal partner so I could help make decisions, because John Wilson had no network marketing experience. John Wilson had an equal partner by the name of Brian Pado who had actually supplied the $800,000 cash down payment for the purchase of Peter's controlling stock. I suggested a three way equal partnership. They said they would take it under advisement.

When I asked how they got Peter to sell them his Eagle stock, they admitted that they had found a $2 million plus shortfall in the books. As part of the sale they had to replace the missing money into Eagle as the down payment. Their goal was still to take Eagle public so they could raise capital in a stock sale to pay off the balance of the purchase price to Peter. Wilson and Pado admitted that they were impressed with the Seattle seminar. And why shouldn't they be? With 800 people in attendance and the brisk sales activity following the meeting, all seemed amicable. Still, I was now alert to any possibility.

In 1995 and 1996, I made every attempt to fix whatever Peter Holliday had perceived was a problem with my marketing style. With the help of Terry Porter, I had made the radio and TV infomercials generic by stripping all references to Eagle and Eagle product names. I had removed all references to Eagle and Eagle products from my "Dead Doctors Don't Lie" audio and video tapes. All of our attendant literature was made squeaky clean and claim-free. They had placed my son Steve on the Eagle board of directors to keep the communications channels open.

They had not given him any indication that there was any trouble brewing. On the surface everything at Eagle seemed to be going more smoothly.

In addition to the 300 seminars per year, I started doing regular radio talk shows as a guest. Sometimes these were just generic programs where our 1-800 number was given out. At other times, these shows were a prelude to an actual seminar. The Eagle business grew rapidly as a result of the New Vision mailings of DDDL, so much so that by January 1997, Eagle was grossing over $4 million per month. Eagle was also signing up 7,000 new distributors per month.

Twenty-two million DDDL tapes were sold by licensed duplicators and mailed out. The message was getting out. Other companies were paying for Eagle advertising—what a concept! Air strikes, road kills, and *Dead Doctors Don't Lie* were winning the war.

The Mineral Toddy, however, was beginning to change. One day you could drink a quart of Toddy minerals like water because the astringent character of the minerals was gone. The next batch of Mineral Toddy was black like India Ink. The next batch was green. The obvious changes in the Mineral Toddy negatively affected all of the products that used the minerals as a base. A quick investigation revealed that Eagle had not bought minerals from T.J. Clark for over two months. John Wilson and Brian Pado had obviously gone to a yet third and even more variable product. They had been promised that they could get the same minerals from another source for a dollar a gallon cheaper before bottling. Typical of accountants, they sacrificed quality for the "bottom line."

Terry Porter and I were on the road in Texas when we called Wilson and Pado from Terry's car phone and complained about the variation in the Toddy Minerals. They denied there was any change in the source of minerals. Terry and I knew better so we anticipated trouble in the near future. With all of Eagle's historical problems in lack of payment of commissions, poor administration, bad service, back orders, and a generally unfavorable atmosphere for distributors, we had always gone back to the fact that we had the best plant derived colloidal minerals. Now we couldn't say that any longer.

21

THE GREAT AMERICAN ADVENTURE

By January of 1997, Eagle's monthly sales had soared to $4.1 million on the back of the "Dead Doctors Don't Lie" tape hysteria. Our successes in marketing and recruiting were compounding rapidly! My dream of Eagle being a major force in nutrition education and in the nutrition revolution was coming true. On one hand, I felt like the little red hen who had started with the grain of wheat and persevered until she wound up with her loaf of bread despite all of the rejection and lack of support from her barnyard friends. On the other hand, I still had feelings of ominous foreboding. Because of our concern, Ma Lan and I continued to build more and more downline distributors and increase infrastructure in self-defense.

The Toddy minerals were not what they used to be. The mineral source was changing. People were beginning to complain that "the minerals didn't work anymore."

My son Steve picked me up from the San Diego Airport at midnight February 22, 1997. I was returning to California after giving 12 highly successful Texas seminars in a row. We'd netted 1,200 new distributors for Terry Porter's downline, and I was in high spirits. Steve reached out shook my hand and said, "Dad, Eagle took away your distributorship! They said you are too controversial, and they wanted a more quiet image for the company so they could take Eagle public."

Ma Lan and I had built the Eagle company up from $17,000 a month to $4 million a month against all odds and predictions and in spite of

Peter's insane management tactics. We had put in uncounted hours and had literally poured in millions of our own dollars, including $1.3 million in 1996 in advertising to build Eagle, and now I was rewarded by having my distributorship terminated. It was the cystic fibrosis story all over again. This time, however, I was in better shape mentally and financially and I had prepared for such an event.

As soon as I got home that night I called John Wilson and asked if he was sure he knew what he was doing. If he didn't return my distributorship, I would be forced to become Eagle's competitor. John said, "There is no turning back. You should talk to my lawyers in the morning."

To make a long story short, we came to three settlements, including stock buy-backs and putting my distributorship that was netting $100,000 per month into a trust. The proposed settlements were win/win agreements. After each agreement, they would suddenly back peddle the next day and refuse to consummate the arrangements. Wilson also claimed that my sales efforts only amounted to less than five percent of the company sales. He was counting on the fact that I was the company's second largest stockholder and told me I wouldn't dare do anything to attack the company and devalue my stock. Wilson finished by saying, "There's no way you can get high quality plant derived colloidal minerals and start a viable company in less than a year. By then Eagle will be sold on the stock market. Why would I risk losing millions of dollars?"

John Wilson obviously didn't know Joel Wallach very well. After exhausting all avenues of reconciliation with the John Wilson gang and Eagle in March of 1997, I started my own company, American Longevity. I called Elmer Heinrich from Rockland the next day and told him that Eagle had terminated my distributorship. Would he sell me minerals? Elmer blurted out, "What? That was the most stupid thing they could have done. Sure, Wallach, I'll sell you minerals!"

By the end of the week I was working on our logo and label designs for our new line of "Virgin Earth" plant derived colloidal minerals, the original mineral source that Eagle had started with in 1991. We immediately started working with the same computer software company that had carried New Vision to over $400 million in sales per year. Several tablet and capsule suppliers were contacted and bids for various products requested. Our long time printer, Vince Marasigan, created brochures for each new Virgin Earth product. Price lists, order forms, and distributor applications were created and ordered. I hired Jerry Nehra the famed MLM attorney and David Stuart, legendary MLM trainee and consultant. My long time friends and associates called and asked about the new company. Without exception, they were tired of the antics of Eagle's management and were ready to sign up with our new company as soon as we could get an American Longevity application in their hands.

By April of 1997—after only one month, not one year—American Longevity was in business. June 15, 1997, American Longevity paid its first commissions. American Longevity has paid commission checks on time, every month, since its inception. This one factor alone has had the most positive affect on American Longevity distributors; we actually paid on time like a network marketing company was supposed to! I would have never started my own company had I not been forced to do so, but now the die was cast and we were on the road to the great American adventure. I was truly in business for myself now.

We developed a half dozen various liquid multiple type products with the Virgin Earth minerals as a base. We had the tools, staff, computers, and the software. Using the same old military tactical approach to a crisis that I had used so many times before, we relentlessly built American Longevity. We employed air strikes using our regular weekly radio programs and daily syndicated radio programs that were already under contract. We took ground by using road kills. We had perfected the technique and relentlessly duplicated them. It was like a homecoming game—we were the underdogs yet energy was high, everybody was up, and we were on our own turf retaking ground inch by inch.

Using our in-house database, mailings announcing the birth of American Longevity went out to anyone who had bought a book, tape, or video. American Longevity was launched and on its way!

Sixty Seconds Worth of Distance Run

There are many factors that contribute to America's greatness. Certainly the Constitution, religious freedom, equal treatment for all in the eyes of the law, the freedom to think and dream and hope, a highly developed technical infrastructure, and personal safety all rank high on the contributing factors list, but the cherry on the cake is the people of America and their yearning for free enterprise—the freedom to be creative, to contribute a service, to start their own businesses, to be able to control their own time and not let the clock be their master—is the magnet that drew "the teeming masses" to America.

Everyone in America has the opportunity for success, they only need an entrepreneurial spirit, a dream, a vehicle to reach that dream and a plan. Age, sex, race, and being born on the "wrong side of the tracks" are non-factors in achieving success in America. The desire to be free and in control of one's own destiny is the bottom line requirement for success, an inner voice that says, "I'd rather be the captain of my own rowboat than a crewmember on an ocean liner!"

Mountain men, frontiersmen, farmers, small business owners, and families with small home-based businesses have many attributes in common. First of all, they are brave and courageous; they take control of their own destiny and dare to venture away from that protective umbrella of friends and community for "something better." It is their spirit of adventure, their daring-do, and their willingness to take calculated risks that give Americans that notorious "cowboy" reputation.

Entrepreneurs are internally motivated; they are self-starters, problem solvers, never giving up, always finding a way to accomplish their task, goal or dream. They go around, over, under, and if necessary through any brick wall or barrier that might present itself—they never, never, never give up.

To be successful, entrepreneurs must be guided in their daily personal lives as well as their business lives by principal and integrity—nobody wants to be associated with schemers, crooks, or charlatans. One's word must be one's bond. Fairness and just settlements are absolute requirements in dealing with people if you want to be a leader. People are inherently attracted to leaders who steadfastly represent and defend their followers.

As far back as I can remember my mother and father were entrepreneurs; they worked hard. They farmed, recycled, bought and sold their goods, and raised their kids—they were good neighbors. They were very honest and intensely proud even though they were poor and uneducated. My mother and father were always positive about our futures and opportunities, and they never stopped believing in the American Dream.

My mother finished high school, but my father never finished 10th grade. Not being college educated or a sophisticated man of letters my father transmitted all of his Missouri wisdom relating to God, honesty, duty to family and country, and courage to me through the spoken word at the kitchen table, while chopping wood, during morning milking, truck trips to the market, and sitting at the campfire. He also encouraged me to read books that he believed were important. The Bible, *My Early Life* by Winston Churchill, and the complete works of Rudyard Kipling led the list.

When I turned nine years old my father gave me a framed copy of Kipling's poem "If" which summarized my father's personal philosophy and outlined his hopes and expectations of me. The poem has been a mentor, an extension if you will of my father's wisdom in times of crisis, growth, and opportunity. Second only to the Bible, Kipling's poem "If" is the most concise truth that a business man or woman can abide by and pass on to their associates or employees. It has certainly been the philosophical compass which has guided me through all of my travails and opportunities in life.

If

If you can keep your head when all about you
Are losing theirs and blaming it on you;
If you can trust yourself when all men doubt you,
But make allowance for their doubting too;
If you can wait and not be tired by waiting,
Or, being lied about, don't deal in lies,
Or, being hated, don't give way to hating,
And yet don't look too good, nor talk too wise;

If you can dream and not make dreams your master;
If you can think and not make thoughts your aim;
If you can meet with triumph and disaster
And treat those two imposters just the same;
If you can bear to hear the truth you've spoken
Twisted by knaves to make a trap for fools,
Or watch the things you gave your life to broken,
And stoop and build 'em up with worn out tools;

If you can make one heap of all your winnings
And risk it on one turn of pitch-and-toss,
And lose, and start again at your beginnings
And never breathe a word about your loss;
If you can force your heart and nerve and sinew
To serve your turn long after they are gone,
And so hold on when there is nothing in you
Except the Will which says to them: "Hold on;"

If you can talk with crowds and keep your virtue,
Or walk with kings nor lose the common touch;
If neither foes nor loving friends can hurt you;
If all men count with you, but none too much;
If you can fill the unforgiving minute
With sixty seconds' worth of distance run
Yours is the Earth and everything that's in it,
And—which is more—you'll be a Man my son!

I picked the name American Longevity for my new company to convey several truths: first, that it was, in fact, an American company; second, that it was to be a symbol that the American Dream was still alive and well; third, that it was an opportunity for everyone who had an entrepreneurial spirit; fourth, that it was formed and designed to promote health and longevity and be an honest business opportunity at the same time. Through the vehicle of American Longevity I could help many Americans with their health while teaching them to help others, I could help people pay off their mortgages, send their kids to college, buy a new car, take a cruise, or finance their dream projects. I love this country!

We had the computers, shipping facilities, trained personnel, and the only genuine source of plant derived colloidal minerals available, but I knew that I needed additional expertise and infrastructure to get a viable network marketing company off the ground and sustain it as a legacy that everyone would be proud to associate with.

David Stewart, a network marketing consultant, Jerry Nehra, a former Amway attorney, Steve Haskins, my personal attorney, my printer Vince Marasigan, and my computer guru John Sarazua were gathered together for a crisis meeting the first week of April 1997. David Stewart brought pre-fabricated policy and procedure manuals, a variety of compensation plans to choose from, and generic material on network marketing. We chose the 20-21 software package and charged John Sarazua with installing the program into our hardware while our printer Vince Marasigan, one of the artists, and I worked overtime on product brochures, labels, sign-up and order forms, and a trade-marked logo. We were adamant that the American Longevity logo should reflect the originality of the company concept.

We didn't have product right away. The first three weeks we were open we displayed and showed empty bottles with computer generated paper labels. We took advance orders and set the official American Longevity launch date for June 1, 1997.

While the concept of starting up American Longevity seemed simple enough, the actual birthing process had complications. For convenience and economics our first meetings were held in Santa Cruz, San Jose, Monterey, and Watsonville, California. Infiltrators from Eagle covered each of the 500 chairs in the Monterey meeting with stacks of their material, they had video cameras present in hopes of catching Eagle distributors that they believed might be cooperating with me, and they handed out anti-Wallach audiocassettes with Eagle's 800 number on the label. Video cameras were used by Eagle loyalists to record the presentation. The police were called, and we had them removed for trespassing.

The Santa Cruz meeting took place in the Coconut Grove meeting hall. It was raining a typical coastal spring rain that evening, and at first it did not seem strange that people were wet when they came upstairs to the seminar room. Then it dawned on me that they were all holding the audiocassette and reading the thick anti-Wallach package that Eagle was handing out. I grabbed one of the handouts from a very startled and very wet little old lady, and when I asked her were she had gotten the material she said, "A man was standing in the door and wouldn't let us in out of the rain unless we took the material."

I rushed to the front door and found a large man, over six feet tall and weighing well over 220 pounds, and several of his cohorts blocking the door. There was a long line of confused seniors standing in the rain looking like drowned rats. I directed the local distributor to call the police. Rather than sit passively by and wait for them, I took action to get the attendees out of the rain—if it's to be, it's up to me! I tried to grab the larger man's supply of brochures; he wouldn't let go so we had a brief tug-of-war until I brought my wrestling skills into play. I stepped on his foot and twisted him to the ground, and while he was trying to get up, I succeeded in getting the Eagle literature away from him.

In moments the police arrived and began writing up a trespassing complaint. The police inquired as to their home address and they said, "San Diego." The police asked why they were 800 miles north of their home trespassing and causing problems and he replied, "John Wilson hired us to disrupt Wallach's meetings." The same team of goons followed and harassed us for four weeks through our entire series of central California, San Francisco, and San Diego seminars and trade shows!

By September 1997, in only five months, American Longevity had recruited almost 20,000 distributors and paid out, *on time*, almost $1 million in commission checks. We went back to the original plant derived

Virgin Earth colloidal minerals discussed in the "Dead Doctors Don't Lie" tape, and we continue to use them as the flagship American Longevity product.

By September of 1997, Eagle's monthly revenues had sunk 50 percent from the January high of $4.1 million. The Eagle infrastructure was beginning to unravel as a result of their self-inflicted wounds. Network marketing can be as fragile as the stock market, perhaps more so because for most individuals their investment is small. John Wilson continued to send anti-Wallach letters and faxes into the Eagle downline, creating an exit stampede. I had directly or indirectly through the "Dead Doctors Don't Lie" tape recruited all 100,000 Eagle distributors, and if Eagle didn't want Wallach, the distributors didn't want Eagle.

According to Brian Pado, by March of 1998, Eagle's (since renamed SupraLife International) monthly sales were down to $1.3 million per month and the new distributor recruitment was down from a high of 7,000 new distributors per month in January of 1997 to well below 300 per month.

The Eagle policy and procedure manual only allowed for arbitration to deal with distributor disagreements, so arbitration complaints were filed against Eagle for wrongful termination of my distributorship. Subsequently, Ma Lan and Steve Wallach's distributorships were terminated by Eagle. Other leading distributors were also terminated by Eagle. More arbitration claims were filed against Eagle for wrongful terminations.

A lawsuit was filed in Federal Court against Peter Holliday, John Wilson, and other Eagle officers and staffers for breaking both the federal and the state of California's anti-trust laws and for conversion (embezzlement). Because of the fraud and racketeering aspects of their activities associated with the purchase of Eagle, the suit asked for application of the RICO Laws and triple damages amounting to $92 million. A derivative suit had been filed by stockholders controlling almost 40 percent of SupraLife stock against SupraLife International, its officers, Peter Holliday, John Wilson, and John Wilson's former accounting firm.

American Longevity at the 10 month mark had 30,000 distributors and was doing about $1 million in monthly sales. By November of 1998, American Longevity had over 50,000 distributors and was headed for $2 million in monthly sales and paid out $5 million in commissions.

On December 17, 1998, the arbitration panel voted in my favor. The AAA arbitration ruling resulted in vindication for myself and resulted in the following press release:

"Dead Doctors Don't Lie" Author Dr. Joel Wallach Wins Arbitration Against Soaring Eagle, Panel Finds He Was Wrongfully Terminated As An Eagle Distributor; Eagle Settles Case With Other Wallach Family Members.

San Diego, Calif.—In a decision released on December 17, 1998, the American Arbitration association ruled that Dr. Joel Wallach was **wrongfully terminated** as a distributor and held that Supralife International, Inc., formerly known as Soaring Eagle ("Eagle") violated its distributor agreement with Dr. Wallach as a result of his termination. The arbitration panel in a published ruling held: "We conclude that principles of good faith and fair dealing are inherent in an Eagle distributorship agreement. **We have determined that it is not only unfair, but legally unacceptable to abruptly terminate Dr. Wallach's distributorship agreement** in reliance upon matters which were previously the subject of demands for corrective action, with which, according to the evidence, Dr. Wallach complied."

"The ruling was a 100 percent victory for both Dr. Wallach and American Longevity," said Steve Wallach, Dr. Wallach's son and a consultant for American Longevity. "It not only vindicated Dr. Wallach from any wrongdoing and showed that Eagle management had acted in bad faith in terminating him, but it also showed how important Dr. Wallach was to Eagle as a company and how Eagle's demise is certain without him."

"Today was also a victory for all distributors of multi-level marketing companies. It shows that large companies can not cheat their distributors out of commissions and get away with it," said Dr. Wallach. "This case was never about money, it was about standing up for what is right. Eagle had no excuse for the terrible way in which they treated me and numerous other distributors. Now they are paying for their actions. Here at American Longevity we want to be known as the company that cares about its distributors and leads the industry in providing its distributors with the best support. Every American Longevity distributor is part of the family, and we take care of our family."

The panel of three arbitrators awarded Dr. Wallach a total of $230,000 in damages. The panel ruled that, due to Dr. Wallach's great success with American Longevity, his damages as a result of the wrongful termination should be reduced, hence the $230,000 award.

American Longevity was created by Dr. Wallach in April of 1997, after he was terminated as an Eagle distributor on February 23. Eagle's attorneys had argued to the arbitration panel that due to the great financial success of American Longevity and the fact that Soaring Eagle was no longer a viable company without Dr. Wallach, Dr. Wallach's damages should be reduced as he was making more money with American Longevity than he had been with Eagle. One of Eagle's attorneys even proclaimed that Eagle was "insolvent."

"It shows how important Dr. Wallach was to that company and how incompetent and greedy Eagle management was for terminating him," stated Steve Wallach. "Dr. Wallach built Eagle from a company with zero sales to one with monthly earnings close to $5 million dollars at the time of his termination. They should have commended him for his effort, but instead they got greedy, saw dollar signs and terminated him. However, they did not realize how important he was to Eagle's existence. He **was** Eagle. Now they are paying the price." Since Dr. Wallach's termination in February of 1997, Eagle's sales have plummeted from approximately $5 million per month to a mere $800,000 per month according to testimony by Eagle's current Customer Service Manager, Sally Osborne.

Earlier in the week several former Eagle distributors, led by Dr. Wallach's wife Dr. Ma Lan and son Steve, settled in their case for wrongful termination for a total of $338,000. The other claimants in the case were Richard and Roxanne Renton, John and Jonnie Taylor, and Thomas Adcock. Michelle Wallach also had a claim for Eagle to allow a transfer of her downline to an investment group.

"There is no point in beating a dead horse," said

Steve Wallach. "Eagle made it quite obvious that they did not feel they would be around much longer, and it was difficult to counter that evidence given their terrible financial condition. They lost approximately $1,000,000 in the first half of 1998 alone, and the second half does not look any better for Eagle."

One of the main arguments of Soaring Eagle's attorneys at the arbitration hearing was that Eagle was no longer a viable company, primarily due to the departure of Dr. Wallach and the creation of American Longevity. Eagle presented strong evidence that it was in a financial tailspin that it could not recover from, therefore limiting the amount the plaintiffs could have recovered.

An additional issue that came to light during Dr. Ma Lan's arbitration was Eagle's failure to compress their distributor's downlines as had been promised in Eagle's marketing materials. Eagle's in-house counsel Mike Shea admitted that, except in 1996, Eagle had failed to perform compressions of its distributors' downlines until 1998. "All along, between 1992 and 1997, Eagle was promising its distributors that annual compressions would be performed," said Steve Wallach. "Just think of all the money Eagle has cheated their distributors out of for their failure to perform compressions as promised. This is no way to treat your distributors."

"We realize that distributors are the backbone of our company," said Dr. Wallach. "Unfortunately, Eagle management has never realized this which has lead to their downfall. If Eagle spent half as much time educating its distributors as it did creating a so called 'Compliance Department' to terminate them it would not be in the financial hole today." After Dr. Wallach's termination Eagle literally spent hundreds of thousands of dollars creating and implementing a Compliance Department lead by in-house counsel Michael Shea and Jason Murphy to police the activities of Eagle distributors. Numerous distributors were terminated by Eagle as a result of alleged "investigations" by Eagle's compliance department.

"It turned into a witch hunt," says Roxanne Renton, a former Eagle distributor. "I was getting daily phone calls from undercover Eagle employees trying to pry into my business and how I was running my distributorships. They were just looking for excuses to terminate me. I was treated terribly when I should have been commended for my efforts in building Eagle's distributor base. I was amazed during my arbitration at the number of files Eagle maintained on so many of its distributors. It's like they had nothing better to do than spy on the activities of hard working business builders. They were watching everything we did, and it was ridiculous. I am so glad to be dealing with American Longevity, a company which appreciates my efforts and does not tell me how to run my own business."

American Longevity was founded by Dr. Joel Wallach in April of 1997 and is committed to providing its distributors with the finest products and support without interfering in their everyday activities. American Longevity paid out $5.3 million in distributor commissions in 1998, its first full year of business.

Appendix A

The New Alphabet of Wellness

Some 79 minerals have been detected in animal and human tissue (i.e. blood, liver, muscle, brain, etc.). Their presence in the tissues fulfills the first criteria for calling a mineral an "essential nutrient." Literally thousands of studies provide additional support for considering 60 of these 79 nutrients to be essential. These studies were done on animals at every stage of life: pregnant, suckling, weanling, and mature. Furthermore, these studies were carried out on animals of virtually every description: laboratory mice, rats, rabbits, hamsters, guinea pigs, rabbits, dogs, cats, pigs, sheep, cattle, chickens, turkeys, ducks, etc. These minerals are considered essential because they are known to act as cofactors for DNA, RNA, enzyme systems, or cofactors for vitamins. As a Boy Scout, I collected rocks and mineral ores because they were easy to classify and were pretty to look at, but had learned little of their value as disease preventing and curing elements essential for animals and man. Now, even a simple look at minerals presented with an eye to their nutritional value should lead even the disinterested skeptic to appreciate their importance and essentiality to animal and human health. The following list is presented in alphabetical order according to the chemical symbols of each element.

Ac—Actinium originated in igneous rocks and is usually found at extremely low concentrations of 5.5 x 10 (-16) ppm. Actinium is readily absorbed by plant roots, but very little is transported to the stem, leaves, and shoots of the plant. Actinium accumulates in and presumably has metabolic functions in the bones and liver.

Ag—Silver originates from igneous rocks and sedimentary rocks. It's found at the rate of 0.07 ppm in rocks, 0.01 ppm in soils, 0.00013 ppm in fresh water, and 0.0003 ppm in seawater. It's present in marine algae at 0.25 ppm, land plants from 0.06 ppm to 1.4 ppm in accumulator plants growing near silver ore. Epiogonum ovalifolium is a silver indicator plant. Silver is found at 3.0 to 11.0 ppm in marine animals, 0.05 to .7 ppm in land mammals, and at 0.16 to 0.8 ppm in muscle tissue. Even tortoise shell contains silver at 0.05 to 0.7 ppm. Silver has been employed in human health care and in the search for immortality since the time of the Chinese alchemist 8,000 years ago. Many feel that silver is in fact an essential element, not because it is required by an enzyme system, but rather because it serves as a systemic disinfectant and immune system stimulator.

Sir Malcom Morris reported in the *British Medical Journal* (May 12, 1917) that colloidal silver is free from the drawbacks of other preparations of silver, viz. pain caused and discoloration of the skin. Instead of producing irritation, it has a distinctly soothing effect. It rapidly subdues inflammation and promotes healing of the lesions. It can be used with remarkable results in enlarged prostate with irritation of the bladder, in pruritis ani and perineal eczema, and in hemorrhoids.

J. Mark Hovell reported in the *British Medical Journal* (December 15, 1917) that, "colloidal silver has been found to be beneficial for permanently restoring the patency of the Eustachian tubes and for reducing nasopharyngeal catarrh. Colloidal silver has also been used successfully in septic conditions of the mouth (including pyorrhea alveolysis—Rigg's disease), throat (including tonsilitis and quincies), ear (including Menier's symptoms and closure to Valsalva's inflation), and generalized septicemia, leucorrhea, cystitis, whooping-cough and shingles."

Taken internally, the particles of colloidal silver are resistant to the action of dilute acids and alkalis of the stomach and intestine. Consequently they continue their catalytic action and pass into the intestine unchanged.

T.H. Anderson Wells reported in *Lancet* (February 16, 1918) that a preparation of colloidal silver was "used intravenously in a case of puerperal septicemia without any irritation of the kidneys and with no pigmentation of the skin."

Silver sulfadiazine (Silvadene, Marion Laboratories) is used in 70 per cent of the burn centers in America. Discovered by Dr. Charles Fox,

Columbia University, sulfadiazine has been used successfully to treat syphilis, cholera, and malaria; it also stops the Herpes simplex virus responsible for cold sores and fever blisters.

Silver is an anti-bacterial, anti-viral, anti-fungal, anti-metabolite that disables specific enzymes that microorganisms use for respiration. Silver is such an efficient bactericide that our great-grandmothers put silver dollars into fresh milk to keep it from spoiling at room temperature. Humans can consume 400 mg of silver per day. A silver "deficiency" results in an impaired immune system. In *The Body Electric* Dr. Robert Becker identified a relationship between low levels of tissue and dietary silver and the rate of illness. He stated, "Silver deficiency was responsible for the improper functioning of the immune system" and "silver does more than just kill disease causing organisms; it was also causing major growth stimulation (another criteria for essentiality) of injured tissue." Human fibroblast cells were able to multiply at a greater rate, producing large numbers of primitive, embryonic cells in wounds. These cells are able to differentiate into whatever cell types that are necessary to heal the wound.

Dr. Bjorn Nordstrom of the Carolinska Institute, Sweden has used silver in his alternative cancer therapy programs. According to *Science Digest* (Silver: Our Mightiest Germ Fighter. March, 1978) silver is an antibiotic. Silver kills over 650 disease-causing organisms. Resistant strains fail to develop as they do with normal antibiotics. Silver is absolutely non-toxic to humans at standard rates of consumption.

Al—Aluminum is found in igneous rocks at 5,000 ppm, 82,000 ppm in shales, 25,000 ppm in sandstone, 4,200 ppm in limestone, and 71,000 ppm in clay. Aluminum represents 12 percent of the earth's crust and is the most common metal in the earth's crust. Aluminum is found in high concentrations in all plants grown in the soil, including common food crops such as squash, tea, wine, and wheat. Aluminum is found in large biological quantities in every plant grown in the soil. You can't eat any grain, vegetable, fruit, or nut or drink any natural water source or juice without taking in large quantities of aluminum.

The aluminum found in plants is organically bound colloidal aluminum and appears not to have any negative affect and in fact appears to be an essential element in human nutrition. Acid soils yield highest amounts of soil aluminum to plants. It is found in marine plants at 60 ppm and is especially high in plankton and red algae. Aluminum is found in land plants at an average of 500 ppm, with a range of 0.5 to 4,000 ppm. It is found in marine mammals at 19 to 50 ppm. In mammals, the highest levels are found in the hair and lungs.

Aluminum's known biological function is to activate the enzyme succinic dehydrogenase. It increases the survival rate of newborns, and, according to professor Gerhard Schrauzer, former professor of chemistry at UCSD, is "probably an essential mineral for human nutrition." A single faulty study over 25 years ago suggested a link between chronic aluminum exposure and Alzheimer's disease.

In a study that appeared November 5, 1992 in the journal *Nature*, Frank Watt, et al (Oxford University) used a highly accurate technique to quantify the levels of aluminum in the brains of Alzheimer's patients. To their surprise, they found the same levels of aluminum in the brains of the non-Alzheimer's controls as they did in their Alzheimer's patients. The June 1997 issue of the Berkley Newsletter reported that there is no link between Alzheimer's disease and aluminum.

Am—Americum are radioactive isotopes and have a half life of 7,950 years. Americum accumulates in mammalian bone.

Ar—Argon is found in igneous rocks at 3.0 to 5.0 ppm and can be used to date ancient rocks using the potassium/argon dating system. It is found in fresh water and sea water at 0.06 ppm and mammalian blood at 0.75 ppm.

As—Arsenic is found in igneous rock at .0 to 8.0 ppm, shale at 13.0 ppm, sandstone and limestone at 1.0 ppm, fresh water at 0.0004 ppm, seawater at 0.003 ppm, and soils at 6.0 ppm. Argentina and New Zealand actually have toxic levels of arsenic in some soil regions. Arsenic also accumulates in marine plants at the rate of 30.0 ppm, land plants at 0.02 ppm, marine animals at 0.005 to 0.3 ppm, and land animals at a rate of less than 0.2 ppm concentrating in hair and nails. It is essential for survivability of newborn and neonatal growth.

Arsenic in combination with choline prevents 100 percent of perosis ("slipped tendon") in poultry. Arsenic deficiency in humans results in a "carpal tunnel syndrome," "TMJ," and other "repetitive motion" type degeneration. Arsenic metabolism is affected by tissue and blood levels of zinc, selenium, arginine, choline, methionine, taurine, and quaniacetic acid, all of which affect methyl-group metabolism and polyamine synthesis which is the site of arsenic function in human physiology.

The French Academy first identified arsenic in dead human bodies in 1834. Arsenic normally appears in human female blood at 0.64 ppm. Levels rise to 0.93 ppm during menstruation and 2.20 ppm during months five and six of pregnancy. At 90 to 120 ppm, arsenic promotes the growth rate of chicks. The rate of growth and metamorphosis of tadpoles is enhanced by the presence of arsenic as well.

At—Atatine is a radioactive isotope with an extremely short half-life of 7.2 to 8 hours. Astatine is accumulated by the mammalian and human thyroid following ingestion, but is rapidly excreted.

Au—Gold is found in igneous and sedimentary rocks at 0.004 ppm, fresh water at 0.00006 ppm, sea water at 0.000011 ppm, marine plants at 0.012 ppm, land plants 0.0005 to 0.002 ppm, marine animals at 0.0003 to 0.008 ppm, land animals at 0.00023 ppm, and in mammalian liver forms, as a colloid. Gold concentrates in the horse tail plant. Gold compounds (gold sodium thiomalate, gold thioglucose also known as aurothio-glucose) are frequently administered by orthodox physicians as an add on therapy with salicylates (aspirin) for arthritis when added pain relief is required. Gold has been reported only to be effective against active joint inflammation and is not usually helpful for treating advanced destructive rheumatoid arthritis.

B—Boron is found in igneous rocks at 10 ppm, shale at 100 ppm, sandstone at 35 ppm, limestone at 20 ppm, fresh water at 0.013 ppm, sea water at 4.0 to 6.0 ppm, soil from 2.0 to 100 ppm (highest in saline and alkaline soils), marine plants 120 ppm (highest in brown algae), land plants at 150 ppm (chenopodiaceae and plumboginaceae are indicator plant families), marine animals at 20 to 50 ppm, and land animals at 0.5 ppm. Boron is essential for bone metabolism including efficient use of calcium and magnesium and proper function of endocrine glands (i.e.— ovaries, testes, and adrenals).

Pure boron is hard and gray and melts at over 4,000 degrees F. Boron, a non-metallic mineral, occurs as a combination in nature (i.e.- borax, boric acid or sassolite, ulexite, colemanite, boracite, and tourmaline).

Prior to 1981, boron was not considered an essential nutrient. Boron was first shown to be an essential mineral for growing chicks. It was not until 1990 that boron was accepted as an essential nutrient for humans.

Boron is required for the maintenance of bone density and normal blood levels of estrogen and testosterone. Within eight days of supple-menting boron, women lost 40 percent less calcium, 33 percent less magnesium, and less phosphorus through their urine. Women receiving boron supplementation had blood levels of estradiol 17B doubled to "levels found in women on estrogen replacement therapy." Levels of testosterone also double with Boron supplementation.

Ba—Barium is found in igneous rocks at 425 ppm, shale at 580 ppm, sandstone at 50 ppm, limestone at 120 ppm, fresh water at 0.054 ppm, sea water at 0.03 ppm, soil at 500 ppm, marine plants at 30 ppm (highest in brown algae), land plants at 14 ppm (the fruit of Bertholletia excelea can have up to 4,000 ppm), marine animals 0.2 to 3.0 ppm (highest in hard tissue such as bone and shell), and land animals at up to 75 ppm (highest in bone, lung, and eyes). Barium was considered essential to mammals in 1949.

Be—Beryllium is found in igneous rocks at 2 to 8 ppm, shale at 3 ppm, sandstone and limestone at < 0.1 ppm, fresh water at 0.001 ppm, sea water at 0.0000006 ppm, soil at 0.001 ppm, marine plants (highest in brown algae), land plants at less than 0.1 ppm (highest in plants grown on volcanic soils), and land animals at 0.0003 to 0.002 ppm in soft tissue.

Bi—Bismuth is found in igneous rocks at 0.17 ppm, shale at 1.0 ppm, seawater at 0.000017 ppm, land plants at 0.06 ppm, marine animals at 0.09 ppm, and land animals at 0.004 ppm. Stress has historically been blamed as the boogy-man as the cause of gastric, peptic, and duodenal ulcers. Human studies have in fact demonstrated that the true cause of ulcers is an infection with a bacterium known as Helicobacter pylori. Australian gastroenterologist Barry Marshall, M.D. and pathologist J. Robbin Warren proposed their theory for the bacterial cause of gastric ulcers in 1983. The bacterial cause for gastric ulcers was known in pigs in 1952. The treatment of choice for ulcers is ten days to four weeks on tetracycline antibiotics, antacids, and bismuth subsalicylate. You've heard of bismuth treating stomach symptoms if you've heard of a pink liquid with the name of Pepto Bismol™.

Br—Bromine is a "halogen" related to iodine. It is found in igneous rocks at 3.0 to 5.0 ppm, shale at 4.0 ppm, sandstone at 1.0 ppm, limestone at 0.2 ppm, fresh water at 0.2 ppm, sea water at 65 ppm, soil 5.0 ppm, marine plants at 740 ppm (highest in brown algae), land plants at 15 ppm, marine animals at 60 to 1000 ppm, and land animals at 6.0 ppm. Bromine functions in the form of brominated amino acids. There is strong evidence for Bromine's essentiality in mammals.

C—Carbon is found in igneous rocks at 200 ppm, shale at 15,300 ppm, sandstone at 13,800 ppm, limestone at 113,500 ppm, fresh water at 11 ppm, sea water at 28 ppm, soils at 20,000 ppm (up to 90 percent of carbon in soil is bound in the humus), marine plants at 345,000 ppm, land plants at 454,000 ppm, marine animals at 400,000 ppm, and in land animals at 465,000 ppm (280,000 ppm in bone). Carbon functions as an essential structural element for all organic molecules (i.e.- carbohydrates, fats, amino acids, enzymes, vitamins, etc.).

Carbohydrates normally furnish most of the energy required to move, perform work, and for the basic biochemical functions of life itself.

The chief sources of carbohydrates include grains, vegetables, fruits and sugars. Carbohydrates in their simplest form have the formula CH_2O. Hydrogen and oxygen are present in the same ratio that is found in water with one carbon for each molecule of water.

Plants are able to manufacture carbohydrates (sugar and starch), vitamins, amino acids, and fatty acids. To manufacture carbohydrate, plants take CO_2 and H_2O and subject them to a chemical process called photosynthesis. In the presence of chlorophyll, a magnesium/carbon ring structure, carbohydrate is produced using the energy from sunlight. O_2 is released as a by-product of the reaction. Carbohydrates are classified as monosaccharides (glucose or "grape sugar," fructose), disaccharide's (sucrose = glucose and fructose, maltose = glucose and glucose, lactose = glucose and galactose), oligosaccharides, and polysaccharides (starch, dextrin, fiber, cellulose, and glycogen or "animal starch" are all complexes of glucose units).

Lipids or fats, like carbohydrates, are composed of carbon, hydrogen and oxygen. Fats have the common property of being insoluble in water, soluble in organic solvents such as ether and chloroform, and can be utilized as energy by living organisms. Fats as a group of carbon compounds includes ordinary fats, oils, waxes, and unrelated compounds. The primary food sources of lipids are butter, flax seed oil, olive oil, animal fat, nuts, seeds, whole grains, olives, avocados, egg yolks, dairy, etc. Fats serve as a source of immediate or stored energy. A gram of fat contains 9 calories per gram compared with 4.5 calories per gram.

Triglycerides (the primary component of fats and oils) are composed of carbon, hydrogen, and oxygen. Structurally, they are esters of a trihydric alcohol (glycerol) and fatty acids. The fatty acids can have from four to 30 carbon atoms and constitute the bulk of the triglyceride mass. One hundred grams of fat or oil will contain 95 grams of fatty acids.

A fatty acid or hydrocarbon chain is described with regard to three characteristics: chain length, degree of "saturation" with hydrogen, and location of the first "double bond." The length is a reference to the number of carbon atoms in the chain (i.e.- C(16) has 16 carbons in the chain). The term "short" (less that 6 carbons), "medium" (7 to 11 carbons), and "long" (12 or more carbons) are used to describe the chains of fatty acids in the structure of triglycerides.

The degree of hydrogen "saturation" in fatty acids is defined by the number of double bonds between carbon atoms in the fatty acid chains. A chain can contain all the hydrogen it can hold and have no double bonds, in which case it is referred to as a saturated fatty acid. It can contain one double bond (monounsaturated fatty acid) or it may contain several double bonds (polyunsaturated fatty acids).

The location of the first double bond as counted from the "tail" or methyl end of the fatty acid is referred to as the "omega" number (i.e.- omega 3, omega 6, etc.).

Three polyunsaturated fatty acids (linoleic, linolenic, and arachidonic acids) are known as essential fatty acids (EFA). Three percent of the total daily calorie intake is required from EFA. However, only two (linoleic and linolenic) are designated as Essential Fatty Acids. Arachidonic acid can be synthesized by humans from lenolenic acid. EFA's have essential vitamin-like functions in fat transport and metabolism, and in maintaining the integrity of cell walls (bilipid layer membranes). They are also part of the fatty acids of cholesterol esters and phospholipids in plasma lipoproteins and mitochondrial lipoproteins. Serum cholesterol can be lowered by the consumption of EFA. EFA's are also the raw material for the human body to manufacture prostaglandins that help regulate blood pressure, heart rate, vascular dilation, blood clotting, bronchial dilation, and central nervous system (brain and spinal cord) function. EFA deficiency in human infants results in a poor growth rate, eczema, and lowered resistance to infectious diseases.

Cholesterol is a member of a large group of fats known as sterols. They all have a complex carbon ring structure. Cholesterol is only found in animal tissue, but similar sterols are found in plants. Cholesterol is an essential part of the structure of cell walls, brain and spinal cord (myelin), the raw material for the production of vitamin D in the human body, bile acids, adrenal cortical hormones, estrogen (a cholesterol deficiency makes menopause a living hell), progesterone, and testosterone (a cholesterol deficiency will turn hubby into a TV watching steer who is totally disinterested in sex).

Proteins are the fundamental structural components of the living cell (cytoplasm). They are essential parts of the cell nucleus and protoplasm. Proteins are the most abundant of all carbon containing organic compounds in the human body. The greatest mass of body protein is found in the skeletal muscle, the remainder is found in other organs (liver, kidney, heart, stomach, etc.), bones, teeth, blood, and other body fluids (lymph). Enzymes are proteins that work to facilitate chemical reactions in the body.

Proteins, like carbohydrates and fats, contain carbon, hydrogen, and oxygen. In addition they also contain 16 percent nitrogen (the amine group) sometimes in conjunction with other elements such as phosphorus, iron, sulfur and cobalt. The basic structural unit of a protein is the amino acid. Amino acids are united by "peptide bonds" into long chains of various geometric structures to form specific proteins. Digestion of proteins breaks the peptide bonds to release individual amino acids. Use of protein for energy provides 4.5 calories per gram.

Classically there are nine essential amino acids that are required in the daily diet as they cannot be manufactured by the human body. Forty-three percent of the dietary protein for human infants must be the essential amino acids. Growing children require 36 percent essential amino acids and adults require 19 percent for maintenance. To the classic list of essential amino acids, I would add arginine, taurine, and tyrosine. Over the long haul, these three amino acids help prevent certain specific diseases. Respectively, those diseases are cancer, macular degeneration, and goiter.

The classic essential amino acids are:

Amino acid	Function
Valine	protein production
Lysine	protein production
Threonine	protein production
Leucine	protein production
Isoleucine	protein production
Tryptophane	precursor of niacin and serotonin
Phenylalanine	precursor of thyroxin and epinephrine
Methionine	formation of choline and creatine phosphate
Histidine	formation of histamine

An individual consuming protein at even 300 gm per day (almost 3/4 of a pound of meat a day) will have no adverse effects as long as they do not have kidney or liver disease.

Vitamins are a major carbon group of unrelated organic carbon compounds needed by the human body in minute quantities each day. They are essential for specific metabolic reactions of the cell and are required for normal growth, development, maintenance, health, longevity, and life itself. Vitamins work as coenzymes or activating side groups for essential subcellular enzyme systems. Vitamins regulate metabolism, facilitate the conversion of fat and carbohydrate to energy, and are required for the formation and repair of tissues in embryos, children, teens, adults, and seniors.

Taking optimum levels of essential vitamins goes a long way to preventing birth defects and solving the problems of reduced physical effectiveness and debilitating degenerative diseases.

Ca—Calcium is found in igneous rocks at 41,500 ppm, shale at 22,100 ppm, sandstone at 39,100 ppm, limestone at 302,000 ppm, fresh water at 15 ppm, sea water at 400 ppm, soils at 7,000 to 500,000 ppm (lowest in acid soils and highest in limestone or alkaline soils), marine plants at 10,000 to 300,000 ppm (highest in calcarious tissue—red, blue-green, and green algae and diatoms), land plants 18,000 ppm, marine animals 1,500 to 20,000 ppm, 350,000 ppm in calcarious tissue (sponges, coral, molluscs, echinoderms), land animals at 200 to 85,000 ppm, 260,000 ppm in mammalian bone, 200 to 500 ppm in soft tissue, and at levels lower than 5ppm in red blood cells. Calcium is essential for all organisms and is found in the cell walls of plants, all calcareous tissues, and mammalian bones. Calcium also helps regulate electrochemical functions in cells and activates several enzymes.

Calcium is the fifth most abundant mineral element in the earth's crust and biosphere. There is evidence that clearly shows humans are designed to consume and use high calcium diets. The late Paleolithic period of 35,000 to 10,000 years ago was the most recent time that our human forebears lived in the environment for which they had been biochemically designed. The agricultural revolution occurred 10,000 years ago and it reduced the wide variety of wild foods in the human food chain while increased food energy (calories). These dietary changes universally and forever decreased man's dietary intake of minerals, trace minerals, and rare earths. The uncultivated food plants and wild game commonly available to Stone Age humans would supply 1600 mg at basal energy intakes and between 2,000 and 3,000 mg of calcium at the energy levels required to support hunting and work.

During the 20th century, American adults have a calcium intake of only one-fifth to one-third as much as did Stone Age humans. The National Health & Nutrition Examination Survey II reported a median calcium intake for American women of between 300 and 508 mg per day and only 680 mg for men.

Common Calcium Deficiency Diseases

Osteoporosis
Kyphosis
Dowager's hump
Lordosis
Legg-Perthe's disease
Compression fractures
Spontaneous fractures
Receding gums
Osteomalacia
Osteoarthritis
Degenerative arthritis
Ankylosing spondylitis
Hypertension
Insomnia
Kidney stones
Bone spurs (heel spurs)
Calcium deposits
Cramps and twitches
PMS
Sciatica
Low back pain
Bell's Palsy
Tinnitis
Wallach's vertigo
Trigeminal neuralgia
Spinal stenosis
Nutritional secondary hyperparathyroidism
Osteofibrosis
Tetany
Panic attacks
Elevated blood calcium
Prolonged clotting time

Other nutrients that are commonly found in the American diet aggravate the national calcium deficiency. Diets rich in salt and phosphates (protein and soft drinks) result in an increased calcium "cost." In effect these foods increase the requirements for calcium. Urinary calcium loss increased from 96 mg per day to 148 mg per day when food was heavily salted. As phosphate intake is doubled the output of urinary calcium increases 50 per cent.

There are no less than 147 deficiency diseases that can be attributed to calcium deficiencies or imbalances. The most recent clinical research clearly points out that the entire scope of American diets are critically deficient in calcium. The only practical way to get enough calcium is through supplementation. Interestingly, the allopathic physicians who did the study failed in their duty. Instead of simply recommending effective calcium supplementation, they recommended eating five cups of broccoli a day as a valuable source of calcium. Try and get a kid to eat that!

The more common calcium deficiency diseases are easy to recognize and run from poor clotting time of the blood when you nick yourself shaving (calcium is a cofactor in the clotting mechanism), arthritis (which physicians traditionally treat with pain killers), to the dozens of variations of osteoporosis.

Famous people who have suffered from calcium deficiency include Pope John Paul II (fractured hip/osteoporosis), Elizabeth Taylor (osteoporosis/hip replacement surgery), "Bo" Jackson (fractured hip/osteoporosis), Bill Walton, a vegan of professional basketball fame (knee, foot, and bone spurs), Ted Williams of baseball fame (osteoporosis and arthritis), etc.

Calcium is the most abundant mineral in the human body. The average male has 1,200 grams and the average female has 1,000 grams. Calcium makes up two percent of the adult body weight (water makes up 65 to 75 percent). Calcium also composes up to 39 percent of the total mineral reserves of the body (ash). Ninety-nine percent of body calcium is found in the bones and teeth. The other one percent is found in the blood, extracellular fluids, and within cells where it is a cofactor and activator for numerous enzymes.

Calcium in bones is in the form of hydroxyapatite salts composed of calcium phosphate and calcium carbonate in a classic crystal structure bound to a protein framework called "bone matrix." Put a chicken "drumstick" bone in a quart of vinegar for two weeks and the calcium will be leached out of the bone leaving the protein matrix. Similar types of hydroxyapatite are found in the enamel and dentine of teeth; however, little is available from teeth to contribute to rapidly available Ca to maintain blood levels.

In addition to being a major structural mineral, Ca is also required for the release of energy from ATP for muscular contraction, and blood clotting. In the blood clotting process ionized Ca stimulates the release of thromboplastin from the platelets and converts prothrombin to thrombin. Thrombin helps to convert fibrinogen to fibrin, and fibrin is the protein web that traps red blood cells to make blood clots. Calcium mediates the transport function of cell and organelle membranes. Ca effects the release of neurotransmitters at synaptic junctions. It also mediates the synthesis, secretion, and metabolic effects of hormones and enzymes. Ca helps to regulate the heart beat, muscle tone, and muscle receptivity to nerve stimulation.

Calcium is mainly absorbed in the duodenum, where the environment is still acid. Once the food in the intestine becomes alkaline, absorption drops. Calcium is absorbed from the small intestine by active cellular transport and by simple diffusion. Metallic calcium absorption may be limited to 10 percent or less and is affected by many substances in the gut. Calcium is highly absorbable, up to 98 percent in the organically bound plant derived colloidal mineral and water soluble chelated form.

Causes of calcium deficiency include a lack of vitamin D. So does a deficiency of stomach acid. Often the lack of stomach acid or hypochlorhydria results from a restricted NaCl (salt) intake. Lactose intolerance, celiac disease, high fat diet, and low protein intake and high phytate consumption can lead to calcium deficiency. Phytic acid is a phosphorus containing acid compound found in the bran of grains and seeds as well as the stems of many plants. Oatmeal and whole wheat especially contain phytic acid. When phytic acid combines with calcium it forms an insoluble product called calcium phytate which cannot be absorbed by the body. Oxalic acid in rhubarb, spinach, chard, and mustard greens combines with Ca to form an insoluble calcium oxalate, which is not absorbed. Fiber itself, besides the phytate content, prevents calcium absorption. Alkaline intestine, gut hypermobility (too rapid transit time brought on by too much fiber fruit, etc.), and pharmaceuticals (antiseizure drugs, diuretics, etc.) result in decreased absorption and retention. Excesses of sugar and caffeine from coffee, tea, colas, etc. will leach calcium from the bones.

Parathormone secreted by the parathyroid gland and calcitonin secreted by the thyroid gland maintain a serum calcium of 8.5 to 10.5 mg percent by drawing on calcium reserves from the bones. The parathormone can also affect the kidney so that it retains more calcium. The same hormone can cause the gut to be more efficient in absorption. When the blood calcium begins to rise from too much parathyroid activity, calcitonin reduces availability of calcium from the bones.

In 1980, McCarron et al theorized that chronic calcium deficiency probably led to hypertension. More than 30 subsequent studies supported the original theory of calcium deficiency as the cause of hypertension. In addition, recent studies have shown that serum ionized calcium is consistently lower in humans with untreated hypertension. In a recent review article, Sower and others noted that the association of calcium intake and high blood pressure is most clear in people with daily calcium intakes of less than 500 mg a day.

The phenomenon of salt sensitive hypertension consists of a rise in blood pressure and sustained increase in urinary loss of calcium in response to salt consumption. Among black and elderly whites with essential hypertension, restricted intakes of calcium and potassium, rather than elevated salt consumption is responsible for salt sensitivity. In a four-year study of 58,218 nurses, hypertension was more likely to develop in females who took in less than 800 mg of Ca per day.

Up to 75 percent of consumed calcium is lost in the feces. Two percent is lost in the urine and sweat (15 mg per day is lost in normal sweating—this can double or triple in active athletes or individuals engaged in physical labor). In cases of excess urine loss of calcium (osteoporosis, excess phosphorous, etc.), kidney stones, bone spurs, and calcium deposits will develop. Bone and heel spurs and calcium deposits always develop at the sites of insertions of tendons and ligaments during a raging osteoporosis. Bone spurs, heel spurs, and calcium deposits can be reversed and eliminated by supplementing with significant amounts of chelated and colloidal calcium sources.

Not only are our soils and food deficient in calcium, additionally the American diet is rich in phosphorous, which is found in just about everything we eat. Ideally, the calcium to phosphorous (or Ca:P) ratio in our daily diet should be 2:1. This ideal ratio is not possible by simply eating food. You would have to eat 25 pounds of broccoli every time you ate a 16 oz. steak! The only possible way to approach the 2:1 ideal is to avoid as much as possible the food items containing high amounts of phosphorous (I hate calling colas, processed "cheese," etc., food) and supplement with plant derived colloidal and chelated calcium.

Cd—Cadmium is found in igneous rocks at 0.2 ppm, shale at 0.3 ppm, sandstone at 0.05 ppm, limestone at 0.035 ppm, fresh water at 0.08 ppm, sea water at 0.00011 ppm, soils at 0.06 ppm, marine plants at 0.4 ppm, land plants at 0.6 ppm, marine animals at 0.15 to 3.0 ppm, and in land animals at 0.5 ppm (accumulates in kidney tissue). Functions in nature by stimulating the hatching of nematode (round worm) cysts. Cadmium-bound proteins have been isolated from mollusks and the horse kidney.

Ce—Cerium, a rare earth, is found in igneous rocks at 60 ppm, shale at 59 ppm, sandstone at 92 ppm, limestone 12 ppm, sea water 0.0004 ppm, soil 50 ppm, land plants accumulates to 320 ppm, and land animals 0.003 ppm (accumulates in bone). Cerium nitrate is used as a topical disinfectant for severe burn victims.

Cl—Chlorine is found in igneous rocks at 130 ppm, shale at 180 ppm, sandstone at 10 ppm, limestone at 150 ppm, fresh water 7 to 8 ppm, sea water at 19,000 ppm, soil at 100 ppm (higher in alkaline soils, near the sea and in deserts—a major exchangeable anion in many soils), marine plants at 4,700 ppm, land plants at 2,000 ppm, marine animals at 5,000 to 90,000 ppm (highest in soft coelenterates), and land animals at 2,800 ppm. In land animals, Cl's highest concentration is found in mammalian hair and skin. Chlorine is essential for all living species' electrochemical and catalytic functions, activates numerous enzymes, and is the basic raw material for our stomachs to make stomach acid (HCl) for protein digestion by pepsin, B12 absorption (intrinsic factor activation), and absorption of minerals. Sodium chloride (NaCl) or salt is the universal source of chloride ions for all living things.

Cm—Curium is found in igneous rocks at 0.0001 ppm. All isotopes are radioactive with a 2.5 x 108 years half-life. Cm exists in some molybdenites. This radioactive mineral will accumulate in mammalian bone.

Co—Cobalt is found in igneous rock at about 25 ppm, shales at 19 ppm, sandstone at 0.3 ppm, limestone at 0.1 ppm, fresh water at 0.0009 ppm, sea water at 0.00027 ppm, soils at 8 ppm (higher in soils derived from basalt or serpentine; vast areas of the earth are known to be absolutely devoid of cobalt), marine animals at 0.5 ppm, and in land animals at 0.03 ppm (greatest concentrations in bone and liver).

Cobalt is essential for all forms of life including blue green algae, some bacteria and fungi, some plants, insects, birds, reptiles, amphibians, and mammals including man. Cobalt functions as a cofactor and activator for enzymes, fixes nitrogen during amino acid production, and a single cobalt atom is the central metal component of vitamin B12 which itself is a cofactor and activator (cobamide coenzymes) for several essential enzymes.

B12 cobalt is chelated in a large tetrapyrrole ring similar to the phorphyrin ring found in hemoglobin and chlorophyll. The original B12 molecule isolated in the laboratory contained a cyanide group, thus the name cyanocobabalamine. There are several different cobalamine compounds that have vitamin B12 activity, with cyanocobalamine and hydroxycobalamine being the most active.

Vitamin B12 is a red crystalline substance that is water soluble. The red color is due to the cobalt in the molecule. Vitamin B12 is slowly deactivated by exposure to acid, alkali, light, and oxidizing or reducing substances. About 30 percent of B12 activity is lost during cooking (electric, gas, or microwave).

In 1948, B12 was isolated from liver extracts and demonstrated anti-pernicious anemia activity. The essentiality of cobalt is unusual in that the requirement is for a cobalt complex known as cyanocobalamine or vitamin B12. A pure cobalt requirement is only found in some bacteria and algae and the need for B12 cobalt is thought by some to represent a symbiotic relationship between microbes which generate and manufacture B12 from elemental cobalt and vertebrates that require B12.

Ruminants (i.e. cows, sheep, goats, deer, antelope, buffalo, giraffe, etc.) can use elemental cobalt because the microbes fermenting and digesting plant material in their first stomach (rumen) convert elemental cobalt into vitamin B12, which the animal then uses. Carnivores can get their B12 from the ruminant by consuming stomach contents, liver, bone, and muscle from their kills. Poultry, lagomorphs (rabbits and hares), and rodents actively eat feces during the night (coprophagy) and in the process obtain vitamin B12 manufactured by intestinal microorganisms.

Metallic cobalt itself is absorbed at the rate of 20 to 26.2 percent by mice and in humans if intrinsic factor is present in the stomach and the stomach ph is 2.0 or less. Intrinsic factor is a mucoprotein enzyme known as Castle's intrinsic factor and is part of normal stomach secretions. If a person has hypochlorhydria (low stomach acid—usually a NaCl deficiency) the intrinsic factor will not work and B12 cobalt is not absorbed—this is why doctors frequently give B12 shots to older people on salt restricted diets. Sublingual (under the tongue) and oral spray B12 is available. Plant derived cobalt is very bioavailable; however, because of low salt diets and cobalt depleted soils, vegetarians frequently have B12 deficiencies.

The B12 intrinsic factor complex is primarily absorbed in the terminal small intestine or ileum. Calcium is required for the B12 to cross from the intestine into the bloodstream as well as an active participation by intestinal cells. Simple diffusion can account for only one to three percent of the vitamin's absorption. There is an enterohepatic (intestine direct to the liver) circulation of Vitamin B12 that recycles B12 from bile and other intestinal secretions which explains why B12 deficiency in vegans may not appear for five to ten years after giving up meat.

The maximum storage level of B12 is 2 mg, which is slowly released to the bone marrow as needed. Excess intake of B12 above the body's storage capacity is shed in the urine (expensive urine). Vitamin B12/cobalt joins with folic acid, choline, and the amino acid methionine to transfer single carbon groups (methyl groups) in the synthesis of the raw material to make RNA and the synthesis of DNA from RNA. DNA and RNA are directly involved in gene function; remember the concept of preconception nutrition to prevent birth defects. Growth, myelin formation (converts cholesterol into the insulating material myelin found around nerves in the brain, spinal cord, and large nerve trunks), and red blood cell synthesis are dependent on B12. Cobalt is also required as a necessary cofactor for the production of thyroid hormone.

The discovery of the essentiality of cobalt came from observing a fatal disease ("bush sickness") in cattle and sheep from Australia and New Zealand. It was observed that "bush sickness" could be successfully treated and prevented by cobalt supplements. Bush sickness was characterized by emaciation (unsupplemented vegans), dull stare, listless and starved look, pale mucus membranes, anorexia, and pernicious anemia (microcytic/hypochromic).

In humans, a failure to absorb B12/cobalt results in a deficiency disease. This can result from a surgical removal of parts of the stomach (eliminates areas of intrinsic factor production), or surgical removal of the ileum portion of the small bowel, small intestinal diverticulae, parasites (tapeworm), celiac disease (allergies to wheat gluten and cows milk albumen), and other malabsorption diseases. Pernicious anemia and demyelination of the spinal cord and large nerve trunks are classic diseases that result from a B12/cobalt deficiency.

Less than 0.07 ppm Co in the soil results in cobalt deficiency in animals and people who eat crops grown from those soils. 0.11 ppm Co in the soil prevents and cures Co deficiency.

The human RDA for B12/cobalt is 3 to 4 mcg per day, but 250 to 400 mcg gives more safety. Pregnant and nursing mothers should especially take care to supplement with optimum amounts of B12. A baby being nursed by a deficient mother has their deficiency extended over a long period of time. This may result in serious permanent nerve damage.

Cobalt excess in man (20 to 30 mg/day) may create an accelerated erythropoiesis (RBC – red blood cell – production) by stimulating an increased production of the kidney hormone erythropoiten.

Cr—Chromium is found in igneous rocks at 100 ppm, shale at 90 ppm, sandstone at 35 ppm, limestone at 11 ppm, fresh water at 0.00018 ppm, sea water at 0.00005 ppm, soils at 5 to 3,000 ppm (higest in soils derived from basalt and serpentine), marine plants 1 ppm, land plants at 0.23 ppm, marine animals at 0.2 to 1.0 ppm, and in land animals at 0.075 ppm where it is found accumulated by RNA and insulin.

Chromium activates phosphoglucosonetase and other enzymes and is closely associated with GTF or glucose tolerance factor. GTF is a combination of chromium III, dinicotinic acid, and glutathione. The reported plasma levels of chromium in humans over the past 20 years has ranged from 0.075 to 13 ng/ml. Concentrations of chromium in human hair are ten times greater than in blood, making hair analysis a much more accurate view of chromium tissue stores and function in the human. There is 1.5 mg in the human body.

Very little inorganic chromium is stored in the body. Once inorganic chromium is absorbed, it is almost entirely excreted in the urine (therefore urine chromium levels can be used to estimate dietary chromium status). Dietary sugar loads (i.e. colas, apple juice, grape juice, honey, candy, sugar, fructose, etc.) increase the natural rate of urinary Cr loss by 300 percent for 12 hours. The average intake of 50 to 100 µg of inorganic chromium from food and water supplies only 0.25 to 0.5 µg of usable chromium. By contrast 25 percent of chelated chromium is absorbed. The chromium RDA for humans is a range of 50 to 200 µg per day for adults.

The concentration of chromium is higher in newborn animals and humans than it is at older ages. In fact, the chromium levels of unsupplemented human tissue steadily decreases throughout life. Of greater concern has been the steady decline in the average American serum chromium since 1948:

Mean Chromium Blood Levels (µg/l)	Year
28—1000	1948
13	1971
10	1972
4.7 to 5.1	1973
0.73 to 1.6	1974
0.16	1978
0.43	1980
0.13	1985

The fasting chromium plasma level of pregnant women is lower than that of nonpregnant women. Increasing impairment of glucose tolerance in "normal" pregnancy is well documented and reflects a chromium deficiency that oftentimes results in pregnancy onset diabetes. One study demonstrated abnormal glucose tolerance in 77 percent of clinically "normal" adults over the age of 70. According to Richard Anderson, USDA, "Ninety percent of all Americans are deficient in chromium."

Gary Evans, Bemidji State University, Minnesota, very clearly showed an increased life span in laboratory animals by 33.3 percent when they were supplemented with chromium. Prior to this study gerontologists, led by Roy Walford, felt a severe restriction of calories was the only way to extend life past the expected average. Deficiencies of chromium in humans are characterized by a wide variety of clinical diseases as well as a shortened life expectancy. The clinical diseases of chromium deficiency are aggravated by concurrent vanadium deficiencies.

Diseases and Symptoms of Chromium Deficiency

Low blood sugar
Prediabetes
Diabetes (adult onset, Type II)
Hyperinsulinemia
Hyperactivity
Learning disabilities
ADD/ADHD
Hyperirritability
Depression
Manic depression
Bi-polar disease
Anxiety attacks

Panic attacks
Dr. Jekyll/Mr. Hyde rages –"Bad seeds"
Impaired growth
Peripheral neuropathy
Negative nitrogen balance—protein loss
Elevated blood triglycerides
Elevated blood cholesterol
Coronary blood vessel disease
Aortic cholesterol plaque
Infertility
Decreased sperm count
Shortened life span

Cs—Cesium is found in igneous rocks at 1 ppm, shale at 5 ppm, sandstone at limestone at 0.5 ppm, fresh water at 0.0002 ppm, sea water at 0.00005 ppm, soils at 0.3 to 25 ppm, marine plants at 0.07 ppm, land plants at 0.2 ppm, and in land animals at 0.064 ppm. In land animals the highest concentrations were found in muscle.

As an alkaline mineral, cesium behaves similarly to sodium, potassium, and rubidium chemically. Cesium and potassium enter into a solute complex, which participates in ion antagonism, osmosis, permeability regulation, and maintenance of the colloidal state in the living cell. The increase in supplemental potassium increases the rate of excretion or loss of cesium. Cesium chloride is used as part of alternative cancer therapy programs. Cesium provides "high ph therapy" for cancer by entering the cancer cell and producing an alkaline environment. It has been recommended for all types of cancers including sarcomas, bronchiogenic carcinoma, and colon cancer.

Cu—Copper is found in igneous rocks at 55 ppm, shale at 45 ppm, sandstone at 5 ppm, limestone at 4ppm, fresh water at 0.01 ppm, sea water at 0.003 ppm, soils at 2 to 100 ppm (copper is strongly absorbed by humus, but there are known areas of the world with extreme copper deficiency), marine plants 11 ppm, land 14 ppm, marine animals at 4 to 50 ppm (accumulates in the blood of annelid worms, crustaceans and mollusks, especially cephlopods), and in land animals at 2 to 4 ppm with highest levels in the liver. Copper is essential to all living organisms and is a universally important cofactor for many hundreds of metalloenzymes. Copper deficiency is widespread and copper deficiency diseases are quite common.

Copper Deficiency Symptoms and Diseases

⟨ White, grey, and silver hair
⟨ Dry brittle hair ("steely wool" in sheep)
⟨ Ptosis (sagging tissue—eye lids, "crow's feet," skin, breasts, stomach, etc.)
⟨ Hernias (congenital and acquired)
⟨ Varicose veins (including hemorrhoids)
⟨ Spider veins
⟨ Aneurysms (cerebral artery, coronary artery, and large artery blowouts)
⟨ Kawasaki disease (congenital aneurysms with streptococcal infection)
⟨ Anemia (especially common in high milk and vegan diets)
⟨ Hypo and Hyperthyroid dysfunction
⟨ Arthritis (especially where bone growth plates are involved)
⟨ Ruptured vertebral discs
⟨ Liver cirrhosis
⟨ Violent behavior, blind rage, explosive outbursts, and "criminal behavior"
⟨ Learning disabilities
⟨ Cerebral palsy and hypoplasia of the cerebellum (congenital ataxia in sheep)
⟨ High blood cholesterol
⟨ Iron storage disease (hemosiderosis)
⟨ Reduced carbohydrate tolerance
⟨ Neutropenia (low neutrophil count)

Copper is required in many physiological functions: RNA, DNA, Lysil oxidase cofactor, melanin production (hair and skin pigment), electron transfer for subcellular respiration, tensile strength of elastic fibers in blood vessels, skin, vertebral discs, etc. Neonatal enzootic ataxia (sway back, lamkruis) was recognized as a clinical entity in 1937 as a copper deficiency in pregnant sheep. Copper supplements prevented the syndrome, which was characterized by demyelination of the cerebellum and spinal cord. Cavitation or gelatinous lesions of the cerebral white matter, chromatolysis, nerve cell death and myelin aplasia (failure to form during embryonic life) were also identified as copper deficiency diseases in sheep. These are identical to the classical changes of human cerebral palsy.

Famous people affected or dying of an obvious copper deficiency include: Albert Einstein (ruptured aneurysm), Paavo Airola (ruptured cerebral aneurysm), Conway Twitty (ruptured abdominal aneurysm), and George and Barbara Bush (thyroid disease and white hair). Four to six of every 100 Americans autopsied have died of a ruptured aneurysm. An additional 40 percent have aneurysms that had not ruptured.

The average well-nourished adult human body contains between 80 and 120 mg of copper. Concentrations are higher in the brain, liver, heart, and kidneys. Bone and muscle have lower percentages of copper but contain 50 percent of the body total copper reserves because of their mass. It is of interest that the greatest concentration of copper is found in the newborn. Their daily requirement is 0.08 mg/kg, toddlers require 0.04 mg/kg and adults only 0.03 mg/kg.

The average plasma copper of women ranges from 87 to 153 mg/dl. For men it ranges from 89 to 137 mg/dl. About 90 percent of the plasma copper is found in ceruloplasmin.

Copper functions as a cofactor and activator of numerous cupro-enzymes that are involved in the development and maintenance of the cardiovascular system. Deficiency of Cu in the pregnant female results in congenital defects of the heart and brain, and Kawasaki disease, cerebral palsy, and hypoplasia of the cerebellum. Deficiency of Cu also results in reduced lysyl oxidase activity causing a reduction in conversion of proelastin to elastin causing a decrease in the tensile strength of arterial walls and ruptured aneurysms. Deficiency of copper also results in lower skeletal integrity including a specific type of arthritis in children that forms bone spurs in the bone growth plate. Lack of Cu can result in myelin defects, anemia, poor hair keratinization, and loss of hair color. Nutropenia (reduced numbers of neutrophillic WBC's or white blood cells) and leukopenia (reduced total WBC count) are the earliest indications of a copper deficiency in an infant. Infants whose diets are primarily cows milk frequently develop anemia and/or iron storage disease.

Menkes' Kinky Hair Syndrome is thought to be a sex-linked recessive defect of copper absorption. The affected infants exhibit retarded growth, defective keratin formation of the hair, loss of hair pigment, low body temperature, degeneration and fractures of aortic elastin (aneurysms), arthritis in the growth plates of long bones, and a progressive mental deterioration. Mental deterioration results from brain tissue being totally devoid of the essential enzyme cytochrome oxidase.

Because of absorption problems of metallic copper, injections of copper and liver extracts are useful for these children. Serum and plasma copper increases 100 percent in pregnant women and women using oral contraceptives. Serum copper levels are also elevated during acute infections, liver disease, and pellagra (niacin deficiency). Accumulations of copper in the cornea form Kayser-Fleischer rings.

Dy—Dysprosium, a rare earth, is found in igneous rocks at 3.0 ppm, in shale at 4 to 6 ppm, sandstone at 7.2 ppm, and limestone at 0.9 ppm. Concentrations in terrestrial animals (0.01 ppm) are highest in the bones.

Er—Erbium, a rare earth, is found in igneous rock at 2.8 ppm, shale at 1.9 ppm, sandstone at 1 ppm, limestone at 0.36 ppm, land plants up to 46 ppm in Carya spp. (a variey of plant), marine animals at 0.02 to 0.04 ppm, and land animals primarily in bone.

Eu—Europium is a "light" rare earth found in igneous rocks at 1 to 2 ppm, shale at 1.1 ppm, sandstone at 0.55 ppm, limestone at 0.2 ppm, land plants at 0.021 ppm (accumulates up to 16 ppm in Carya spp.), marine animals at 0.01 to 0.06 ppm, and land animals at 0.00012 ppm in soft tissue and 0.2 ppm in bone.

Europium has extended the life of laboratory species over their normal expected lifespan by 100 percent. Europium is found in higher concentration in breast milk from women in third world countries than in American women.

F—Fluorine is found in igneous rocks at 625 ppm, in shale at 740 ppm, sandstone at 270 ppm, limestone at 330 ppm, fresh water at 0.09 ppm, sea water at 1.3 ppm, and soils at 200 ppm (flouride can be "fixed" or tightly bonded in several types of clay.) Certain types of F rich soils in Madras, Spain, and South America are toxic to grazing livestock. Fluorine is found in marine plants at 4.5 ppm, land plants at 0.5 to 40.0 ppm (accumulates in Dichapetolum cymosum), marine animals at 2.0 ppm (accumulates in fish bones), and land animals at 150 to 500 ppm in mammalian soft tissue and 1,500 ppm in teeth and bones.

Prior to 1972, fluoride was considered essential in animals because of its apparent benefit for tooth enamel in warding off dental caries ("cavities"). In 1972, Schwarz proved that fluoride was in fact an essential mineral for animals and humans.

The skeletal reserves of fluoride in an adult man can reach 2.6 grams; the average daily intake by Americans is 4.4 mg from combined sources of food and water.

Fluoridation of drinking water is still highly controversial. Some studies show that fluoridated water helps reduce fractures from osteoporosis, while other studies showed an increase in hip fractures. Clinical toxicity is observed as dental fluorosis at fluoride concentrations of 2 to 7 ppm and osteosclerosis at 8 to 20 ppm. Chronic systemic toxicity appears when the fluoride levels reach 20 to 80 mg per day over several years.

Approximately 10,000 American towns and cities serving 100 million people have added fluoride to their drinking water at the rate of 1 mg/L which has reportedly reduced dental caries by 60 to 70 percent. In certain western states in the United States, there is an excess of fluoride, reaching levels of 10 to 45 ppm with resultant mottling of teeth in children.

As a result of epidemiological studies by Yiamouyiannis and Burk in 1977, full scale congressional hearings were held to examine the charge that 10,000 excess cancer deaths were caused by fluoridation of certain public water systems. As a result of those hearings, the committee mandated that the U. S. Public Health Service conduct animal studies to confirm or refute the theory that fluoridated water increased cancer deaths. The studies were carried out by the National Toxicology Program under the supervision of the U.S. National Public Health Service with special focus on oral, liver, and bone cancers.

In 1990, the results of the fluoride study showed an increase in rat precancerous lesions in mucus membrane cells. There was an increase in cancers of the oral mucus membranes (squamous cell carcinoma). A rare form of osteosarcoma appeared at double the rate in males as females, and there was an increase in thyroid follicular cell tumors and liver cancer (hepatocholangio carcinoma).

Fe—Iron is found in igneous rocks at 56,000 ppm, shale at 47,200 ppm, sandstone at 9,800 ppm, limestone at 3,800 ppm, fresh water at 0.67 ppm, sea water at 0.01 ppm, and soils at 38,000 ppm (iron content is responsible for most soil color). Iron is most available in acid soil and availability is greatly determined by bacterial activity in the soil. It's found in marine plants at 700 ppm (very high in plankton), land plants at 140 ppm, and marine animals at 400 ppm (high in the blood of annelid worms), echinoderms, fish, and in the eggs of cephalad moluscs. Fe is essential to all land animals.

Boussingault in the 1860s was the first to regard iron as an essential nutrient for animals. During the 1920s, feeding rats on an exclusive milk diet created an animal model for iron deficiency research.

In a healthy adult human there is three to five grams of iron. The newborn infant has nearly double the amount of iron per kg than adults. Sixty to 70 percent of tissue iron is classed as essential or functional iron, and 30 to 40 percent as storage iron. The essential iron is found as an integral part of hemoglobin, myoglobin (muscle oxygen storing pigments—particularly rich in deep diving animals such as whales, walrus, seals, etc.), and subcellular respiratory enzymes involved with oxidation and electron transfer processes.

Functions of iron include cofactor and activator of enzymes and metallo enzymes, respiratory pigments (iron is to hemoglobin what magnesium is to chlorophyll), and electron transfer for utilization of oxygen.

Iron is stored in bone marrow and liver (i.e. hemosiderin and ferritin). Heme iron from meat is 10 percent available for absorption while iron from fresh plant sources are only one percent available because of phytates. Iron absorption takes place primarily in the duodenum where the intestinal environment is still acid.

Experimental evidence shows very clearly that "pica" is a specific sign of iron deficiency. Pica can drive children and adults to eat ice (pagophagia), dirt (geophagia), or lead paint. Iron deficiency results from pregnancy, menstruation, chronic infections, hypochlorhydria (low stomach acid from salt restricted diets), chronic diarrhea, chronic bleeding (i.e. cancer, ulcers, parasites, blood clotting problems, etc.), and impaired absorption (i.e. high fat diets, high fiber diets, celiac disease, etc.). Symptoms of iron deficiency include listlessness, fatigue, heart palpitations on exertion, reduced cognition, memory deficits, sore tongue, angular stomatitis dysphagia, and hypochromic microcytic anemia. Stomach hydrochloric acid is required for optimal absorption of iron. Ascorbic acid increases the absorption of iron; clays and phytates decrease the absorption of iron. The RDA of 18 mg per day as metallic iron is too low for those eating high fiber, high phytate diets.

Excesses of iron can cause cirrhosis of the liver, fibrosis of the pancreas, diabetes, and heart failure. These diseases are not the direct toxic affects of iron, but rather the increased iron results in the increased needs of selenium, copper, zinc, etc.

Fr—Francium is found only as radioactive isotopes. The longest lived has a half life of 22 minutes.

Ga—Gallium is found in igneous rocks at 15 ppm, shale at 19 ppm, sandstone at 12 ppm, limestone at 4.0 ppm, fresh water at 0.001 ppm, sea water at 0.00003 ppm, soils at 0.4 to 6.0 ppm to 30.0 ppm, marine plants at 0.5 ppm, land plants at 0.06 ppm, marine animals at 0.5 ppm, and in land animals at 0.006 ppm. Gallium was claimed to be an essential nutrient in 1938 and again in 1958. Gallium has specific areas of metalloenzyme activity in the human brain and has been reported to specifically reduce the rate of brain cancer in laboratory animals. British research shows that supplemented diets of pregnant women reduces the rate of brain cancer in children.

Gd—Gadolium, a rare earth, is found in igneous rocks at 5.4 ppm, shale at 4.3 ppm, sandstone at 2.6 ppm, limestone at 0.7 ppm, land plants can concentrate Gd up to 70 ppm by Carya spp, and in marine animals at 0.06 ppm. Land animals accumulate gadolium in bone and liver very quickly after absorption.

Ge—Germanium is found in igneous rocks at 5.4 ppm, shale at 1.6 ppm, sandstone at 0.8 ppm, limestone at 0.2 ppm, sea water at 0.00007 ppm, soil at 1.0 ppm in humus, especially in alkaline soils, and marine animals at 0.3 ppm. The existence of the element germanium had been predicted by Mendeleev in his periodic table, but it was not until 1886 that a German scientist, Clemens Winkler, isolated this element and named it Germanium. Radio-do-it-yourself kits from the 40s and 50s utilized the germanium diode crystal to attract the radio signal to your radio. The germanium atom is structured so it accepts and transmits electrons, thus acting as a semiconductor. It is therefore not too surprising that germanium is closely related to silica and carbon. Biologically, germanium is a highly effective electrical impulse initiator intracellularly and acts as a metallic cofactor for oxygen utilization.

In 1950, Dr. Kazuhiko Asai, a Japanese chemist, found traces of germanium in fossilized plant life. Russian researchers quickly attributed anti-cancer activity to germanium. Dr. Asai was able to connect the healing properties of certain herbs to relatively high levels of germanium. Many of these herbs are germanium accumulator plants. Germanium is known to enhance the immune system by stimulating production of natural killer cells, lymphokines such as IFN(y) interferon, macrophages, and T-suppresser cells.

Asai synthesized GE-132, carboxyethyl germanium sesquioxide, in 1967 by a hydrolysis method. This organic germanium structure forms a cubic structure with three negative oxygen ions at the base of a cubic triangle. As an organic or chelate form of germanium, GE-132 is absorbed at the rate of 30 percent efficiency and the total intake is excreted in one week.

Food plants and animals contain small amounts of germanium (i.e. beans—4.67 ppm, tuna—2.3 ppm). Healing herbs such as garlic, aloe, comfrey, chlorella, ginseng, watercress, Shiitake mushroom, pearl barley, sanzukon, sushi, waternut, boxthorn seed, and wisteria knob contain germanium in amounts ranging from 100 to 2,000 ppm. The "holy waters" at Lourdes, known world wide for their healing properties, contains large amounts of germanium.

A severely reduced immune status, arthritis, osteoporosis, low energy, and cancer typify deficiencies of germanium.

Twenty to 30 mg per day is the recommended maintenance dose for germanium. Fifty to 100 mg per day doses are commonly used when an individual has a serious illness that requires an increased oxygen level in the body.

H—Hydrogen is found in igneous rocks at 1,000 ppm, shale at 5,600 ppm, sandstone at 1,800 ppm, limestone at 860 ppm, fresh water at 111,000 ppm, sea water at 108,000 ppm, soil at 600 to 24,000 ppm (in very acid soils it can become the major exchangeable cation), marine plants at 41,000 ppm, land plants at 55,000 ppm, marine animals at 52,000 ppm, and in land animals at 70,000 ppm. Additionally hydrogen makes up a small portion of the gaseous atmosphere. Hydrogen functions as a major constituent of water and all organic molecules. Seventy percent of the human body is water. The regulation of the acid-base balance in the human body is in fact the regulation of the hydrogen ion (H+) levels of cellular and extracellular fluids.

The acidity of the body is critically regulated within a narrow range by numerous and complex homeostatic mechanisms. The pH of healthy blood ranges from 7.36 to 7.44. When the pH falls below 7.30, the patient has acidosis. When the pH rises above 7.44, the person has alkalosis.

Blood pH below 6.8 and above 7.8 is rapidly fatal. Intracellular pH ranges between 6.0 and 7.4. Rapid metabolism (hyperthyroid) or decreased blood flow (heart attack) increases the carbon dioxide levels and therefore decreases pH or acidifies the blood. In contrast to the internal body, the pH of secretions and excretions can be more variable and range from 1.0 in stomach acid to 8.2 in pancreatic juice and alkaline urine in vegans.

Hydrogen ions circulate in the body in two forms, volatile and non-volatile (metabolic hydrogen ions). Volatile hydrogen ions are found as a weak acid (carbonic acid), which must continuously be excreted from the lungs as carbon dioxide and water.

Non-volatile (metabolic) hydrogen ions are produced by the normal metabolic processes of the body or are consumed as part of food. The largest amounts of hydrogen ions are produced by normal and abnormal metabolism. Large amounts of hydrogen ions may be generated and/or retained as part of a disease activity (i.e. emphysema, diabetes, anxiety or loss of chloride ions, NaCl deficiency, cystic fibrosis, Addison's

Disease, etc.).

Hydrogen ion concentration (pH) is controlled by the body by means of dilution, buffering respiratory control of volatile hydrogen ion concentrations and kidney control of non-volatile hydrogen ions. Buffer systems react to hydrogen ion concentrations in fractions of seconds, respiratory controls react in minutes, and the kidneys may require as much as an hour to several days to respond.

Metabolic hydrogen ions must be excreted by the kidney in one of three forms: 60 percent as ammonium ions, 40 percent as weak acids, or trace amounts as free hydrogen ions. It is the amount of free hydrogen ions in the urine that determines the urine's pH. Acidifying the urine with unsweetened cranberry juice can often times control bladder infections (cystitis).

He—Helium is found in igneous rocks at 0.008 and seawater at 0.0000069 ppm.

Hf—Hafnium is found in igneous rocks at 3 ppm, shale at 2.8 ppm, sandstone at 3.4 ppm, limestone at 0.3 ppm, sea water at 0.000008 ppm, soil at 3.0 ppm, marine plants at 0.4 ppm, land plants at 0.01 ppm, and in land animals at 0.04 ppm.

Hg—Mercury is found in igneous rocks at 0.08 ppm, shale at 0.4 ppm, sandstone at 0.03 ppm, limestone at 0.04 ppm, fresh water at 0.00008 ppm, sea water at 0.00003 ppm, soil at 0.03 to 0.8 ppm (lowest in the surface layers of the soil because it is leached and also it is volatilized), marine plants at 0.03 ppm, land plants at 0.015 ppm (Arenaria setacea is an accumulator plant), land animals at 0.046 ppm (accumulates in the brain, kidney, liver, and bone), and marine animals at 0.0009 to 0.09 ppm.

Mercury occurs universally in the bios and has long been known as a toxic element, even though the early Chinese alchemists insisted that the regular consumption of mercury or "potable gold" was the path to immortality. Mercury is concentrated in the environment by industry, mining operations, agriculture, dental repairs (amalgams), and microorganisms that methylate mercury in the sediments at the bottoms of fresh water or salt water rivers, lakes, oceans, and seas. Mercury has been detected in all tissues of accident victims, with no known mercury exposure except dental mercury amalgam fillings.

Mercury in fish is present as methyl mercury. People who rarely eat fish have very low levels of mercury (2–5 µg/kg). Moderate fish consumers have 10 µg/kg. High fish consumers (especially if they eat shark, tuna, or swordfish) have higher values of 400 µg/kg.

Mercury mineworkers accumulate mercury, which can reach levels that produce disease.

The biological half life of methyl mercury in humans is 70 days and four days for inorganic mercury. The placenta acts as a barrier against the passage of inorganic mercury but not methyl mercury. Methyl mercury transfers very easily to the fetus ("congenital" Minamata Disease in Japanese infants).

The main industrial source of mercury is the chloralkali industry. Additional major sources include the manufacture of electrical appliances, paint, dental amalgams, pharmaceuticals slimicides and algicides (paper and pulp industry), seed treatments as agricultural fungicides— especially dangerous as methyl mercury, and burning of fossil fuels.

The metabolic antagonism between mercury and selenium results in the protection from selenium poisoning by mercury and the protection from mercury poisoning by selenium supplementation. Because a mutual antagonism between Hg and Se exists, Se protects the human kidney from necrosis (tissue death) by mercury poisoning and the placental transfer of mercury. Mercury vapor from dental amalgam has been shown to increase the percent of antibiotic resistant bacteria in the gut from 9 percent to 70 percent in monkeys given dental mercury fillings. The drug resistant bacterial population dropped to 12 percent when the fillings were removed.

Mercury poisoning from inhalation of mercury vapors was reported during the Victorian Age in "hatters" who used mercury nitrate paste to prevent molds from growing on felt hats, hence the expression "mad as a hatter" from Alice in Wonderland. Goldsmiths and mirror workers could also suffer from inhalation poisoning. In modern times dentists have developed several disease syndromes including multiple sclerosis, ALS (Lou Gehrig's Disease), and Parkinson's Disease depending on what part of the brain was most severely affected by mercury toxicity. Annette Funicello contracted multiple sclerosis, which is believed to be caused by vapors from dental mercury amalgams.

The manifestations of direct Hg poisoning are primarily neurological (i.e. tremors, vertigo, irritability, moodiness [suicidal], depression), salivation, inflammation of the mouth, stomatitis, and diarrhea.

In poisoning with inorganic mercury, the liver and kidneys are the target organs primarily affected. Poisoning with the more toxic alkyl mercury results in progressive lack of coordination, loss of vision, heart palpitations, loss of hearing, and mental deterioration caused by a toxic neuroencephalopathy in which the neuronal cells of the cerebral and cerebellar cortex are selectively affected.

In 1962, Minamata, Japan, mercury contaminated factory effluent (waste water) was dumped into the bay, which in turn contaminated aquatic plant material which was eaten by fish. The contaminated fish were eaten by the bay residents with disastrous results. The Minamata disaster was characterized by a high incidence of "congenital" damage to the newborn (i.e. mental retardation, cerebral palsy, and high infant mortality).

In Iran, large scale methyl mercury poisoning was reported when large numbers of people were fed bread made with mercurial fungicide treated seed grain and meat (liver and kidneys) from animals fed the treated grain. The result of consuming the mercury contaminated grains was thousands of babies born retarded and a high incidence of congenital brain defects including cerebral palsy.

Ho—Homium, a rare earth, is found in igneous rocks at 1.2 ppm, in shale at 0.6 ppm, sandstone at 0.51 ppm, limestone at 0.17 ppm, land plants at 16 ppm in Carya spp., marine animals at 0.005 to 0.01 ppm, and land animals at 0.5 ppm in bone.

I—Iodine is found in igneous rocks at 0.5 ppm, in shale at 2.3 ppm, sandstone at 1.7 ppm, limestone at 1.2 ppm, fresh water at 0.002 ppm, sea water at 0.06 ppm, soil at 5 ppm (strongly bound in humus—large areas of earth are known to be devoid of I), land plants at 0.42 ppm, marine animals at 1.0 to 150 ppm, and in land animals at 0.43 ppm (concentrates in the thyroid gland and hair). Iodine is known to be essential to red and brown algae and all vertebrates. In combination with the amino acid tyrosine, iodine is manufactured into the thyroid hormone thyroxin. Iodine intake is usually low to begin with, but since Americans have begun restricting their salt intake at the advice of their doctors, goiter and hypothyroidism has become epidemic.

The average American takes in 170–250 mcg/day of iodine. Humans lose considerable amounts of it in their sweat—up to 146 mcg/day with only moderate exercise. Metallic iodine is not toxic up to 2,000 mcg/day. Goiter develops in Japanese living along the seacoast despite high daily iodine consumption. Japanese subjects being fed Chinese cabbage, turnips, buckwheat, noodles, 2.0 mcg iodine, soybean, or seaweed developed goiter in all groups except the seaweed eating group.

Northern parts of the Adictis Islands had more clinical goiter than the southern areas while the southwest was goiter-free. Forty-six percent of the population of Pisila, 40 percent of the population of Polje, and only 3 percent of the population of Milahnici were affected. There is identical iodine content of the soil in all three locations. A severe copper deficiency in the soils of the north and the south cause the deficiency state because copper is a required cofactor to utilize iodine.

Some one million Americans have either a hypothyroid (low, under-active) or a hyperthyroid (overactive) condition. Thyroid hormones control and regulate digestion, heart rate, body temperature, sweat gland activity, nervous and reproductive system, general metabolism, and body weight.

Symptoms of Hypothyroidism

Hashmoto's disease
Fatigue
Cold intolerance
Muscle aches and pains
Heavy or more frequent periods
Low sex drive
Brittle nails
Weight gain
Hair loss
Muscle cramps
Depression
Constipation
Elevated blood cholesterol
Puffy face
Dry skin and hair
Inability to concentrate
Poor memory
Goiter

Symptoms of Hyperthyroidism

Grave's disease
Insomnia
Heat intolerence
Excessive sweating
Lighter/less frequent periods
Hand tremors
Rapid pulse
Exophthalmos ("bug-eyes")
Weight loss

Increased appetite
Muscle weakness
Frequent bowel movements
Irritability
Nervousness
Goiter

Many foods and food additives are known as "goitrogens" because they interfere with the thyroid metabolism and produce thyroid disease. These foods and food additives are nitrates, broccoli, cabbage, Brussels sprouts, etc.

In—Indium is found in igneous rocks at 0.05 to 1.0 ppm, land plants at 0.62 ppm, and land animals at 0.016 ppm.

Ir—Iridium is found in igneous rocks at 0.001 ppm, land plants at 0.62 ppm, and land animals at 0.00002 ppm.

K—Potassium is found in igneous rocks at 20,000 ppm, shale at 26,000 ppm, sandstone at 10,700 ppm, limestone at 2,700 ppm, fresh water at 2.3 ppm, sea water at 380 ppm, soil at 14,000 ppm (a major exchangeable cation in all, but most in alkaline soils), marine plants at 52,000 ppm, land plants at 14,000 ppm, marine animals at 5,000 to 30,000 ppm, and land animals at 7,400 ppm (highest levels in soft tissue).

Potassium is essential to all organisms and is the major cation in cell cytoplasm with a wide variety of electrochemical and catalytic functions for enzyme systems. Potassium constitutes five percent of the total mineral content of the body. It is the major cation of the intracellular fluid and there is a small amount in the extracellular fluid. With sodium, the other "electrolyte," K participates in the maintenance of normal water balance, osmotic equilibrium, and acid-base balance. Potassium participates with Ca in the regulation of neuromuscular activity.

Potassium is easily absorbed. Ninety percent of ingested K is excreted through the urine. There is essentially no storage of K in the human body, thus requiring a significant daily intake of 5,000 mg.

Muscular weakness and mental apathy are features of K deficiency. Hypokalemic cardiac failure is the most serious K deficiency event. Diuretics, both natural and prescribed, sweating, colds and flu, vomiting, and diarrhea increase the rate of loss of all minerals, including K, compared with the normal expected excretion rate.

Kr—Krypton is found in igneous rocks at 0.0001 ppm and sea water at 0.0025 ppm. Krypton is legendary as the home planet of "Superman" and the source of the mineral "kryptonite" which had a crippling effect on "Superman." In fact krypton is totally harmless to humans and may in fact be an essential element.

La—Lanthanum is a "light" rare earth and is found in igneous rocks at 30 ppm, shale at 20 ppm, sandstone at 7.5 ppm, limestone at 6.2 ppm, sea water at 0.000012 ppm, soil at 30 ppm, marine plants at 10 ppm, land plants at 0.085 ppm, marine mammals at 0.1 ppm, and in land animals at 0.0001 ppm in soft tissue and 0.27 ppm in bone. Notably the yeast Candida albicans accumulates up to 370 ppm/day. This may be how Candida causes a debilitating energy sapping "chronic fatigue" disease by "stealing" lanthanum from the patient.

The growth of the protozoa Blepherisma and Tetrahymena pyriformis is stimulated and their life span doubled by the presence of the rare earth lanthanum at concentrations of 0.32 ppm.

Li—Lithium is found in igneous rocks 20 ppm, shale at 66 ppm, sandstone at 15 ppm, limestone at 5 ppm, fresh water at 0.0011 ppm, sea water at 0.18 ppm, soil at 30 ppm (Li + is freely mobile in the soil), marine plants at 5 ppm, land plants at 0.1 ppm, marine animals at 1 ppm, and in land animals at 0.02 ppm. Since 1915, the risk of clinical depression nearly doubles with each succeeding generation. Myrna M. Weissman, a psychiatrist at Columbia University, New York City, says that, "Depression is a world wide phenomenon happening at younger and younger ages." In 1935, the age of early onset of depression was during the early 20s. By 1955 onset of depression dropped to between 15 and 20 years of age. One in four women and one in ten men will develop depression. Prozac, America's "leading" antidepressant pharmaceutical, was introduced in 1987. Sales soared to $350 million in 1989, more than was spent on all antidepressants just two years earlier. Prozac sales topped $1 billion in 1995 as a result of 650,000 prescriptions per month!

While the professional psychiatrist says that depression and manic depression are due to feelings that we are out of control of our lives, negative thinking, and self recrimination ("I'm a loser"), they treat depression successfully with the trace mineral lithium. Depression and manic depression with all that implies are simply a lithium deficiency aggravated by high sugar consumption.

Animal studies show that a deficiency of lithium results in reproductive failure, infertility, reduced growth rate, shortened life expectancy, and behavioral problems. In humans, manic depression, depression, "bi-polar" disease, rages, road rage, Dr. Jekyll/Mr. Hyde behavior, hyperactivity, ADD, ADHD, and "bad seeds" are hallmarks of Li deficiency aggravated by a high sugar intake.

Chelated Li supplemented at 1,000 to 2,000 µg/d {micrograms per day?} causes a dose dependent increase in hair Li levels. Hair Li levels increased after four weeks of supplementation and leveled off and became stationary after three months. When the Li supplementation was stopped, hair Li levels dropped to presupplement values in two months. This scenario does not extend to metallic lithium carbonate. A comparison of 2,648 subjects showed that 65 percent had hair Li values ranging between 0.04 to 0.14 µg/G, 16 percent contained more than 0.14 µg/G and 18.4 percent had less than 0.04 µg/G. The highest levels of Li were found in university students from Tijuana, Mexico. The lowest were found in Munich, Germany.

Normal controls showed almost 400 times more hair Li than do the violent criminals from California, Florida, Texas, and Oregon. The estimated daily intake of Li by the EPA ranges from 650 to 3,100 µg/d, however, much of the ingested Li is metallic and not biologically available.

Lu—Lutecium, a rare earth, is found in igneous rocks at 0.5 ppm, shale at 0.33 ppm, sandstone at 0.096 ppm, limestone at 0.067 ppm, land plants at up to 4.5 ppm by Carya spp., marine animals at 0.003 ppm, land animals at 0.003 ppm, and land animals at 0.00012 ppm in soft tissue and 0.08 ppm in bone.

Mg—Magnesium is found in igneous rocks at 23,300 ppm, in shale at 15,000 ppm, sandstone at 10,700 ppm, limestone at 2,700 ppm, fresh water at 4,1 ppm, seawater at 1,350 ppm, and in soil at 5,000 ppm (highest in soil derived from basalt, serpentine, or dolomite). Mg is the second most common exchangeable cation in most soils. Mg is found in marine plants at 5,200 ppm, land plants at 3,200 ppm, marine animals at at 5,000 ppm, and in land animals at 1,000 ppm where it accumulates in mammalian bone.

Magnesium is essential to all living organisms and has electro-chemical, catalytic, and structural functions. It activates numerous enzymes and is a constituent of all chlorophylls.

The adult human contains 20 to 28 grams of total body Mg. Approxi-mately 60 percent is found in bone. Twenty-six percent is associated with skeletal muscle and the balance is distributed between various organs and body fluids. Serum levels of Mg range from 1.5 to 2.1 mEq/L (a measure of electrolytes) and it is second to K as an intracellular cation. Half of the Mg, including most that is bound in the bone, is not exchangeable.

Magnesium is required for the production and transfer of energy for protein synthesis, for contractility of muscle and excitability of nerves, and as a cofactor in myriad enzyme systems. AN EXCESS OF MAGNESIUM WILL INHIBIT BONE CALCIFICATION. Calcium and Mg have antagonistic roles in normal muscle contraction, calcium acting as the stimulator and Mg as the relaxer. An excessive amount of Ca can induce signs of Mg deficiency.

Perhaps the most important manifestation of Mg deficiency in modern times is "malignant calcification." Malignant calcification appears as calcium deposits in soft tissue, especially the media or middle layer of arterial walls. Magnesium deficiency appears to be the basic root cause of arteriosclerotic calcium deposits, not elevated blood cholesterol!

Magnesium Deficiency Diseases

Asthma
Anorexia
Menstrual migraines
Growth failure
ECG changes
Neuromuscular problems
Tetany (convulsions)
Depression
Muscular weakness
Muscle "ties"
Tremors
Vertigo
Calcification of arterial media
"Malignant calcification" of soft tissue

The rate of absorption of Mg ranges from 24 to 85 percent. The lesser absorption rate is for metallic sources of Mg, the higher rates of absorption are associated with plant derived colloidal mineral sources. Vitamin D has no effect on Mg absorption. The presence of fat, phytates, and calcium reduces the efficiency of absorption. High performance athletes lose a considerable amount of Mg in sweat.

The RDA for Mg is 350 mg/day for adult males, 300 mg/day for adult females, and 450 mg/day for pregnant and lactating females. If the kidneys are healthy there is no evidence of toxicity at up to 6,000 mg/day.

Mn—Manganese is found in igneous rocks at 950 ppm, shale at 850 ppm, sandstone at 50 ppm, limestone at 1,100 ppm, fresh water at 0.012 ppm, sea water at 0.002 ppm, soil at 850 ppm (can be a major exchangeable cation in very acid soil), marine animals at 1.0 to 60 ppm (lowest in fish), and in land animals at 0.2 ppm with the highest concentration in mammalian liver and kidney. Total body content of Mn in humans is only 10 to 20 mg. Manganese is essential to all known living organisms. It activates numerous enzyme systems including those involved with glucose metabolism, energy production, and superoxide dismutase. It is a major constituent of several metalloenzymes, hormones, and proteins of humans. Manganese is part of the developmental process and the structure of the three fragile ear bones and joint cartilage. Excessive levels of Mn found in certain community water supplies and in some industrial processes can produce a Parkinsonian syndrome or a psychiatric disorder (locura manganica) resembling schizophrenia.

Deficiency diseases of Mn are very striking, ranging from severe birth defects (congenital ataxia, deafness, chondrodystrophy), asthma, convulsions, retarded growth, skeletal defects, disruption of fat and carbohydrate metabolism to joint problems in children and adults (i.e. TMJ, Repetitive Motion Syndrome, Carpal Tunnel Syndrome).

Deficiency Diseases of Manganese

Congenital ataxia
Deafness (malformation of otolithes)
Asthma
Chondromalacia
Chondrodystrophy
"Slipped Tendon"
Defects of chondroitin sulfate metabolism (poor cartilage
   formation)
TMJ
Repetitive motion syndrome
Carpal tunnel syndrome
Convulsions
Infertility (failure to ovulate, testicular atrophy)
Still births/spontaneous abortions (miscarriages)
Loss of libido in males and females
Retarded growth rate
Shortened long bones

Repetitive stress injury or repetitive motion syndrome now costs corporate America twenty billion dollars per year and accounts for 56 percent of the 331,600 gradual onset work related illnesses. In 1991, orthopedic surgeons performed 100,000 carpal tunnel operations (at $4,000 per surgery) with lost work, wages, and medical cost of over $29,000 per case.

At risk for the repetitive motion syndrome are those working in the world of computers: journalism, airline reservations, directory assistance, law, data entry, graphic design, and securities brokerage. Chief among the blue collar victims are the auto assembly workers, chicken pluckers, meat cutters, postal employees, dock workers, etc. Repetitive motion syndrome was observed three centuries ago in monks who were scribes and was described in 1717 by Bernardo Ramazzini, an Italian physician (considered the father of occupational medicine).

Repetitive motion syndrome victims have reached such numbers that federal legislation has been passed in the form of OSHA and Americans with Disabilities Act (ADA) to ensure work place safety. Large numbers of ergonomically correct keyboards and devices have been developed. We see literally millions of people at work with Velcro wrist, neck, elbow, finger, knee, back, and hip supports—all for manganese deficiencies!!!

Mo—Molybdenum is found in igneous rocks at 1.5 ppm, shale at 2.6 ppm, sandstone at 0.02 ppm, limestone at 0.4 ppm, fresh water at 0.00035 ppm, sea water at 0.01 ppm, soil at 2 ppm (strongly concentrated by humus, especially in alkaline soils; a few soils worldwide are rich enough in molybdenum to cause Mo poisoning in animals consuming the plants). Numerous soils are known for Mo deficiency. Mo is found in marine plants at 0.45 ppm, land plants at 0.9 ppm, marine animals at 0.6 to 2.5 ppm, and in land animals at 0.2 ppm with the highest levels in the liver and kidney.

Molybdenum is essential to all organisms as a constituent of numerous metalloenzymes. Molybdenum is known to be an integral part of no less than three essential enzymes: Xanthine oxidase, Aldehyde oxidase, and Sulfite oxidase.

The average American daily intake in food ranges from 76 to 1109 mcg per day. The RDA for Mo is 250 mcg per day. Toxicity occurs at 10 mg per day as a gout-like disease and interference with copper metabolism.

N—Nitrogen is found in igneous rocks at 20 ppm, fresh water at 0.23 ppm, sea water at 0.5 ppm, soils at 1,000 ppm (99 percent present as non-basic N bound in humus), marine plants at 15,000 ppm, land plants at 30,000 ppm, marine animals at 75,000 ppm, and in land animals at 100,000 ppm.

Nitrogen functions as a structural atom in protein, nucleic acids (RNA, DNA), and a wide variety of organic molecules. Dietary N (as protein) furnishes the amino acids for synthesis of tissue protein and other special metabolic functions:

1. Proteins are used to repair worn out body tissue.
2. Proteins are used to build new tissue (muscle, infant growth, childhood development, teenagers, pregnancy, maintenance, and repair).
3. Proteins can be an emergency source of heat and energy (albeit more expensive in biological terms than fat or carbohydrate).
4. Proteins make up essential body secretions and fluids (i.e. enzymes, hormones, mucus, milk, semen, etc.).
5. Blood plasma proteins maintain osmotic fluid balance. Hypoproteinemia results in edema.
6. Proteins maintain acid-base balance of blood and tissue.
7. Proteins aid in transport of other essential substances (i.e. minerals, fats, vitamins, etc.).
8. Proteins make up basic immunoglobulins (antibodies).
9. Proteins provide a nitrogen pool for the synthesis of amino acids and new proteins.

Classic protein deficiency results in infertility, poor growth, lowered immune status, edema, and Kwashiorkor (potbellied, thin children of Third World countries). The availability and usability of N from various foods are quite different and must be considered when choosing N sources.

Nitrogen/Protein Utilization Values of Common Foods

Nitrogen Source (Protein)	Chemical Score	% Utilization
Whole egg	100	94
Human milk	100	87
Cow's milk	95	82
Soy bean	74	65
Sesame	50	54
Peanut	65	47
Cotton seed	81	59

Nitrogen/Protein Utilization Values of Common Foods *(cont.)*

Nitrogen Source (Protein)	Chemical Score	% Utilization
Maize (corn)	49	52
Millet	63	44
Rice	67	59
Wheat	53	48

Mixing protein sources such as beans and rice, wheat and legumes, or vegetable and animal tends to improve the utilization of the vegetable protein source and make up for missing amino acids.

Na—Sodium is found in igneous rocks at 23,600 ppm, shale at 9,600 ppm, sandstone at 3,300 ppm, limestone at 400 ppm, fresh water at 6.3 ppm, sea water at 10,500 ppm, soil at 6,300 ppm (is a major exchangeable cation in soils, especially alkaline soil), marine plants at 33,000 ppm, land plants at 1,200 ppm, marine animals at 4,000 ppm, and in land animals at 4,000 ppm. "Salt hunger" dates back to the very beginning of animals and man and is one of the very basic cravings of living organisms. Carnivores (man or beast) do not show the great craving for salt because meat contains relatively large amounts of NaCl. Herbivores and human vegetarians demand large amounts of NaCl in grains, vegetables, nuts, and fruits. The average sodium dietary intake per day in western cultures is five to twelve grams per day while the Japanese, who outlive Americans by an average of four years, consume an average of 28 grams per day!

Sodium, chlorine, and potassium are three indispensable "electrolytes" so intimately associated in the body that they can be presented together. Sodium makes up two percent, potassium five percent, and chlorine three percent of the total mineral content of the human body. All three are widely distributed throughout the body tissues and fluids, however, Na and Cl are primarily extracellular (outside the cell), while K is an intracellular (inside the cell) mineral. Sodium, potassium, and chlorine are involved in at least four important physiological functions in the body:

1. Maintenance of normal water balance and distribution.
2. Maintenance of normal osmotic equilibrium.
3. Maintenance of normal acid-base balance.
4. Maintenance of normal muscular irritability.

Hormonal control of Na, K, and Cl balance is regulated by the adrenal cortex hormones as well as by the anterior pituitary gland. Addison's

Disease, a loss of function of the adrenal cortex, results in the loss of Na and K retention with clinical signs of general weakness, muscle cramps, weight loss, and a marked "salt hunger." The symptoms can be relieved with the supplementation of NaCl or by administering adrenal cortical hormones.

Deficiencies of NaCl occur primarily in hot weather (e.g. the American heat wave of 1993), heavy work in a hot climate, or exercise when large volumes of sweat are produced for body cooling. "Water intoxication" occurred in infants fed low sodium formulas because of doctors' insane paranoia with Na has been known to result in brain swelling causing death from a simple Na deficiency. The treatment for Na deficiency is water and salt, either orally or IV (saline 0.9 per cent).

Nb—Niobium is found in igneous rocks at 20 ppm, shale at 11 ppm, sandstone at 0.05 ppm, limestone 0.3 ppm, sea water at 0.00001 ppm, land plants at 0.3 ppm, and marine animals at 0.001 ppm.

Nd—Neodymium, a rare earth, is found in igneous rock at 28 ppm, shale at 16 ppm, sandstone at 11 ppm, limestone at 4.3 ppm, marine plants at 5 ppm, land plants accumulates up to 460 ppm in Carya spp., marine animals at 0.5 ppm, and accumulates in the liver and bone of land animals. Neodymium is a "light rare earth" proven to enhance normal cell growth and double the life span of laboratory species.

Ne—Neon is found in igneous rocks at 0.005 ppm and sea water at 0.00014 ppm.

Ni—Nickel is found in igneous rocks at 75 ppm, shale at 68 ppm, sandstone at 2.0 ppm, limestone at 20 ppm, fresh water at 0.01 ppm, sea water at 0.0054 ppm, soils at 40 ppm (higher in soils derived from serpentine), marine plants at 3 ppm, land plants at 3 ppm (accumulated by Alyssum bertalonii), marine animals at 0.4 to 25 ppm, and land animals at 0.8 ppm (is found in RNA).

Symptoms of Nickel Deficiency

⟨ Poor growth
⟨ Anemia
⟨ Depressed oxidative ability of the liver
⟨ Increased newborn mortality
⟨ Rough/dry hair
⟨ Dermatitis
⟨ Delayed puberty
⟨ Poor zinc absorption

Less than 10 percent of ingested metallic nickel is absorbed. Nickel deficiency was first reported in 1970. Nickel functions as a cofactor for metalloenzymes and facilitates gastrointestinal absorption of iron and zinc. Optimal tissue levels of vitamin B12 are necessary for the optimal biological function of nickel. Vitamin B12 deficiency results in an increased need for nickel by animals and man.

Np—Neptunium. All isotopes of neptunium are radioactive. The half-life of Np is 2.2 x 10(6). Neptunium accumulates in mammalian bone after ingestion. Neptunium has been found in fresh water organisms in the Hanford River (USA).

O—Oxygen is found in igneous rocks at 464,000 ppm, shale at 483,000 ppm, sandstone at 492,000 ppm, limestone at 497,000 ppm, fresh water at 889,000 ppm, sea water at 857,000 ppm, soils at 490,000 ppm, marine plants at 470,000 ppm, land plants at 410,000 ppm (except anaerobic organisms), marine animals at 400,000 ppm, and land animals at 186,000 ppm. Terrestrial O consists of 99.76 percent (16) O with a half-life of less than two minutes.

Oxygen is a structural atom of water (in and out of living systems) and all organic compounds of biological interest, O_2 is required for respiration by all aerobic organisms. We can live for 30 days without food, three to seven days without water under ideal circumstances, but only four minutes without gaseous oxygen. This critical requirement for oxygen makes it the most important of all elements from the standpoint of immediate survival and maintenance. According to the 1980s U.S. Geological Survey, our earth's atmosphere had 50 percent oxygen at the time when dinosaurs flourished. These oxygen levels were arrived at by inserting microneedles into trapped air bubbles in polar ice and determining the oxygen levels in the prehistoric ice. Some paleontologists claim that the simultaneous and universal demise of the dinosaurs followed the widespread quieting of the earth's volcanoes, which reduced the atmospheric levels of CO_2, which in turn reduced the oxygen levels to 38 percent. It is theorized that the 12 percent drop in the earth's oxygen levels was sufficient to cause the apocalyptic end of the dinosaurs.

The Geographical Survey also reported that the earth's atmosphere still contained 38 percent oxygen as late as one hundred years ago. During the 1950s the percentage of oxygen in our atmosphere dropped to 21 percent and today only 19 percent of our gaseous atmosphere is oxygen. The continued drop in oxygen levels reflects an increase in oxygen consuming species and fossil fuel combustion (i.e. vehicles, electric, and power generating plants). Combined with increased consumption is lower oxygen production (i.e. decreasing acreage of rain forests and aquatic algae). The net result of this continued drop in oxygen levels is a relative "anaerobic state" compared with the 38 percent of just 100 years ago and a very dramatic "anaerobic state" compared with the 50 percent oxygen levels 75 million years ago.

Most pathogenic organisms (diseases producing germs) are by themselves anaerobic. They are "happier," and flourish and reproduce with more vigor in the absence of oxygen. You know them as gangrene organisms, type A Streptococcus, etc. They are able to survive and grow in living cells weakened by low oxygen environments, which are also conducive for the growth of viruses, yeast, fungus, cancer, etc. The question is why have anaerobic diseases "suddenly" appeared in the 80s and 90s, diseases that we have little or no human history or experience? Regardless of the name, tuberculosis, consumption, or scrofula can be found in five thousand-year-old mummies from Egypt and China, one thousand-year-old corpses from Peru, and in ancient writings from the Greeks and Romans. The "new" modern day anaerobic diseases have no history with humans, nor will you find anything in biblical or ancient writings describing HIV, EBV, CMV, Herpes II, Hanta virus, Candida albicans yeast, Toxic Shock Syndrome, E. coli, or "flesh eating" type A Streptococcus.

The most plausible theory is that the anaerobic disease causing organisms laid around in a dormant state as long as the atmospheric oxygen remained high (i.e. 50, 38, or even 21 percent) and inhibited their activity and growth. With the precipitous dip in atmospheric oxygen we are having an "oxygen counter revolution" with a return to an anaerobic bios.

Anaerobic Diseases of Humans

Disease	*Year of Appearance*
VIRAL	
Mycoplasma (rheumatoid arthritis and "Desert Storm Syndrome")	1958
Herpes II (sexually transmitted herpes)	1978
HIV (AIDS virus)	1982
EBV, CMV (Chronic Fatigue Syndrome)	1982
Hanta Virus (Four Corners Disease)	1993

Ebola Virus	1996

BACTERIA

Staphylococcus (Toxic Shock Syndrome)	1982
E. coli (Toxic Shock Syndrome)	1993
Type A Streptococcus ("Flesh-eating" Strep)	1994

YEAST/FUNGUS

Candida albicans ("Candida")	1982
Coccidioidomycosis ("Valley Fever")	1900—35/yr, 1992—1,450/yr
Cancer (all types)	1900—1/10, 1994—2/3

Dr. Otto Warburg of the Max Plank Institute, Germany, was the recipient of two unshared Nobel Prizes. Linus Pauling was the only other individual to be awarded two unshared Nobel Prizes. One of Warburg's Nobel's came for discovering the amino acid and describing the basic composition of proteins and the second for discovering that the metabolism of the cancer cell is fermentative and anaerobic while the normal noncancerous cell is aerobic. During the 1950s, Warburg was able to demonstrate clearly that cancer cells ferment sugar under anaerobic conditions and die in the presence of oxygen.

Neutrophils, a type of white blood cell that help defend us by identifying, engulfing, and destroying invading micro-organisms (i.e. virus, yeast, fungus, etc.), parasites, and cancer cells, use hydrogen peroxide as their "lethal weapon." Neutrophils are packed with small organelles (microscopic organs) called peroxisomes, whose sole function is to produce hydrogen peroxide and inject it onto the captured pathogen or cancer cell for the specific purpose of destroying it. Neutrophils tend to be very sloppy, dribbling their over-production of hydrogen peroxide freely into the blood stream. The potential danger of hydrogen peroxide free in the blood stream could be a loose cannon, but fortunately we humans are blessed with a protective ubiquitous enzyme called catalase. Catalase literally covers our red blood cells and coats the inside walls of our blood vessels. The function of catalase is to rapidly facilitate the decomposition of hydrogen peroxide down to water (H_2O) and singlet oxygen atom (O).

There are concerns by the uninitiated regarding the "free radical" status of singlet oxygen which has a free electron. When singlet or atomic oxygen comes into direct contact with tissue cells outside of the circulatory system (i.e. cell culture, test tube, wounds, etc.) the cells will die. In the whole animal or human other factors come into play to prevent "free radical" damage. When ingested in proper dilution on an empty stomach or administered intravenously under proper conditions, food grade hydrogen peroxide is readily absorbed through the stomach and duodenal walls directly into the blood stream where it is immediately broken down into water and singlet oxygen. The free electron of the singlet oxygen either combines with a free electron of a carcinogenic free electron or with the free electron of another singlet oxygen, becoming O2.

Carcinogenic free electrons frequently remain free electrons under many circumstances. They are actually quite happy with their free electron status. On the other hand, the free electron of the singlet oxygen does not like to be a singlet electron and if it doesn't locate another free electron to attach to, it will grab onto another singlet oxygen in nanoseconds becoming atmospheric O2—the required stuff of respiration.

Ozone O3 —> H2O2+ O-

catalase —> H_2O + O2

Oxygen in the form of hydrogen peroxide has been used topically, intravenously, and orally since the Civil War. It has been used widely in Europe for over 50 years for alternative cancer therapies, circulatory disease, arteriosclerosis, emphysema, asthma, gangrene, and more recently as a therapy for stroke patients.

Stroke patients have inactive but living cells surrounding the stroke site known as "sleeping beauty" cells that can be reactivated or jump started when they are exposed to several atmospheres of oxygen in hyperbaric chambers. Athletic injuries can also be treated by putting the injured athlete into a hyperbaric oxygen chamber. The healing time is shortened significantly so the athlete can return to play in weeks instead of months.

Os—Osmium is found in igneous rocks at 0.0015 ppm. It oxidizes organic matter as OsO4 and is reduced to Os.

P—Phosphorus is found in igneous rocks at 1,050 ppm, shale at 700 ppm, sandstone at 170 ppm, limestone at 400 ppm, fresh water at 0.005 ppm, sea water at 0.07 ppm, and in soil at 650 ppm where it has been "fixed" by hydrous oxides of Al and Fe in acid soil. P is found in marine plants at 3,500 ppm, land plants at 2,300 ppm, marine animals at 4,000 to 18,000 ppm, and land animals at 17,000 to 44,000 ppm.

Phosphorus is an extremely important essential mineral, however, it gets little or no attention from nutritionists because it is widely available in all foods. Phosphorus is a major structural mineral for bones and teeth. It has more functions in the human than any other mineral including its role as a vital constituent of nucleic acids, activating enzymes, and for several steps of the ATP energy cycle, RBC metabolism. A complete discussion of P would require a discussion of every metabolic function in the body. Second in abundance only to calcium in the human body, it comprises 22 percent of the body's total mineral content. The human body contains about 800 grams of P, just short of two pounds, of which 700 grams is found in bones and teeth as insoluble calcium phosphate.

The balance of P in the human body is found as biologically active intra and extracellular colloidal P in combination with carbohydrates, lipids, protein, and a wide variety of other biologically active organic compounds including the blood's major buffer system. B-complex vitamins function as coenzymes to intracellular metabolic functions only when combined with phosphorus.

Phosphorus is part of most proteins and as such becomes problematic because elevated P intake increases Ca requirements when "high protein diets" are consumed. Under those circumstances P can aggravate osteo-porosis, arthritis, high blood pressure, loosen teeth, etc. Phosphorus is present as phytates in cereals and whole grain flours, therefore, if bread is made from unleavened flours, the phytic acid will complex with Ca, Fe, Zn, and other minerals further lowering their absorption rate.

The average adult human dietary intake of P is 1,000 to 1,500 mg/day. In adults and older children, the absorption of metallic P is limited to about three to five per cent and as high as eight to 12 percent in infants. Mixed dietary sources of chelated P may be absorbed at the rate of 40 to 50 percent. Optimal absorption of metallic and chelated P occurs when the dietary Ca:P ratio is 1:1. Organically bound colloidal P is absorbed up to 98 percent.

Deficiencies of P have long been recognized in livestock. Symptoms of P deficiency include the behavior of pica and cribbing and fractures. Phosphorus deficiency has only recently been recognized in humans. The widespread, universal, and ultimately fatal results of P deficiency are the result of its widespread biological functions, significantly as the result of a decrease in ATP synthesis (complete metabolic energy failure) with associated neuromuscular, skeletal, blood, and kidney disease.

Clinical P depletion and resultant low blood P (hypophosphatemia) without P supplementation, excessive use of antacids, hyperparathyroidism (low calcium/high phosphate diets are the cause of this one), improper treatment of diabetic acidosis, use of diuretics, sweating during exercise, and work and alcoholism with and without liver disease. Vegetarians and vegans who do supplement with minerals rarely have P deficiency, however, because of their high phytic acid intake. They tend to always have other mineral deficiencies including Ca, Cu, Cr, V, Li, and Zn.

Pa—Protoactinium is found in igneous rocks at 1.4×10^{-6} ppm and sea water at 2.4×10^{-31} ppm. All isotopes of Pa are radioactive with a half-life of 32,000 years. Protoactinium accumulates in mammalian bone after ingestion.

Pb—Lead is found in igneous rocks at 12.5 ppm, shale at 20 ppm, sandstone at 7 ppm, limestone at 9 ppm, soil at 10 ppm (higher in limestone soils and humus), fresh water at 0.005 ppm, sea water at 0.00008 ppm, marine plants at 8.4 ppm, land plants at 2.7 ppm (many plant species are adapted to grow in Pb-rich soils and accumulate Pb including Amorpha canescens), marine animals at 0.5 ppm (highest in fish bones), and in land animals at 2.0 ppm. The highest Pb levels are found in bone, liver, and kidney. Lead is found as a required part of the RNA/DNA duplicating system.

Mineral deficient animals and children with the symptoms of pica and cribbing, craving for non-food items (i.e. paint, sand, dirt, etc.), are very susceptible to lead poisoning ("plumbism"). Infants and children with pica will chew on their toys, cribs, windowsills, caulking, furniture, and paint. A chip of lead paint the size of a penny can contain as much as 50 to 100 µg of lead. Consuming this much lead daily over a three month period will result in lead poisoning.

The "normal" background blood lead level is below 40 µg/dl. Children with blood lead above 60 to 80 µg/dl have symptoms of vomiting, irritability, weight loss, muscular weakness, headaches, abdominal pain, insomnia, and anorexia. Children with blood levels of lead above 80 µg/dl show anemia, kidney disease, peripheral neuritis, ataxia, and muscular uncoordination, joint pain, and encephalopathy (brain damage, learning disabilities, etc.) with eventual death.

The best approach to treating lead poisoning is to supplement with all 90 essential nutrients to eliminate pica and cribbing and further ingestion of lead, restoring fluid, and electrolyte balance. In addition, the use of IV or IM chelation therapy using EDTA (ethylenediaminetetra-acetic acid) and BAL (British Anti-Lewisite) for a minimum of five days. It is not unusual for as many as 25 percent of Pb poisoned individuals to have residual loss of IQ, loss of coordination, hyperactivity, learning disabilities, and impulsiveness.

Pd—Palladium is found in igneous rocks at 0.01 ppm and land animals at 0.002 ppm. Palladium accumulates in mammalian liver and kidney.

Pm—Promethium isotopes are all radioactive with a half-life of 2.6 years. Promethium is an important fission product that has now entered the biosphere. Prior to man-made nuclear explosions, Pm did not exist in nature. Pm accumulates in mammalian bone and liver after ingestion.

Po—Polonium is found in igneous rocks at $2 \times 10^{(-10)}$ ppm.

Pr—Praseodymium is a "light" rare earth found in igneous rock at 8.2 ppm, shale at 6 ppm, sandstone at 2.8 ppm, limestone at 1.4 ppm, marine plants at 5 ppm, land plants accumulates up to 46 ppm (Carya spp.), marine animals at 0.5 ppm, and in land animals at 1.5 ppm (accumulates in liver and bone).

Pt—Platinum is found in igneous rocks at 0.005 ppm and land animals at 0.002 ppm.

Pu—Plutonium. All plutonium isotopes are radioactive with a half-life of 24,000 years. Plutonium was released into the earth's atmosphere by nuclear explosions. Marine plants show 4,000 times the background level of seawater, land plants record 0.4 to 2.2 disintegrations/sec/kg, land animals show 0.07 to 6.8 disintegrations/sec/kg. Pu accumulates in mammalian bone after contact or ingestion.

Ra—Radium is found in igneous rocks at $9 \times 10^{(-7)}$ ppm, shale at $11 \times 10^{(-7)}$ ppm, sandstone at $7 \times 10^{(-7)}$ ppm, limestone at $4 \times 10^{(-7)}$ ppm, fresh water at $3.9 \times 10^{(-110)}$ ppm, sea water at $6 \times 10^{(-11)}$ ppm, soils at $8 \times 10^{(-7)}$ ppm, marine plants at $9 \times 10^{(-4)}$ ppm, land plants at $10^{(-9)}$ ppm, marine animals at $0.7^{(-15)} \times 10^{(-9)}$ ppm, and in land animals at $7 \times 10^{(-9)}$ ppm. The highest concentrations are found in mammalian bone; all isotopes of Ra are radioactive.

Rb—Rubidium is found in igneous rocks at 90 ppm, shale at 140 ppm, sandstone at 60 ppm, limestone at 3 ppm, fresh water at 0.0015ppm, sea water at 0.12 ppm, soil at 100 ppm ("fixed" by clay soils), marine plants at 7.4 ppm, land plants at 20 ppm, marine animals at 20 ppm, and in land animals at 17 ppm. The highest levels are found in liver and muscle; the lowest levels are found in bone.

Rubidium can replace the electrolyte function of potassium in many species, including bacteria, algae, fungi, and certain invertebrates (echinoderms—starfish).

Re—Rhenium is found in igneous rocks at 0.005 ppm, marine plants at 0.014 ppm, and marine animals at 0.0005 to 0.006 ppm. Land animals accumulate Re in the thyroid.

Rh—Rhodium is found in igneous rocks at 0.001 ppm.

Rn—Radon is found in igneous rocks at 4 x 10(-13) ppm, fresh water at 1.7 x 10 (-15) ppm, and sea water at 6 x 10 (-16) ppm. All isotopes of Rn are radioactive with a half-life of 54 seconds to 3.8 days. Radon is carcinogenic and highly toxic when inhaled. Radon is a common household hazard. It is odorless and colorless. Detection requires the use of kits which are generally available.

Ru—Ruthenium is found in igneous rocks at 0.001 ppm, land plants at 0.005 ppm, and in land animals at 0.002 ppm. RuO4 is highly toxic.

S—Sulfur is found in igneous rocks at 260 ppm, shale at 2,400 ppm, sandstone at 240 ppm, limestone at 1,200 ppm, fresh water at 3.7 ppm, sea water at 885 ppm, soils at 700 ppm, marine animals at 5,000 to 19,000 ppm (highest in coelenterates and mollusks), and in land animals at 5,000 ppm with the highest levels in cartilage, tendons, keratin, skin, nails, and hair. Its lowest concentrations are in the bones. In soils, up to 90 per cent of soil S is bound tightly in humus, SO4 is a major exchange anion in many soils and occurs in soils near volcanoes. In land plants S occurs at a rate of 3,400 ppm with the lowest concentrations in bryophytes and gymnosperms.

Sulfur is an important structural atom in most proteins as sulfur amino acids (cystine, cysteine, and methionine) and small organic molecules. Glutathione, a tripeptide containing cysteine, is essential to cellular reactions involving sulfur amino acids in protein. Sulfur is found in a reduced form (-SH) in cysteine and in an oxidized form (-S-S-) as the double molecule cystine. This "sulfhydrl group" is important for the specific configuration of some structural proteins and for the biological activities of some enzymes (proteins that do work).

Sulfur-containing proteins work in indirect ways to maintain life:
- ⟨ Hemoglobin
- ⟨ Hormones (insulin, adrenal cortical hormones)
- ⟨ Enzymes
- ⟨ Antibodies

Sulfur also occurs in carbohydrates such as heparin, an anticoagulant that is concentrated in the liver and other tissues, and chondroitin sulfate (cartilage, gelatin). The vitamins thiamine (B1) and biotin have S bound in their molecule. The toxic properties of arsenic are the result of its ability to combine with sulfhydryl groups. A deficiency of sulfur results in degenerative types of arthritis involving degeneration of cartilage, osteoarthritis, degenerative arthritis, weakened ligaments, weakened tendons, Systemic Lupus Erythematosis, sickle cell anemia, and various "collagen diseases."

Sb—Antimony is found in igneous rocks at 0.2 ppm, shale at 1.5 ppm, sandstone at 0.05ppm, limestone at 0.2 ppm, sea water at 0.00033 ppm, soil at 2 to 10 ppm, land plants at 0.06 ppm, and in land animals at 0.006 ppm where it concentrates in mammalian heart muscle. Antimony potassium tartrate (tartar emetic) is still used today as the preferred treatment for blood flukes (schistosomiasis or bilharziasis).

Sc—Scandium is found in igneous rock at 22 ppm, shale at 13 ppm, sandstone and limestone at 1 ppm, sea water at 0.000004 ppm, soils at 7 ppm, land plants at 0.008 ppm, and in land animals at 0.00006 ppm where it concentrates in mammalian heart and bone.

Se—Selenium is found in igneous rocks at 0.05 ppm, shale at 0.6 ppm, sandstone at 0.05 ppm, limestone at 0.08 ppm, fresh water at 0.02 ppm, sea water at 0.00009 ppm, soils at 0.2 ppm, marine plants at 0.8 ppm, land plants at 0.2 ppm, and in land animals at 1.7 ppm where the highest concentrations are found in liver, kidney, heart, and skeletal muscle. Keep in mind that Se is not universally distributed. Vast areas of earth are deficient or totally devoid of Se. Se is found in the humus of alkaline soils when present. Selenium is the most efficient antioxidant (anti-peroxident). It's used at the subcellular level in the glutathione peroxidase enzyme system and metalloamino acids (selenomethionine, etc.). Selenium prevents cellular and subcellular lipids and fats from being peroxidized which literally means it prevents body fats from going rancid. "Rancid" body fats are seen externally as "age spots" or "liver spots." The golden brown "pigment of aging" is technically known as ceroid lipofucsin and results from peroxidation that selenium could reverse.

Selenium also functions to protect cellular and organelle bi-lipid layer membranes from oxidative damage. High intakes of vegetable oils, including salad dressing and cooking oils, concurrent with a selenium deficiency is the quickest route to a heart attack and cancer. The polyunsaturated configuration of the oils when heated or treated with hydrogen ("trans fatty acids") literally causes the rancidity ("free radical" damage) of cellular fat. The clinical diseases associated with selenium deficiency are diverse and to the uninformed shrouded in mystery. Selenium deficiency is one of the more costly mineral deficiency complexes affecting embryos, the new born, toddlers, teens, young adults, and seniors alike.

Selenium Deficiency Diseases

Direct Results
Anemia
"Age spots" & "Liver spots"
Fatigue
Muscular weakness
Myalgia (muscle pain and soreness)
Fibromyalgia
Scoliosis
Muscular dystrophy (MD, White Muscle Disease, Stiff Lamb Disease)
Cardiomyopathy (Keshan Disease, "Mulberry heart" Disease)
Heart palpitations
Atrial fibrilation
Liver cirrhosis
Pancreatitis
Pancreatic atrophy
Infertility
Low birth weight
High infant mortality
SIDS (Sudden Infant Death Syndrome)
Cystic Fibrosis (congenital)

Indirect Results
HIV (increased rate of conversion to AIDS and transmission to fetus)
ALS (Lou Gehrig's Disease)
MS (Multiple sclerosis)
Alzheimer's Disease
Cancer (increases cancer risk significantly)

Selenium deficiency can result in infertility in both men and women. Congenital selenium deficiency during pregnancy can result in a wide variety of problems ranging from miscarriage, low birth weight, high infant mortality, cystic fibrosis, muscular dystrophy, cardiomyopathy, and liver cirrhosis. Selenium deficiency in growing children can result in crib death or SIDS (Sudden Infant Death Syndrome). Sixty-five percent of SIDS deaths occur in children on canned infant formulas. Slow growth, small size (failure to reach genetic potential for size and mass), muscular dystrophy, scoliosis, cardiomyopathy (muscular dystrophy of the heart muscle or Keshan Disease), anemia, liver cirrhosis, muscular weakness, lowered immune capacity, and neuromuscular diseases are also linked to Se deficiency.

In young adults, selenium deficiency appears as anemia, chronic fatigue, muscular weakness, myalgia, fibromyalgia, muscular tenderness, pancreatitis, infertility, muscular dystrophy, scoliosis, and cardiomyopathy. Cardiomyopathy is quite common in young athletes such as basketball and football players at the high school, college, university, and professional levels because of Se deficiency, as are multiple sclerosis and liver cirrhosis. Selenium deficiency in adults appears as reduced immune capacity, anemia, infertility, "age spots" or "liver spots", myalgia, fibromyalgia, muscle weakness, MS, ALS, Parkinson's Disease, Alzheimer's Disease, palpitations or irregular heart beat, cardiomyopathy, liver cirrhosis, and cancer.

In a review of the anti-cancer effects of selenium, Dr. Gerhard N. Schrauzer, head of the Department of Chemistry, UCSD, states:

> Selenium is increasingly recognized as a versatile anticarcinogenic agent. Its protective functions cannot be solely attributed to the action of glutathione peroxidase. Instead, selenium appears to operate by several mechanisms, depending on dosage and chemical form of selenium and the nature of the carcinogenic stress. In a major protective function, selenium is proposed to prevent the malignant transformation of cells by acting as a "redox switch" in the activation-inactivation of cellular growth factors and other functional proteins through the catalysis of oxidation-reduction reactions of critical -SH groups or -S-S- bonds.
>
> The growth-modulatory effects of selenium are dependent on the levels of intracellular glutathione peroxidase and the oxygen supply. In general, growth inhibition is achieved by the Se-mediated stimulation of cellular respiration (more oxygen, less cancer). Selenium appears to inhibit the replication of tumor viruses in animals and the activation of oncogenes by similar mechanisms. However, it may also alter carcinogen metabolism and protect DNA against carcinogen-induced damage. In additional functions of relevance to its anticarcinogenic activity, selenium acts as an acceptor of biogenic methyl groups, and is involved in detoxification of metals and certain xenobiotics. Selenium also has immunopotentiating properties. It is required for optimal macrophage and natural killer cell functions.

The school of pharmacy from the University of Georgia released a report in August of 1994 that concludes that a human selenium deficiency is related to the clinical onset of full blown AIDS in chronically infected HIV patients. According to their report, HIV requires large amounts of selenium for replication. In selenium deficient patients, the virus competes with the patient for the limited amounts of available selenium. The HIV patient actually dies of a chronic selenium deficiency encephalopathy, liver cirrhosis, or cardiomyopathy. Long-term HIV patients (20 years or more) that never developed full blown clinical AIDS had supplemented with large amounts of selenium.

Si—Silica is found in igneous rocks at 281,500 ppm, shale at 73,000 ppm, sandstone at 368,000 ppm, limestone at 24,000 ppm, fresh water at 6.5 ppm, sea water at 3 ppm, soils at 330,000 ppm (found as SiO_2, the most abundant form of Si in nature, in silicates and clays), marine plants at 1,500 to 20,000 ppm, marine animals at 70,000 ppm, and in land animals at 120 to 6,000 ppm where it is mainly concentrated in hair, lungs, and bone. Plants accumulating the most Si are diatoms, horsetail, ferns, Cyoeraceae, Graineae, and Juncaceae, and the flowers of Pappophorum silicosum. Silicon supplementation increases the collagen in growing bone by 100 percent. Tissue levels of Si decrease with aging in unsupplemented humans and laboratory species. Dry brittle finger and toenails, poor skin quality, poor calcium utilization, and arterial disease characterize silica deficiency. High fiber diets contain high levels of Si, which leads many investigators to believe that Si helps to lower cholesterol. The recommended intake of Si ranges from 200 to 500 mg/day.

Sm—Samarium is a "light" rare earth found in igneous rocks at 6 ppm, shale at 5.6 ppm, sandstone at 2.7 ppm, limestone at 0.8 ppm, land plants at 0.0055 ppm (accumulates up to 23 ppm), marine animals at 0.04 to 0.08 ppm, land animals at 0.01 ppm in heart muscle and 0.0009 ppm in mammalian bone and liver. Samarium enhances normal cell proliferation and doubles the life span of laboratory species.

Sn—Tin is found in igneous rocks at 2 ppm, shale at 6 ppm, sandstone and limestone at 0.5 ppm, fresh water at 0.00004 ppm, sea water at 0.003 ppm, soils at 2 to 200 ppm (strongly absorbed by by humus), marine plants at 1 ppm, land plants at 0.3 ppm (highest in bryophytes and lichens), marine animals at 0.2 to 20 ppm, and land animals at 0.15 ppm with the highest levels found in the lungs and intestines. Originally the presence of tin in tissue was attributed to environmental contamination; however, careful and detailed studies by

Schwarz demonstrated that tin produced acceleration in growth in rats and further met the standards for an essential trace element. As a member of the fourth main group of chemical elements, tin has many chemical and physical properties similar to those of carbon, silica, germanium, and lead.

Rats fed tin at 17.0 ng/gm show poor growth, reduced feeding efficiency, hearing loss, and bilateral (male pattern) hair loss, while rats fed 1.99 μg/gm were physiologically and anatomically normal. Schwarz demonstrated tin to be an essential element in 1970. Tin has been shown to exert a strong induction effect on the enzyme heme oxygenase, enhancing heme breakdown in the kidney. There is also evidence for tin having cancer prevention properties. A federal study released in November of 1991 showed that men in recent generations have poorer hearing at any given age than men in earlier generations. Men over age 30 lose their hearing more than twice as fast as women of the same age. So much for talk about having a "tin ear"!

Sr—Strontium is found in igneous rocks at 375 ppm, shale at 300 ppm, sandstone at 20 ppm, limestone at 610 ppm, fresh water at 0.08 ppm, sea water at 8.1 ppm, soils at 300 ppm, marine plants at 260 to 1,400 ppm, land plants at 26 ppm, marine animals at 20 to 500 ppm, and in land animals at 14 ppm where it's most highly concentrated in mammalian bone. Strontium can replace calcium in many organisms, including man. There is considerable evidence for essentiality in mammals including man. Deficiencies of strontium are associated with certain types of Ca and boron resistant osteoporosis and arthritis. Strontium 90, the man-made product of fission atomic explosions and the greatest biohazard fear during the cold war, does not occur in nature.

Ta—Tantalum is found in igneous rocks at 2 ppm, shale at 0.8 ppm, sandstone and limestone at 0.05 ppm, sea water at 0.0000025 ppm, and in marine animals accumulates up to 410 ppm.

Tb—Terbium is found in igneous rock at 0.9 ppm, shale at 0.58 ppm, sandstone at 0.41 ppm, limestone at 0.071 ppm, land plants at 0.0015 ppm, marine animals at 0.006 to 0.01 ppm, and land animals at 0.0004 ppm where it accumulates in the bone.

Tc—Technetium. All isotopes of technetium are radioactive and not known to occur in nature. Technetium is poorly absorbed by mammals.

Te—Tellurium is found in igneous rocks at 0.001 ppm, land plants at 2 to 25 ppm, and in land animals at 0.02 ppm.

Th—Thorium is found in igneous rocks at 9.6 ppm, shale at 12 ppm, sandstone and limestone at 1–7 ppm, soils at 5 ppm, marine animals at

0.003 to 0.03 ppm and land animals at 0.003 to 0.1 ppm.

Ti—Titanium is found in igneous rocks at 5,700 ppm, shale at 4,600 ppm, sandstone at 1,500 ppm, sea water at 0.001 ppm, soils at 5,000 ppm, marine plants at 12 to 80 ppm (accumulates in plankton), land plants at 1 ppm, marine animals at 0.2 to 20 ppm, and land animals at 0.2 ppm.

Tm—Thulium is a "heavy" rare earth and is found in igneous rocks at 0.48 ppm, shales at 0.28 ppm, sandstone at 0.3 ppm, limestone at 0.065 ppm, land plants at 0.0015 ppm, and land animals at 0.00004 ppm. Thulium supplementation enhances the growth of normal cells and has doubled the life span of laboratory species.

U—Uranium is found in igneous rocks at 2.7 ppm, shale at 3.7 ppm, sandstone at 0.95 ppm, limestone at 2.2 ppm, fresh water at 0.001 ppm, sea water at 0.003 ppm, soil at ppm (absorbed by humus, especially in alkaline soils), land plants at 0.038 ppm (Astragalus spp. is an accumulator plant), marine animals at 0.004 to 3.2 ppm, and animals at 0.013 ppm. All natural isotopes are alpha emitters and may also decay by fission. Uranium is accumulated by mammalian kidney and bone after ingestion.

V—Vanadium is found in igneous rocks at 1135 ppm, shale at 130 ppm, sandstone at 20 ppm, limestone at 20 ppm, fresh water at 0.001 ppm, sea water at 0.002 ppm, soils at 100 ppm (V is absorbed by humus, especially in alkaline soils), marine plants at 2 ppm, land plants at 1.6 ppm (accumulated by the fungus Armanita muscaria), marine animals at 0.14 to 2.0 ppm, and in land animals at 0.15 ppm. Metallic vanadium (vanadyl sulfate) is absorbed from the intestinal tract very poorly at only 0.1 to 1.0 percent, vanadium chelates are absorbed at 40 percent, and plant derived colloidal forms at up to 98 percent.

Vanadium was proven to be essential in 1971. Vanadium stimulates blood sugar (glucose) oxidation and transport in fat cells and glycogen (animal starch) synthesis in liver and muscle, and inhibits liver gluconeogenesis (production of glucose from fat) and absorption of glucose from the gut. Vanadium enhances the stimulating effect of insulin on DNA synthesis. Despite low serum insulin, the blood glucose levels of diabetic rats fed vanadium was the same as normal controls. Vanadium appears to function like insulin by altering cell membrane function for ion transport. Therefore vanadium has a very beneficial effect for humans with glucose and carbohydrate intolerance (i.e. hypoglycemia, hyperinsulinemia, narcolepsy, prediabetes, depression, manic depression, bi-polar disease, "chemical imbalance," ADD, ADHD, violent behavior, etc.) by making the cell membrane insulin receptors more sensitive to insulin.

Several cultures including African Americans, Native American Indians, Hispanics, and Hawaiians have an increased rate of diabetes when they eat their ethnic foods and consume canned, processed foods that are fried and high in sugar. Vanadium supplementation can have a major positive economic impact by reducing or even eliminating most cases of adult onset diabetes. Diabetes alone costs American taxpayers a minimum of $105 billion each year.

Vanadium inhibits cholesterol synthesis in animals and humans; this is followed by decreased plasma levels of cholesterol and reduced aortic cholesterol. Vanadium initiates an increase in the contractile force of heart muscle known as the "inotropic effect." Vanadium has known anticarcinogenic properties. Feeding 25 µg of vanadium per gram of diet blocked induction of mouse mammary tumor growth. The vanadium supplement reduced tumor incidence, average tumor count per animal, and prolonged median cancer-free time without inhibiting overall growth or health of the animals.

Clinical Diseases Associated with Vanadium Deficiency

Slow growth
Increased infant mortality
Infertility
Elevated cholesterol
Elevated triglycerides
Hypoglycemia
Hyperinsulinemia
Narcolepsy
Prediabetes
Diabetes
ADD, ADHD
Depression
Manic depression, Bi-polar disease
Tourette's syndrome
Cardiovascular disease
Obesity

W—Tungsten is found in igneous rocks at 1.5 ppm, shale at 1.8 ppm, sandstone at 1.6 ppm, limestone at 0.6 ppm, seawater at 0.0001 ppm, soils at 1 ppm, marine plants at 0.0035 ppm, marine animals at 0.0005 to 0.05 ppm, and in land animals at 0.005 ppm. Tungsten accumulates in heart muscle and teeth at 0.00025 ppm.

Xe—Xenon is found in igneous rocks at 0.00003 ppm and in seawater at 0.000052 ppm. Xenon binds to mammalian hemoglobin and myoglobin producing an anesthetic effect.

Y—Yttrium is a "heavy" rare earth found in igneous rocks at 33 ppm, shale at 18 ppm, sandstone at 9.1 ppm, limestone at 4.3 ppm, sea water at 0.0003 ppm, soils at 50 ppm, land plants at 0.6 ppm (accumulates in ferns), marine mammals at 0.01 to 0.2 ppm, and in land animals at 0.04 ppm where it is found in mammalian bone, teeth, and liver. Yttrium enhances normal cell growth and doubles the life span of laboratory species. Exposure of pregnant mice to yttrium leads to rapid placental transfer. Fourteen percent of ingested yttrium can be detected in the newborn mice.

Yb—Ytterbium is a rare earth found in igneous rocks at 3 ppm, shale at 1.8 ppm, sandstone at 1.3 ppm, limestone at 0.43 ppm, land plants at 0.0015 ppm, marine animals at 0.02 ppm, and in land animals at 0.00012 ppm where it accumulates at up to .3 ppm in bone, teeth, and liver. Exposure of pregnant mice leads to rapid placental transfer. Fourteen percent of ingested ytterbium can be detected in newborn mice.

Zn—Zinc is found in igneous rocks at 70 ppm, shale at 95 ppm, sandstone at 116 ppm, limestone at 20 ppm, fresh water at 0.01 ppm, seawater at 0.01 ppm, soils at 50 ppm, marine plants at 6 to 1,500 ppm, land plants at 100 ppm, marine animals at 6 to 1,500 ppm, and in land animals at 160 ppm. Zinc accumulates in mammalian kidney, prostate, and eye. Zinc was known to be an essential growth factor for bread mold 100 years ago, essential for rats 50 years ago, and essential for humans 20 years ago. Zinc deficiency produces a wide range of diseases including congenital birth defects and degenerative diseases of all age groups.

Congenital Birth Defects Associated with Zinc Deficiency

⟨ Down's Syndrome
⟨ Cleft lip
⟨ Cleft palate
⟨ Brain defects (dorsal herniation, hydroenchalocoel)
⟨ Micro or anopthalmia (small or absent eyes)

⟨ Agnathia (small lower jaw)
⟨ Spina bifida
⟨ Clubbed limbs
⟨ Syndactyly (webbed toes and fingers)
⟨ Polydactyly (extra limbs and digits)
⟨ Atresia (failure to develope limbs, digits,organs, anal
    opening,etc.)
⟨ Hernias (hiatal, diaphragmatic, umbilical, inguinal, etc.)
⟨ Heart defects
⟨ Lung defects
⟨ Urogenital defects (horseshoe kidney, small kidney, intersex
    malformations of the male and female genitalia)

There are 1.4 to 2.3 grams of Zn in the adult human. The liver, pancreas, kidney, bone, and skeletal muscles have the greatest reserves of Zn. Lesser amounts are found in the eye, prostate gland, semen, skin, hair, fingernails, and toenails. There are no less than 70 metalloenzymes that require Zn as a functional cofactor. These include carbonic anhydrase, alkaline phosphatase, lactic dehydrogenase, and carboxypeptidase. Zinc helps to bind enzymes to substrates by maintaining spatial and configurational relationships. Some enzymes bind Zn so tightly that even during severe Zn depletion they can still function.

Zinc participates in the metabolism of nucleic acids and the synthesis of proteins. Zinc is also an integral part of the RNA molecule itself where Zinc provides the "metallic fingers" and participates in cell division and synthesis of DNA. The DNA-dependent RNA polymerase is a zinc-dependent enzyme, as is thymidine kinase.

Excesses of dietary copper and iron and high phytate diets (vegans) will reduce availability of dietary zinc. Heavy losses of zinc occurs in sweat, therefore unsupplemented athletes are particularly at risk for zinc deficiency with the following symptoms such as anorexia nervosa, muscle weakness, pica and cribbing, etc.

<u>Symptoms and Diseases of Zinc Deficiency</u>

⟨ Pica/Cribbing (geophagia, wool eating, hair eating, etc.)
⟨ Loss of sense of smell
⟨ Loss of sense of taste
⟨ Infertility
⟨ Failure of wounds and ulcers to heal

⟨ Immune status failure
⟨ Poor growth (short stature)
⟨ High infant mortality
⟨ Hypogonadism (small poorly functioning ovaries and testes)
⟨ Perpetual prepubic state
⟨ Anemia
⟨ Alopecia (hair loss)
⟨ Acrodermatitis enteropathica (parakeratosis)
⟨ "Frizzy" hair
⟨ Diarrhea
⟨ Depression
⟨ Paranoia
⟨ Oral and perioral dermatitis
⟨ Weight loss (anorexia nervosa)
⟨ Benign prostatic hypertrophy (noncancerous prostatic enlargement)
⟨ Severe body odor ("smelly tennis shoe" syndrome)
⟨ Anorexia and Bulimia

Zr—Zirconium is found in igneous rocks at 165 ppm, shale at 160 ppm, sandstone at 220 ppm, limestone at 19 ppm, fresh water at 0.0026 ppm, seawater at 0.000022 ppm, soils at 300 ppm, marine plants at 20 ppm, land plants at 0.64 ppm, marine animals at 0.1 to 1.0 ppm, and land animals at 0.3 ppm.

Appendix B

LET'S PLAY DOCTOR

References for *Dead Doctors Don't Lie*, including those for this chapter, are found at the end of the book for two reasons: 1) to prevent the book from being so large you couldn't carry it, and 2) to keep the cost down. One reason medical books cost $120 is that there are more pages of references than there are pages of facts and "how to" information.

The information here represents five college degrees (Dr. Ma Lan and myself). It also reflects a total of 24 years of college and 50 years of combined research and clinical experience. In addition, no less than 200 books and literally thousands of journal articles have been "predigested" for you in hopes of saving you time and expense. Those who wish to spend the time and effort to follow up one or more points in more detail will be able to do so with some ease as we have chosen a few books that are comprehensive reviews. From there you can go to thousands of journal articles if you so desire.

A last bit of advice is to avoid problems in diagnosis and treatment by spending some time reading this chapter and confirming your "diagnosis" and reviewing the "treatments." Don't become like the "orthodox" doctors and "shoot from the hip" in a trial and error type of "practice." More than 400 diseases and the veterinary/alternative medicine approach to dealing with them are listed in alphabetical order. Now armed with all this information, you are in a position to take back control of your own health.

Note: These suggestions are *in addition* to consuming adequate amounts of the other 90 essential nutrients daily.

ABRASIONS (scrapes): clean wounds with soap and water to remove gross dirt and debris. Disinfect wounds with H2O2 (hydrogen peroxide). Wounds may be bathed in a variety of herbal washes or poultice. Our choice is aloe, plantain (Plantago major), or comfrey (Symphytum officinale). Colloidal silver is useful here. Take Vitamin C orally to bowel tolerance (anywhere from 1–5 grams). Covering abrasions with nonstick dressings will help prevent infection.

ABSCESS (boil): bring abscess to "a head" (a soft point in the center) with a hot water and boric acid compress or poultice (sitz bath if near the anus or buttock) using a 3 percent solution of boric acid. Herbal alternatives include echinacea (Echinacea angustifolia) or sand sagebrush (Artemisia fififolia). Once the abscess opens (by itself or with a sterile needle or blade) it can be flushed clean using a syringe filled with any of the above herbal solutions.

If large enough, the resulting cavity can be filled with gauze (umbilical "tape" is particularly good for this purpose) soaked with any of the above solutions. If the abscess cavity contains bits of puss or dead tissue, it can be flushed with H2O2. The cavity will gradually fill with "granulation tissue" leaving no trace of the cavity. Take Vitamin C orally to bowel tolerance.

ABSENCE ATTACKS (*petit mal*): patient stops what he is doing and rapidly blinks eyes then starts the activity again where he left off. Treatment should include choline 4 gm/day, taurine 500 mg t.i.d., dimethyl glycine 100 mg b.i.d., phosphytidyl choline, and B6 100–300 mg/day. A high fat diet to rebuild myelin and a plant derived colloidal trace mineral mix will often be of benefit.

ACHALASIA (megaesophagus): enervation of the esophagus resulting in failure of cardiac (lower sphincter) sphincter to open. A tendency to regurgitate undigested food is a common sign. Small liquid meals and air swallowing can sometimes relieve this condition. Nighttime elevation of head of the bed will reduce risk of vomiting while asleep. Surgery may be required to relieve severe cases.

ACHLORHYDRIA (loss of stomach acid—hydrochloric acid): Contrary to popular belief, stress will result in <u>loss</u> of stomach acid production. Achlorhydria is also a natural process of aging and perhaps the most significant aging phenomenon. Seventy-five percent of people over the age of 50 years require supplementation of stomach acid. Sodium chloride is the raw material required to manufacture stomach acid, so it follows that people on a salt restricted diet are more likely to develop achlorhydria.

Symptoms include "burp, belch, and bloat" after eating. The reduction or absence of acid in the stomach allows intestinal bacteria and yeast (Candida albicans) to enter the stomach and ferment high carbohydrate foods (i.e. juice, fruit, breads, etc.). Failure to deal with achlorhydria will result in B12, calcium, and protein deficiencies and the onset of new food allergies acquired later in life as a result of absorption of partially digested polypeptides (relatively large protein fragments) which trigger an allergic response.

Treatment of achlorhydria includes salting your food to taste and supplementation of betaine HCl at the rate of 75–250 mg 15–20 minutes before each meal. In the absence of betaine HCl, 1–2 oz. of vinegar with English bitters (Gentian) may be taken before meals. Additionally, plant derived colloidal minerals tone the stomach and increase its ability to produce stomach acid.

ACNE (acne rosacea/acne vulgaris) is a frequent skin disease in teenagers and is sometimes associated with PMS and estrogen supplements during menopause. Papules, pustules, superficial puss-filled cysts, and deep puss-filled canals characterize acne. Acne is primarily the result of an essential fatty acid deficiency with a concurrent intake of too much saturated fat and polyunsaturated fatty acids (fried foods and margarine). Eliminate "fast" foods and other sources of fat and sugar. Check out the probability of food allergies (i.e., wheat, milk, soy) as a contributing factor. Betaine HCl and pancreatic enzymes are of considerable benefit. Essential fatty acids are a must and should be consumed at the rate of 3 percent of your total daily calorie consumption or supplemented at the rate of 9 grams per day in capsule form. A regimen of Vitamin A 300,000 units/day (as beta-carotene) for five months, then reduce to 25,000 i per day B6 100 mg t.i.d., zinc 50 mg t.i.d. for 30 days, and vitamin E oil may be applied topically to acne lesions is also recommended. Exposing areas affected by acne directly to ultra violet light directly for 1–6 minutes may also prove helpful.

ADRENAL GLAND EXHAUSTION (stress) characterized by fatigue and inability to cope with diseases or every day stresses. Adrenal exhaustion directly affects your ability to resist disease or heal a current disease. An adrenal function test can be performed in the following manner. Take base blood pressure in a lying down position after five minutes then stand up suddenly. Pulse should increase by a minimum of ten points. If the pulse does not increase by that amount, your adrenals need help. Concurrent signs and symptoms may include colitis, ulcers and low WBC (white blood cell) count.

Treatment of adrenal exhaustion includes ACE (adrenal cortical extract). Take ten drops of a standard solution sublingually or 3–5 ml IV, vitamin C to bowel tolerance, and zinc 25–50 mg t.i.d. Don't forget to remove the stress. Dietary recommendations: no fried foods, no margarine, no caffeine, and no sugar.

AGE SPOTS: (Liver spots, pigment of aging): These unsightly brown spots are caused by rancid fat (ceroid lipofucsin or trans fatty acids)from cell walls accumulating under the skin. If you have ten on the back of your hand, you have millions in your brain, heart, liver, kidney, lungs, etc. They interfere with cell function, shorten your life, and are a red flag warning for high risk of cancer and heart disease (i.e. cardiomyopathy). The nice thing about age spots is that they are reversible. When they go away on the outside, they are going away on the inside.

Treatment includes eliminating all fried foods, vegetable oils (i.e. salad dressing, cooking oils, margarine, etc.), and sugar from the diet. Take selenium at 500 mcg per day, vitamin E at 1,200 IU and all the other 90 essential nutrients.

AGREEABLE ATTITUDE: usually a disagreeable attitude is the result of food allergies, ADD, ADND, or hypoglycemia (sometimes from poor social training while growing up!) If so these must be dealt with specifically.

Treatment should include plantain (Plantago lanceolata) orally t.i.d., avoidance of sugar in all forms (i.e., alcohol, desserts, sugar, juices, fruits, etc.), avoidance of caffeine, essential fatty acids 9 grams per day, chromium, and vanadium at 50–100 mcg each t.i.d.

AIDS (autoimmune deficiency syndrome) is thought to be caused by the HIV virus. This disease may lay dormant for three to ten years before causing overt symptoms and death. Signs are very low white blood cell counts especially T-cells, coughing, and susceptibility to a variety of diseases including Pneumocystis carnii pneumonia, Karposi's Sarcoma, and a variety of secondary bacterial and viral infections. This disease is transmitted by oral, vaginal, and anal sex, common needles used for IV drugs, contaminated hospital and dental equipment, commercially prepared blood products, and immunotoxic lubricants such as vegetable oils, petrolem jelly, etc.

At this point (1998) prevention is the "magic bullet" for AIDS. Avoid IV "recreational drugs," use unlubricated condoms for sex with partners with unknown sexual histories. Avoid anal sex. Once HIV is contracted, a vigorous program of antiviral medications (i.e. Ribavirin and Isoprinosin) and immune support (Levamisol, hydrazine sulfate) are indicated. Take

Vitamin C to bowel tolerance, 300,000 IU of vitamin A per day as beta carotene, 50 mg zinc t.i.d., ACE (adrenal cortical extract) 10 drops t.i.d. sublingual, selenium 1000 mcg/day orally or by injection, vitamin E 1000 IU/day. Herbs such as garlic (Allium sativum), evening primrose oil (Oenothera biennis), and goldenseal (Hydrastis canadensis) may be of value. Long-term remission can be expected but a "cure" is not available for HIV or AIDS. An unknown in this protocol is Levamisol which may be the immune modulator that everyone is looking for. Also suggested: injectable thymus extract, which can be ordered by your physician from a pharmaceutical company, monthly at 3–5 cc after four initial daily injections of 3–5 cc.

ALCOHOLISM is considered to be an addictive allergy complicated by hypoglycemia and vitamin/mineral malnutrition. Rotation elimination diets and hypoglycemia diets are essential. Don't forget the baseline vitamin/mineral supplements. Take calcium (2000 mg) and magnesium (1000 mg) per day, essential fatty acids 5 mg t.i.d. Vitamin B6 100 mg b.i.d., and chromium and vanadium at 250 mcg/day are essential to solve the hypoglycemia problem. Bioflavonoids (catechin) 1 gram/day and amino acids (i.e. DL-phenylananine) should also be consumed. Take 1 oz. plant derived colloidal minerals diluted in calcium enriched orange juice every time craving for alcohol occurs.

ALLERGIES can be caused by poorly digested food, inhalant allergens (i.e. pollens, smoke, molds, etc.), or chemicals (i.e. perfume, formalin, etc.). Diagnosis can be made using the pulse test, diet diary/challenge, and/or cytotoxic test. Symptoms vary widely from urticaria (skin rash with itching) from strawberries or fish, headaches from perfume, tachycardia (fast heart rate) or palpitations (most allergies-MSG), or paranoia from sugar, etc., to asthma-like syndrome from sulfite (food preservative on raisins, apricots, etc.).

Avoidance is the most effective "cure," however, this may be impractical. Autoimmune urine therapy using five to ten ml of filtered urine subcutaneously every other day for five to eight treatments is suggested. Use a 0.22 micron millipore filter. Take vitamin C to bowel tolerance, bioflavonoids (rutin, catechin, quercetin), 300,000 IU of vitamin A as beta carotene per day, zinc 50 mg t.i.d., essential fatty acids 1 tbsp. b.i.d., rotation diets, and digestive enzymes with betaine HCl before meals.

ALLERGIC SHINERS are the purplish/ black discoloration under the lower eyelids of individuals with allergies. They will appear within minutes of ingestion or inhalation of an allergen. Allergic shiners may take as much as 12 hours to three days to disappear after avoidance of allergenic substance. Allergic shiners are a good diagnostic tool to link allergies as the culprit behind other symptoms i.e., allergic shiners in a hyperactive child, heart disease, cancer, etc. Avoidance of the allergen or allergens is the only "cure" for allergic shiners.

ALZHEIMER'S DISEASE appears to be a physician-caused disease (resulting from cholesterol and saturated fat bashing) in which those afflicted suffer from a progressive loss of memory. Difficulties with arousal and motor function appear in the later stages of the disease. Identified in 1979, it appears to be due to a cholesterol and fat deficiency. Alzheimer's disease is not genetic.

Treatment should include germanium IM 5 ml of standard solution every other day for 24 days followed by oral germanium at 150/mg b.i.d., Hydergine, 6–12 mg/day, piracetam/choline 1.6 grams q.i.d., vasopressin (Diapid) at a rate of one whiff in each nostril q.i.d. which delivers a total daily dose of 12–16 units of U.S.P. Posterior Pituitary, and centro-phenoxine (Lucidril) 6.2–8.0 gram/day. Lecithin at 2,500 mg t.i.d. is very useful at all stages though phosphatydil choline is more efficient. Don't forget the baseline nutritional supplements including colloidal minerals plus betaine HCl and pancreatic enzymes 75–200 mg t.i.d.. Oral and IV H_2O_2 may be helpful, 200 mg vitamin B1 t.i.d., vitamin E at 2000 iu daily, 500 mcg selenium daily and IV chelation will be of value. Eat soft-scrambled (not fried) eggs every day and 72 oz. red meat each month to replace cholesterol needed to rebuild myelin.

ALOPECIA: (baldness): loss of hair, which can occur locally or present as total hair loss. Male pattern baldness, female pattern baldness, and alopecia universalis are examples.

Monoxidil and Retin-A creams will aid some male and female pattern baldness if treated early in the process and use is maintained. Deficiencies of the mineral tin have been shown to cause male pattern baldness in lab animals. I personally have had considerable hair regrowth following the use of plant derived liquid colloidal tin. Alopecia that occurs with eczema is often caused by essential fatty acid deficiency and will respond to IV interlipids and/or oral flaxseed oil at the rate of 9 grams per day. Zinc at 50 mg t.i.d. is also indicated. Elimination of wheat and cow's milk from the diet will increase the rate of recovery. Betaine HCl and pancreatic enzymes at 75–200 mg t.i.d. 15–20 minutes before meals are a must.

AMBLYOPIA is a type of blindness that can be caused by B12 deficiency or tobacco smoking. B12 IM at a rate of 1000 mcg/day for a total of 20,000 mcg usually effects a "cure." Avoid tobacco smoke. Be sure to avoid all fried food and margarine and supplement with all 90 essential nutrients.

AMEBIASIS is an amebic dysentery caused by Entamoeba hystolytica. Diagnosis is dependent upon finding the parasite in a stool examination. Examination of 3–6 samples may be necessary to find the organisms especially if diarrhea has been chronic. The use of the low power lens on the microscope will often allow you to observe the "amebic" movement. Bloody mucus has the highest concentration of the parasite.

Treatment should be to provide symptomatic relief of diarrhea and reduce the loss of protein and electrolytes. Metronidazole at the rate of 750 mg orally t.i.d. for 10 days for adults and 12–17 mg/day t.i.d. orally for children is the treatment of choice.

AMENORRHEA is the lack of, or stopping of, the menstrual period. Many factors are involved in a normal "period" including the requirement of a 20 percent body fat level (trim athletes and very slim ladies stop cycling). Amenorrhea commonly occurs in very slim women athletes, dieters, and anorexics. A weight gain of 10–15 pounds will "jump-start" the cycle and a "period" will result. In many cases, increased levels of zinc at a rate of 50 mg t.i.d. will result in onset of the "period." Essential fatty acids are very useful in the form of flaxseed oil at the rate of 1 tbsp. t.i.d. Herbal stimulus can be effected with saffron (Crocus sativus) as a tea, black cohosh or squawroot (Cimicifuga racemosa) as a fluid extract, and marigold (Calendula officinalis).

ANAPHYLAXIS is an explosive allergic reaction ranging from urticaria to respiratory distress and vascular collapse. This "shock" type of reaction can occur as the result of allergies to foods (i.e. shellfish), insect stings (i.e. bee stings), or drugs (i.e. penicillin) and usually occurs in 1–15 minutes after exposure. Avoidance of exposure is the best preventative.

Immediate injection with adrenaline (epinephrine) from a "bee sting" kit is the treatment of choice and, in many cases, will be lifesaving.

ANAL ABSCESS and anal fissures are caused by constipation and frequent passage of large hard stools. They may occur at the same time with hemorrhoids. Painful red swellings at or near the anal opening are characteristic. These may be opened with a blade or by soaking in hot sitz baths of 3 percent boric acid found at your drug store. A poultice of echinacea (Echinacea angustifolia) may be applied directly to the abscess to disinfect and help to bring it to a "point" so it can be opened. Flushing the opened abscess with 3 percent H2O2 will clean out the puss and disinfect the wound.

ANEMIA is a lack of red blood cells from many possible causes including hemorrhage, infections, and/or nutritional deficiencies. Betaine HCl orally at 75–200 mg t.i.d. 15–20 minutes before meals is required to assure absorption of B12, liver extract orally or IM, nutritional support with iron 20 mg per day, B12 1000 mcg per day for 20 days, folic acid 15 mg for 20 days, copper 2 mg, zinc 50 mg t.i.d., B-2 50 mg b.i.d., B-5 50 mg t.i.d., B-6 50 mg b.i.d. for 20 days, vitamin C to bowel tolerance, vitamin E 800–1200 IU per day, selenium 500 mcg/day, and essential fatty acids at a rate of 9 grams per day. Herbs including sweet cicely (Myrrhis odorata) and marsh marigold (Coltha palustris) are helpful too.

ANEURYSM is a "bubble" or "balloon" in the wall of an artery, much like a "balloon" in a weak tire. This can cause pressure on an organ like a tumor or burst causing stroke or sudden death by hemorrhage. Sudden death by hemorrhage goes by various clinical names such as *subdural hemorrhage, stroke,* or *ruptured aortic aneurysm.* Aneurysms are most frequently caused by copper deficiency which results in weakened elastic fibers. While copper supplementation may not "cure" or repair all aneurysm, it can prevent them when supplemented at the rate of 2–4 mg/day *if it is being properly absorbed.* Surgery will be required for most existing aneurysms, although there is a considerable amount of evidence to show that arterial elastic fibers can be repaired by supplementing diets with copper. We do have one aortic aneurysm that has been corrected with copper supplementation and confirmed by x-ray.

ANGINA is a sharp debilitating pain in the center front of the chest from arterial disease in the heart, which reduces the heart's oxygen supply. Symptoms may appear after strenuous exercise, simply climbing stairs, or after a meal. The allopathic approach is the "coronary bypass" surgery which after 20 years of study has failed to prevent second heart attacks or to extend life. Coronary bypasses *do* however enhance the financial portfolio of the cardiovascular surgeon!

Chelation, either IV with H2O2 and calcium EDTA or orally with vitamin/mineral and herb supplements, or the Dean Ornish diet can effect a cure over a period of time. Avoid sugar, caffeine, and cigarette smoke. Exercise in the form of walking for 30 minutes each day is very helpful. Calcium (2000 mg/day) and magnesium (800 mg/day) and essential fatty acids can help prevent progress of current disease and reduce vitamin D intake from the sun and supplements. Nitroglycerin sublingual capsules and time-release transdermal patches are very useful in relieving symptoms. English hawthorn (Crataegus oxyacantha) and ginko (Ginko biloba) are specific for relieving angina by increasing the blood flow through coronary arteries. Lifestyle changes and supplementation can reverse cardiovascular disease!

ANOREXIA (appetite loss) can be caused by stress, malnutrition, shock, and injury. ANOREXIA NERVOSA is thought by "orthodox" medicine to be a psychiatric disease, however, it now appears that it is a manifestation of a severe food allergy. A common complaint of anorexia nervosa sufferers is "I always feel better when I don't eat and feel bad when I eat." Deficiencies of zinc and lithium are associated with anorexia. Elimination diets and pulse tests are useful in finding the offending food, frequently cow's milk, wheat, eggs, and corn.

Treatment should include betaine HCl and pancreatic enzymes at a rate of 150–250 mg/day t.i.d. and don't forget the baseline vitamin/mineral supplements. Herbs are excellent appetite stimulants. Test herbal preparations of buckbean or marsh trefoil (Menyanthes trifoliata), centaury (Centaurium umbellatum), sweet flag or calamus (Acorus calamus), yellow gentian (Gentiana lutea). All of the herbal preparations should be taken before meals. In the case of ANOREXIA NERVOSA, autoimmune urine therapy may be indicated.

ANOSMIA (loss of smell) can temporarily be caused by colds or rhinitis (nasal inflammation from colds or allergy). Chronic loss of the sense of smell is most frequently the result of a zinc deficiency. In the case of injury, stroke, or tumor, zinc supplementation may not be effective.

Zinc supplement at the rate of 50 mg t.i.d. is very effective in returning the sense of smell.

ANXIETY (panic attacks) affect women twice as frequently as men. When one examines the total hormone biorhythm charts of women, this fact cannot be a surprise. The base cause can be either a food allergy reaction (i.e. corn, cow's milk, etc.) or a severe reactive hypoglycemic reaction often referred to as a "crash and burn" curve because the down slope on the glucose curve is almost vertical. Concurrent PMS can make this a very perplexing situation. Do a pulse test to eliminate allergies and a six-hour GTT.

Treatment should include avoidance of caffeine and sugar in all forms (fruit, juices, processed sugar, candy, etc.). Take chromium and vanadium 200–300 mcg/day, B6 100 mg t.i.d., B3 450 mg t.i.d. as time-release tablets, B1, B2, and B5 at the rate of 50 mg t.i.d., L-tryptophan 10 grams t.i.d., calcium 2000 mg/day, and magnesium at 800 mg/day. Betaine HCl 100–250 t.i.d. before meals and herbs including valerian (Valerian officinalis) can be of value.

APHTHOUS STOMATITIS (canker sores) are often a symptom of food sensitivities (orange juice, tomato juice) or allergies. An elimination/ rotation diet or a pulse test can identify the offending foods. Gluten free diets are frequently effective.

Folic acid at 5 mg t.i.d., B12 at 1000 mcg/day, iron at 15 mg/day and zinc at 50 mg t.i.d. are effective adjuncts to avoidance diets.

ARSENIC TOXICITY is a frequent result of pollution from herbicides, slug poisons, etc. Hair analysis is the best way to determine if toxic levels of arsenic are present. Symptoms are widely varied and include alopecia, constipation, confusion, delayed healing, dermatitis, diarrhea, drowsiness, edema, fatigue, GI complaints, headache, burning and tingling, muscle pain, neuropathy, numbness, pruritis, seizures, stomatitis, and weakness.

Avoid oils during treatment as they promote absorption of arsenic. Identify source of arsenic and eliminate it. IV chelation is very effective in removing the body load of arsenic, as is the oral use of colloidal or chelated selenium.

ARTERIOSCLEROSIS (hardening of the arteries) is the result of fibrosis of the smooth muscle in the walls of elastic arteries, notably the aorta and coronary, pulmonary, carotid, cerebral, brachial, and femoral arteries. The elevated "lesions" produce eddies which produce lipid and calcium depositions. Magnesium deficiencies produce "malignant calci- fication" of elastic arteries and are perhaps "the cause" of arteriosclerosis.

Elevated blood cholesterol is considered to be a significant risk factor for arteriosclerosis. It is of interest that vitamin D is made from cholesterol in our bodies! This becomes significant when we realize that the toxic affect of vitamin D is angiotoxicity. The target tissue of vitamin D toxicity is the elastic arteries and the specific result is fibrosis of the vascular smooth muscle and calcification of the blood vessel wall — fatty deposits soon follow!!! It is a crime that the "orthodox" doctors do not give this as much press coverage as heart transplants. Again this infor- mation would wipe out a medical specialty, so they keep it a secret!!!

Symptoms of arteriosclerosis include angina, headaches, loss of memory, breathlessness, leg cramps ("claudication") in the early stages, and death from stroke and thrombotic type "heart attack" in the final stages.

Treatment includes IV chelation with EDTA and H2O2, oral chelation, oral supplementation with vitamin/mineral supplements that include 800 mg magnesium, and the complete spectrum of plant derived colloidal minerals. In addition to the baseline nutritional supplements, add vitamin C to bowel tolerance, exercise (to increase the caliber of your arteries), and follow a high fiber, low in animal fat diet. Also supplement with essential fatty acids including salmon oil and flaxseed oil 5 gm t.i.d.. Useful herbs include artichoke (Cynara scolymus), bears garlic (Allium ursinum), European mistletoe (Viscum album), cayenne pepper, and garlic (Allium sativum).

ARTHRITIS (rheumatism) is a devastating degenerative disease of the joints. Symptoms of joint noise, joint pain, swelling, and deformative changes are typical. The cause of arthritis is listed as unknown by "orthodox" medicine and treatment is of the "take two aspirins and learn to live with it." Prednisone, a synthetic form of cortisone, is used to treat symptoms. In fact, osteoarthritis and degenerative arthritis are a complex of nutritional deficiencies. In the case of rheumatoid arthritis, a chronic infection with a Mycoplasma spp. is the overt cause. Again, if the truth were released, the "orthodox" doctors would lose an entire specialty in short order, so they keep it a secret.

A dietary calcium/phosphorus ratio of 2:1 is ideal yet impossible to attain in an unsupplemented diet. A vegetarian diet gets close but is complicated by "phytates" (a natural chelating substance found in plants) which makes even supplemented calcium unavailable. The calcium/phosphorus ratios of food items is consistent:

FOOD	CALCIUM	PHOSPHORUS
grain	1	8
red meat	1	12
organ meat (liver, kidney)	1	44
fish	1	12
carbonated drinks	1	8

It is easily seen that none of the calcium/phosphorus ratios of the basic foods are anywhere near correct. These increase the calcium loss from the body including the bones and teeth. The more meat you eat, the more calcium supplementation you need. It is quite simple. Veterinarians know this but we suppose that "orthodox" physicians believe that if a "truth" will wipe out a medical specialty, it must be ignored or kept a secret!

Treatment of arthritis should include calcium at 2000 mg/day and more if you eat meat two or three times per day. Also take magnesium at 800–1000 mg/day, and cartilage (collagen, glucosamine sulfate and chondroitin sulfate) at 1000 mg t.i.d. For rheumatoid arthritis, add tetracycline or minocycline at the low dose acne therapy level daily for one year, or oral food grade H2O2 to deal with the Mycoplasma infection. IV chelation with EDTA and H2O2 is very helpful! Take Vitamin C to bowel tolerance, B6 100 mg b.i.d., B3 450 mg b.i.d. as time-release capsules. Take Vitamin E at 1000 IU/day. Copper at 2 mg/day (may be absorbed from a copper bracelet), selenium 300 mcg/day, zinc 50 mg t.i.d. Plant derived colloidal minerals are 98 percent absorbable and give excellent results!

Rotation elimination diets can help when food allergies aggravate or precipitate symptoms. Dr. Wallach's Pig Arthritis Formula is an easy recipe that can be prepared at home that will economically provide all of the necessary raw material to rebuild cartilage, joint capsules, and bone. Autoimmune urine therapy is very useful for all types of arthritis, especially those aggravated by food allergies. DMSO or pain gels are useful in reducing inflammation and pain when applied topically. Herbs including licorice (Glycyrrhiza glabra), poison ivy (Rhus toxicodendron), and alfalfa (powder or sprouts) are useful adjuncts to arthritis treatment programs.

ASTHMA is a respiratory disease that is characterized by sudden onset with closure of bronchial tubes by spasmodic muscles. ATOPIC ASTHMA has eczema as a feature along with the respiratory disease. Asthma is a disease of malabsorption with essential fatty acid deficiencies and deficiencies of manganese and magnesium. Treatment should include betaine HCl, pancreatic enzymes, and ox bile at 75–200 mg each t.i.d. before meals. Autoimmune urine therapy, essential fatty acids at 5 gm t.i.d., and plant derived colloidal mineral suspensions that contain magnesium and manganese should be taken. Herbs are very useful for treating asthma with some caution when you have allergies to plants. Useful plants include: honeysuckle (Lonicera caprifolium), jaborandi (Pilocarpus jaborandi), leeks (Allium porrum), garlic (Allium sativum), and evening primrose oil or fluid extract (Oenothera biennia). A variety of standard "inhalers" are available to cope with sudden attacks.

ATHEROSCLEROSIS: see arteriosclerosis

ATOPIC DERMATITIS (eczema) is part of the "atopic" patient syndrome which includes asthma, alopecia (hair loss), and lowered immune response. This syndrome is one of malabsorption of essential fatty acids and can include emotional symptoms similar to PMS, hypo-glycemia, asthma, bronchitis, or diabetes as a result of malabsorption of chromium. The malabsorption is usually the result of a "celiac" disease type change in the small intestinal lining rather than dietary deficiency. Do a pulse test to determine food allergies.

Treatment should include a rotation or an elimination diet (usually a pulse test will reveal cow's milk, wheat, or soy products to be the culprits). Autoimmune therapy can be very useful. Supplementation should include essential fatty acids as flaxseed oil at 9 grams per day and vitamin E at 1000 IU/day. If malabsorption is a major problem, the fatty acids may be taken as interlipids IV.

ATHLETES FOOT is actually a form of "ringworm" caused by the fungus Tinea pedis. Treatment includes hydrotherapy in baths of 3 percent boric acid, alternating with vinegar baths. Supplements include zinc at 50 mg t.i.d., 300,000 units of vitamin A/day as beta carotene, and B6 at 100 mg b.i.d.

Various commercial athletes foot products are available as creams, sprays, and powders. We prefer Desenex.

ATTENTION DEFICIT DISORDER (ADD/ADHD, Hyperkinetic, hyperactive) is characterized as hyperactivity and inability to concentrate, cognate, and retain information. Many affected are disruptive, mean and cruel to other children and small animals, wet the bed, have nightmares, and like to play with fire.

ADD and ADHD individuals (children and adults) are sensitive to sugar (natural and processed) the way some people are sensitive to alcohol. This sugar effect ranges from narcolepsy (hyperinsulinemia coma), ADD/ADHD to downright madness (manic depression) and criminal behavior (school violence including shootings).

The standard medical approach to ADD/ADHD is to prescribe Ritalin or Prozac to chemically subdue the ADD/ADHD victim. The side effects of these drugs are significant and include biochemical and emotional addiction, drooling, drowsiness, and explosive emotions (violence, suicide, etc.).

Treatment must include complete removal of alcohol and sugar (natural and processed) from the diet and educating the ADD/ADHD victim that there is a connection between sugar consumption and their negative behavior. The whole family must eat the same way if this dietary approach is to be successful! Plant derived colloidal lithium, chromium, and vanadium are specific supplements to be taken. It is best to take all 90 essential nutrients.

AUTOIMMUNE DISORDERS of all kinds from kidney disease to rheumatoid arthritis (the autoimmune aspect appears as a secondary event rather than the cause as the "orthodox" doctor would have you believe) can be benefited by nutritional support. Essential fatty acids are of great value and may be taken alternately as salmon oil and flaxseed oil at the rate of 9 grams per day along with vitamin E at 1000 IU/day, 300,000 IU of vitamin A as beta carotene, vitamin C to bowel tolerance, zinc at 50 mg t.i.d., and selenium at 300–1000 mcg/day. Injectable thymus at 2–5 cc/day is very useful. Be sure to avoid fried foods, margarine, sugar, and caffeine. (See AIDS)

AUTISM is characterized by resistance to change, repetitive acts, and learning/speech disorders. Concurrent food allergies and hypoglycemia markedly aggravate the presentation of autism. Each must be dealt with as a separate entity if real progress is to be made. (Don't forget the baseline vitamin/minerals.)

Treatment should include avoidance of sugar and food allergens. Supplementation should include calcium and magnesium at double the supplement rate, B6 at five times the RDA for weight and age, and chromium and vanadium for the hypoglycemia. Autoimmune urine therapy can be very useful.

BACKACHE is usually a muscle strain from overwork and/or a "subluxation" (a malalignment of vertebrae) resulting from a fall, osteoporosis, arthritis, bone spurs and calcium deposits, auto accident (whiplash), or improper lifting technique. On occasion, a serious case of constipation will cause a "backache" from impacted stool or pressure from gas. Eighty-five percent of adult Americans get back problems. Plant derived colloidal minerals in the form of Dr. Wallach's Pig Arthritis Formula have been reported to rebuild cartilage, bones, tendons, and ligaments thus relieving back problems without surgery.

Prevention includes proper lifting technique (straight back and bend knees), strengthening exercises, proper nutrition including calcium (2000 mg) and magnesium (800 mg), high fiber diets, and eight glasses of water per day.

Treatment includes massage, chiropractic, hydrotherapy, Dr. Wallach's Pig Arthritis Formula, and poultices of herbs including comfrey (Symphytum officinale) and arnica (Arnica montana).

BAD BREATH (halitosis) can be dealt with by basic care. Use a good anti-tartar toothpaste, hydrogen peroxide tooth gel, floss upon awakening and after meals, use a hydrogen peroxide mouthwash, parsley may be used after each meal, and zinc at 50 mg t.i.d. Digestive enzymes with betaine HCl may be useful.

BALDNESS (thinning hair): see alopecia. Colloidal tin is reported to be effective!

BEDSORES result from pressure of body weight in areas of poor circulation—usually in areas of bony prominence. Massage, sponge baths and ultra violet light are good preventive therapies. Topical applications can include zinc oxide ointment, colloidal silver, plant derived colloidal minerals, aloe vera ointment, vitamin E oil and DMSO, eucalyptus (Eucalyptus globulus), wild carrot (Daucus carota), and comfrey (Symphytum officinale) may all be used topically and/or in poultices to encourage granulation tissue formation and healing.

BEDWETTING is a complex syndrome of children and teenagers. It can be the result of food sensitivities (frequently milk) or hypoglycemia (most often sugar sensitivities). Compare what happens when the "patient" eats complex carbohydrates, animal protein, ice cream, and cookies before bed. Pulse tests and diet diaries with elimination diagnostic diets will be revealing.

Kids who bedwet are also known to play with fire (literally) and are cruel to other kids and animals. They ultimately are potential perpetrators of violence, school violence, mass murder, and serial killings. This is a serious problem not to be treated lightly.

Treatment includes supplementation with all 90 essential nutrients. Pay special attention to chromium and vanadium at 50–150 mcg/day, unsweetened cranberry juice 4 oz. b.i.d., and calcium/magnesium (2000 mg/800 mg). Avoidance of sugar natural and processed, simple sugars (i.e. honey, sweet juices, fruit, etc.), and allergenic foods (i.e. milk and sugar being the most common).

BEE STINGS: A painful "sting" caused by the "injection" of bee venom (formaldehyde) by an agitated bee. Pain gels, DMSO, or Caladryl lotions are very effective in relieving the pain. On occasion an individual becomes sensitive or "allergic" to the bee venom. When this happens a potentially life threatening "anaphylactic shock" situation exists. Prevention is limited to avoidance of bee stings.

Treatment for individuals deemed sensitive to bee stings is limited to the use of adrenaline (epinephrine) from a "bee sting" kit.

BENIGN PROSTATIC HYPERPLASIA is perhaps the most common infirmity of aging in the human male. More than 500,000 American males (85 percent over the age of 50) are afflicted each year. As the prostate enlarges with age (usually the result of a zinc deficiency), the tight outer capsule prevents the gland from expanding outwardly so it squeezes down on the neck of the bladder thus producing the well-recognized symptoms of "frequency" and "urgency" in urination. The prostate is an internal gland that can be "palpated" (felt) with the gloved finger. If you are going to do this exam yourself, it is important to examine the prostate monthly like a woman examines her breast monthly. The normal prostate is firm like an orange and about the size of a walnut. It is found at a depth in the rectum that is just comfortably in reach for the average length index finger.

Benign prostatic hypertrophy produces a uniform enlargement that may be hard in "acute" enlargement or "boggy" in chronic enlargement. Tumors, either benign or malignant, tend to be irregular and nodular. PSA (Prostate Specific Antigen) may be elevated.

Benign prostatic hypertrophy is treated with zinc at 50 mg t.i.d., essential fatty acids as flaxseed oil at 9 grams per day, high fiber diets including pumpkin seeds and alfalfa, 300,000 IU vitamin A as beta carotene per day, vitamin C to bowel tolerance, chlorophyll (best source is alfalfa), amino acids (glycine, alanine, and glutamic acid) at five grams each daily for 90 days, hydrogen peroxide (20 drops per oz. of aloe juice) at 1 oz. b.i.d., unsweetened cranberry juice at two pints per day, herbs including saw palmetto (Sarenoa serrulata), and selenium at 250 mcg t.i.d.

BELL'S PALSY is the sudden drooping of one side of the face due to an inflammation, swelling, or squeezing (the result of osteoporosis) of the "facial" nerve (the 7th cranial nerve as it passes through the skull). Bell's palsy is often mistaken for a stroke because of the sudden onset. Numbness and partial or total loss of muscular control on the affected side of the face are the typical signs and symptoms. Treated properly, there can be as much as an 80 percent chance of significant recovery.

Treatment is B12 at 1000 mcg/day for a total of 20,000 mcg, calcium/magnesium at 2,000 mg and 800 mg per day, essential fatty acids at 5 gm t.i.d., and American ginseng (Panax quinquefolius). Colloidal minerals are useful. Treat for osteoporosis with Dr. Wallach's Pig Arthritis Formula.

BIPOLAR DISORDER (mania/manic depression) is one of those descriptive diagnosis that "orthodox" psychiatry issues. We would estimate that as many as 90 percent of the non-drug dependent patients are totally "curable" at home with home testing and home remedies. Food allergies, sugar sensitivities, environmental sensitivities, hypoglycemia, and hyperglycemia are the major considerations.

Testing for allergies can be accomplished using the pulse test and/or the diet diary and rotation elimination diet. Environmental sensitivities can be identified by the pulse test and avoidance/challenge tests. Hypoglycemia and hyperglycemia require a six-hour GGT. Be sure to record the emotions and behavior of the patient during the entire six hours—the numbers alone are not revealing in and of themselves.

Foods that are common offenders are cow's milk, corn wheat, soy, rye, and sugar. Environmental culprits include house dust, perfume, formaldehyde, and makeup. On the glucose tolerance test, the mania and/or depression may occur on the ascending or the descending arms of the curve so someone must stay with the patients and record emotions and events!!!

Treatment of bipolar disorder requires a considerable effort on the part of the "doctor" and "nurse" because a positive turn around may take some weeks with temporary relapses.

Treatment should include chromium and vanadium at 500 mcg q.i.d., autoimmune urine therapy for five to eight treatments, rotation or avoidance of offending foods, avoidance of sugar, caffeine, environmental allergens, essential fatty acids at 5 gm t.i.d., niacin (B3) 450 mg. q.i.d. in time release tablets, B1, B5, B6 each at 100 mg b.i.d., DL-phenylalanine at 5 gms b.i.d., and choline at 250 mg b.i.d. Plant derived colloidal minerals that contain lithium may be useful.

BIRTH DEFECTS (congenital birth defects) are a national crime in the United States! More than 98 percent are the result of preconception and early pregnancy malnutrition of the embryo! Today there are more teenagers that give birth to Down's Syndrome babies than women over 35. Down's Syndrome, Turner's Syndrome, gay behavior, cleft lips, cleft palates, hernias, heart defects, limb defects, spina bifida, anencephaly, etc. are all examples of preventable diseases that have been eliminated by the veterinary profession by taking great pains to give proper nutrition to the female lab animal, pet, and farm species before and during pregnancy. If you want to see why Americans have such a low rating when it comes to preventing birth defects (32nd in the world!!!), just go to a zoo on a Sunday or a fast food operation and watch what the teenage girls and pregnant women eat!

Prevention of birth defects requires more than "prenatal" vitamins after the second month of pregnancy when the "orthodox" doctor gives his pronouncement "you're pregnant." By then the embryo has formed all organs and tissues (for better or worse!). Conscious attention to preconception vitamins, minerals, and plant derived colloidal trace minerals and avoidance of alcohol is especially important to teenage and middle age mothers-to-be. Don't wait for anyone's advice, it isn't going to come. Do a home pregnancy test as soon as you think you're pregnant. If you haven't been taking supplements, start immediately!!!

BLADDER STONES (kidney stones, cystic calculi) are ironically caused by a calcium and/or a magnesium deficient diet and when you have raging osteoporosis. The minerals in the "stones" come from your own bones!!! Diagnosis may require an x-ray (a flat "plate" of the abdomen). Don't forget the gonadal shield!!! The signal to think "stones" is blood in the urine (use the urine test sticks) and pain or "colic" that gets worse in the bladder or kidney area. "Stones" are potentially very painful and may require Tylenol-3 or morphine to cope with the pain if they are obstructing a ureter (the tube from the kidney to the bladder).

Treatment should include an anti-inflammatory medication such as licorice (Glycyrrhiza glabra) to reduce swelling at the "log jam" so the "stones" can pass. If this isn't strong enough, you may have to resort to prednisone for three (3) days to accomplish this part of the therapy. Calcium and magnesium at 2,000 mg and 1,000 mg is imperative to stop calcium loss from the bones. Reduce meat intake (go more toward the vegetarian scale temporarily) to get your dietary calcium/phosphorus ratio in order. Herbs including dandelion (Taraxacum officinale), khella (Ammi visnaga), madder tea (Rubia tinctorium), and rupturewort tea (Hernia glabra), and unsweetened cranberry juice to acidify the urine can be used.

BLEEDING from superficial wounds is an easy medical problem to deal with by using pressure with a sterile gauze "sponge" or a "Band-Aid" on digits. Bleeding under the skin may indicate vitamin E or vitamin K deficiencies or excessive doses of prescription "blood thinners." Bleeding in the stool, on the other hand, can be a serious symptom indicating hemorrhoids (bright red blood on toilet paper), stomach ulcers (black bloody or "coffee grounds" stool), ulcerative colitis (bloody mucus in stool), colon cancer (bloody mucus in the stool), or coughing blood—lung cancer, etc.

Diagnosis of the serious causes of "bleeding" will require some sophisticated diagnostic techniques performed by a "user friendly" physician (depending on the state, this may include an N.D., D.C., D.O., or M.D.).

Regardless of the cause, superficial bleeding may be treated with poultices of plantain (Plantago major). The specific therapies for the more serious problems will be dealt with as they are discussed.

BLEEDING BOWELS can be part of the irritable bowel syndrome, chronic diarrhea, or intestinal catarrh. Hemorrhoids can show bright red blood on the toilet paper after passing a stool. On a serious note one needs to consider bowel cancer. Amebic dysentery and other parasites should also be considered in the diagnosis.

Treatment for the bleeding bowel should include mullein (Verbascum thapsus), vitamin C at 1,000 mg t.i.d. as time release tablets, alfalfa, and specific therapy per diagnosis.

BLEEDING GUMS are an early warning for several problems, including vitamin C deficiency (scurvy), calcium deficiency (or bad calcium/phosphorus ratio—osteoporosis), receding gums (the gums recede because of underlying bone loss), or vitamin E deficiency.

Treatment should include vitamin C to bowel tolerance, vitamin E at 800 IU/day, correct dietary calcium/phosphorus ratio with supplemental calcium/magnesium at 2,000 mg and 800 mg, herbal therapy including mouthwash with alpine ragwort (Senecio fuchsii), and mouthwash with aloe/hydrogen peroxide or colloidal silver.

BLOATING (gastric) is the accumulation of gas in the stomach. Normally the stomach is sterile because of the acid environment; however, when hypochlorhydria (low stomach acid) occurs, bacteria and yeast from the small intestine migrates up into the stomach. The bacteria in the stomach now "ferments" carbohydrates and sugars that are eaten and produce gas or "bloat."

Treatment of "belch, burp, and bloat" includes oral hydrogen peroxide (20 drops/oz. of liquid to dilute the hydrogen peroxide) at 1 oz. b.i.d., colloidal minerals and betaine HCl, and pancreatic enzymes at 75–200 mg t.i.d. 5 minutes before meals.

BODY ODOR (foot odor, stinky tennis shoes) can occur in anyone, especially teenagers and older people, and often indicates a zinc deficiency. Treatment includes zinc at 50 mg t.i.d., calcium/magnesium at 2,000 mg and 800 mg, plant derived colloidal minerals at 1 oz. per 100 pounds of body weight, lots of green leafy vegetables, alfalfa, and baths and deodorants with hydrogen peroxide. Use bleach to wash socks.

BOILS (carbuncles, abscesses) are usually caused by a "staph" infection of the skin and hair follicles. Boils can occur at a site of irritation. Usually they occur at the neck near a collar line. The tender pus-filled "boil" can be brought to a "head" by poultices of 3 percent boric acid and opened with a blade.

Treatment includes flushing the boil with sand sagebrush (Artemisia fififolia), enchinacea (Echinaca angustifolia) and/or hydrogen peroxide, vitamin C at bowel tolerance, vitamin A at 300,000 IU/day as beta carotene, and zinc 50 mg t.i.d. Antibiotic ointment may be considered if new boils appear until the vitamins and minerals begin to take effect. Don't forget the base line supplements.

BONE PAIN (including "spurs," calcium deposits, Osgood-Slaughter, Legg-Perthes) can be immobilizing and crippling. Bone pain can be part of the "growing pains" especially at the joints or the insertions of tendons into bones (which is where "spurs" occur). Bone pain is a self-diagnosing problem. If it persists, x-rays should be taken to confirm diagnosis of fracture, arthritis, "spurs," or rule the more severe problem of primary or metastatic bone cancer.

Treatment of bone pain and "spurs" includes Dr. Wallach's Pig Arthritis Formula, vitamin C to bowel tolerance, vitamin E at 800–1,200 IU/day, and magnesium at 500 mg t.i.d. for as long as one to two years. Correct the calcium/phosphorus ratio with calcium at 2,000 mg/day and reduce meat intake. Herbs including comfrey (Symphytum officinale) may be helpful. Plant derived colloidal minerals have reversed spurs and calcium deposits without surgery by remodeling the bone.

BREAST CYSTS (fibrocystic breast disease) are a painful and cosmetic disease, yet benign. The normal breast tissue is overgrown with scar tissue and cyst formation (usually multiple cysts). Prevention is simple enough and is related to avoidance of methyl xanthines (i.e. caffeine, coffee, tea, soft drinks, chocolate, etc.).

Treatment includes elimination of methyl xanthines from the diet, essential fatty acids 5 gm t.i.d., and vitamin E at 800–1,200 IU per day.

BREAST TENDERNESS (PMS) is a common symptom of PMS and early pregnancy. The tenderness of PMS is cyclical and that of early pregnancy will be associated with missed periods and a positive home pregnancy test.

Treatment includes vitamin E topically and essential fatty acids orally at 5 gm t.i.d., 2000 mg of absorbable calcium, avoid methyl xanthines, and remember the base line supplements.

BRITTLE NAILS are a common ailment, especially in vegetarians, teenagers, pregnant women, and individuals with food allergies. The causes of brittle nails are malabsorption or deficiencies of essential fatty acids, amino acids (low protein-vegetarian diets), collagen, keratin, calcium, iron, or zinc.

Treatment of brittle nails includes dealing with food allergies to improve absorption, gelatin (unflavored and unsweetened or diabetic brands), essential fatty acids at 5 gm t.i.d., vitamin E at 800–1,200 IU/day, the base line supplementation, and betaine HCl and pancreatic enzymes at 75–200 mg each t.i.d. 15 minutes before meals. To diagnose food allergies,use the pulse test—it's cheap and accurate.

BRONCHIAL ASTHMA: see asthma

BRONCHITIS (grippe, catarrh, chest colds) can be caused by viral or bacterial infections. Allergies, both food and inhalant, will aggravate bronchitis as will essential fatty acid, magnesium, and manganese deficiencies. If bronchitis persists after treatment for five to ten days, consider cystic fibrosis in children and lung cancer in adults. X-rays will be necessary to determine diagnosis of chronic processes.

Treatment includes steam vaporizers at night, essential fatty acids at 5 gm t.i.d., digestive enzymes and betaine HCl at 75–200 mg each, vitamin C to bowel tolerance, vitamin A at 300,000 IU as beta carotene, zinc at 50 mg t.i.d., and herbs including slippery elm (Ulmus fulva), coltsfoot (Tussilago farfara), cowslip (Primula veris), eucalyptus (Eucalyptus globulus) as a poultice/chest rub and/or place in vaporizer, Irish moss (Chondrus crispus), pansy (Viola tricolor), pleurisy root (Asclepias tuberose), and holly hock (Althaea rosea).

BRUISES are the result of a bump or blow that ruptures blood vessels and releases blood into the surrounding tissue including the skin. The fragility (tenderness) of capillaries can result from overdoses of blood thinners, copper deficiency, vitamin K, vitamin C, or vitamin E deficiencies.

Treatment includes vitamin C to bowel tolerance, vitamin E at 800–1,200 IU per day, vitamin K at 30 mcg per day, and pancreatic enzymes at 200 mg t.i.d. between meals. Take enzymes between meals so they get into your bloodstream and dissolve blood clots. Take DMSO topically, pain gel, and herbs including arnica (Arnica montana), marigold (Calendula officinalis), witch hazel (Hamaelis virginiana), and yellow sweet clover (Metilotus officinalis).

BRUXISM (teeth grinding) is the clenching or grinding of teeth. Bruxism usually occurs during sleep and is, therefore, often overlooked until wear of the dental enamel is observed. Bruxism can be the result of food allergies (use the pulse test to find out—sugar, milk, and wheat tend to be the offenders), hypoglycemia (bed-wetting and nightmares may occur with bruxism if hypoglycemia is involved), or deficiencies of calcium, magnesium, and/or B6.

Treatment includes avoidance or rotation of offending food and elimination of sugar from the diet especially before bed. Also take calcium and magnesium at 2,000 mg and 1,000 mg per day and B6 at 50 mg t.i.d.

BURNS are the painful result of contact with radiant (sun) or thermal heat (fire or hot materials). Prevention of sunburn is easy with modern "sun screen" products. The nose may need the special protection of zinc oxide ointment.

1st degree—red, painful surface burns from "sunburn," steam, etc. Dilute white vinegar 1:1 with water and cover burn surface twice daily.

Aloe vera or vitamin E oil can be applied locally.

2nd degree—some degree of damage into the second layer of skin with blisters. Bathe the burn area with vitamin E oil, colloidal silver, or cover with zinc oxide. Supplementation of vitamin C to bowel tolerance will be of value.

3rd and 4th degree burns are characterized by loss of skin, blisters, and, in the case of the 4th degree, actual charring takes place. These types of burns require professional help to prevent infection and fluid loss, and the patient may require "plastic surgery."

BURSITIS is an inflammation of bursal sacs that cushion tendons as they pass over joints (i.e. shoulder, "housemaid's knee," "miner's elbow," and "bunions"). Overwork of an "out-of-shape" joint can bring on a flare up. Don't forget the base line vitamins and minerals as a preventative along with moderate exercise.

Treatment of bursitis includes topical pain gels, DMSO, or liniments with eucalyptus to bring more circulation to the area and remove swelling (which is the source of bursitis pain). Oral support includes B12 at 1,000 mcg/day, vitamin C to bowel tolerance, bioflavonoids 1,200 mg/day, rutin 50 mg t.i.d., vitamin E at 800–1,200 IU/day, calcium and magnesium at 2,000 mg and 1,000 mg per day respectively, gelatin, cartilage 5 gm t.i.d., and alfalfa. Be sure to include Dr. Wallach's Pig Arthritis Formula in your bursitis program.

CALCULUS (tartar) is a build up of calcium carbonate on the tooth, usually at the gingival junction where the gum attaches to the tooth. The source of the calcium is the patient's own bony calcium which is being lost in the saliva. That's why tartar is worst on the back of the lower incisors. When this happens you may need more magnesium to hold calcium in the bones and correct a severe dietary calcium/ phosphorus ratio problem. Reduce red meat, soft drinks, and any other major source of phosphorus in the diet. The use of hydrogen peroxide tooth gels and antitartar toothpastes will help reduce existing tartar and prevent build up.

Treatment of calculus and tartar includes flossing, use a "dental pick" that you can purchase from a pharmacy to pop off large "plates" of hardened material from the back of and between teeth, use a firm tooth-brush and hydrogen peroxide tooth gels and tartar control toothpaste. Treat for osteoporosis with Dr. Wallach's Pig Arthritis Formula.

CANCER (carcinoma, sarcoma, neoplasm, tumor, and malignancy) is one of the more formidable syndromes (a disease is "one diagnosis/ one cause") of today. Prevention is the "magic bullet" that is effective against all forms of cancer.

Prevention of cancer (CA) takes a considerable conscious effort, but then, aren't you worth the same or more effort than the maintenance of your Porsche!!! Don't forget the base line vitamins and colloidal minerals. Be sure to incorporate dietary fiber in each meal. Try to OD on beta-carotene (almost impossible—first sign is dry skin) at about a vitamin A equivalent of 300,000 IU per day. Use selenium at 250 to 500 mcg per day. Avoid fried foods and margarine. Consume a lowfat diet, but don't forget the essential fatty acids for your immune system. Eat four to six cups of vegetables each day and drink eight glasses of water per day. Preferably drink filtered water; drinking distilled water on a regular basis will demineralize your bones! Don't smoke and only drink alcohol in moderation or better yet—not at all. Make sure you have at least two bowel movements per day (better yet, three). Use sunscreens in intense sunlight. Take alfalfa daily in some form as a detoxifier. Do a liver flush once or twice each month by drinking apple juice for three days. Do a hair analysis each year to monitor toxic metal load as well as absorption capability. If you are not absorbing very well, all your nutrient minerals will be low. Check for food allergies using the pulse test. Use biodegradable household cleaners. Avoid foods fried in fat or oil and use organic foods as much as possible. The diagnosis of cancer usually requires an ultrasound exam, biopsy, x-ray, or the use of endoscopic exams. Elevated CEA or PSA are signals to look farther. You are your own first line of defense, therefore, if you find an unusual lump, ulcer, bleeding, extended diarrhea, pain, change in urination or bowel habit, or mole that changes character you should consider cancer as a possible cause. If you do suspect cancer, start with your own therapies right away. It may be weeks before you can get to the "orthodox" doctor for a "rule-in" or "rule-out" diagnosis. Don't go for six months without treatment because the "doctor was too busy." What's more important, your health or his golf game? Once cancer has been "ruled-in" you should intensify your efforts in your own behalf as no one cares as much about you as much as you do!

Treatment of cancer is a busy procedure at best and until you get it "under control" it will take your full time effort whether you opt to take the "CUT, BURN, and POISON" route as well or if you opt totally for alternative therapies. A useful fact to help your thinking process is that the United States government says that THE FIVE-YEAR SURVIVAL RATE OF CANCER PATIENTS HAS NOT CHANGED OVER THE LAST 20 YEARS DESPITE NEW TECHNIQUES IN SURGERY, RADIATION, AND

CHEMOTHERAPY—IN FACT, UNTREATED PATIENTS, AS A GROUP, SURVIVED LONGER! What the government doesn't tell you is that the "untreated" patient group includes those treated with alternative therapies!!

As with any therapy, you will want to educate yourself to benefits and limits of alternative therapies. Using one system or medication for cancer therapy is like limiting the United States defense system to ground forces (this would be a totally absurd line of thinking in these days of nuclear warfare, ICBMs, submarines, etc.). Fortunately, other countries do not have an FDA and, as a result, they have more pharmaceutical companies willing to search for, and make available, medications that our FDA forbids. As a result, our health in terms of dollars spent (1997—$1.2 trillion) and return places us 23rd in the world—kind of frightening, isn't it! A list of medications follow with a brief discussion of the action of each and for what cancer they are recommended. Most can be administered to yourself on a maintenance level once the cancer is under control.

HYDRAZINE SULFATE inhibits the production of glucose from lactic acid in the liver, which literally starves the rapidly growing cancer cells. Hydrazine can prevent metastasis (spreading) and will reduce the size of large tumor masses. The shrinkage of tumor mass has all kinds of benefit including increase in appetite, feeling of well being, reduction in pain, mood improvement, and an improvement in circulation (blood and lymph). This compound is nonspecific and can be used for any tumor type cancer.

CESIUM CHLORIDE provides "high pH therapy for cancer" by entering the cancer cell and causing an alkaline environment. It is recommended for all types of cancer but is particularly effective for SARCOMA, BRONCHOGENIC CARCINOMA (with bone metastasis), and a spectacular 97 percent improvement of COLON CANCER.

LAETRILE, in short, releases small amounts of cyanide which normal cells can detoxify but cancer cells can't. The cyanide from the laetrile then kills the cancer cell. Laetrile may be taken as a preventative measure or a therapy.

GERMANIUM is found in significant amounts in a variety of plants including imported Shiitake mushrooms, ginseng, garlic, etc. Germanium functions by increasing the oxygen flow into cells from the blood (cancer cells do not like high levels of oxygen), increases macrophage (scavenger cells) activity, increases the numbers of antibody forming cells, T-cells, B-lymphocytes, and killer cells, and induces the body to produce interferon! This can be used as prevention or in therapy programs.

CLODRONATE is especially useful for preventing and controlling bone metastasis (spread of cancer from original site to the bone) which is common place in BREAST and PROSTATIC CANCER. Bone metastasis is very painful and difficult to treat with conventional chemotherapy. Clodronate works by stopping the loss of calcium from the bone so that the cancer can be effectively walled off.

FLUTAMIDE: and luteinizing hormone-releasing hormone (LHRH) together are more effective than surgical or chemical castration in cases of PROSTATIC CANCER as well as more aesthetically accepted. Flutamide therapy works well against the original cancer as well as the metastatic bone cancer. Flutamide produces an 81 percent remission against 0 percent remission for two years when compared with "orthodox" approaches.

HOXEY HERBAL FORMULA, a red clover herbal mix, is one of the granddaddies of the modern cancer remedies. It is nonspecific and may be used like Laetrile as a preventive or remedy.

LEVAMISOL is a new product (actually a sheep wormer) that has shown excellent results for cancer by preventing metastisis in general and specifically for colon, breast, brain, throat, esophagus, stomach, liver, and pancreas. LEVAMISOL could be a cancer "magic bullet" for the 1990s!!!

POLYERGA inhibits tumor growth by reduction of glycolysis. Polyerga is effective against tumor forming cancer and can be easily administered at home. It is, therefore, very economical.

There are many adjunctive therapies for cancer programs. Remember it is absurd to use single mode programs. Among adjunct therapies, hydrogen peroxide stands out. "Orthodox" medicine used H2O2 IV in the 1800s so there is lots of history with no bad side effects as well as lots of positive evidence that increasing oxygen in the blood has beneficial effects in your fight against cancer. Rremember cancer doesn't like elevated oxygen levels.

CO Q0 increases the immune fighting ability of your phagocytes as well as increases the efficiency of tissue detoxification.

DMSO is useful for the treatment of LEUKEMIA in that it causes the maturation of the "premature" WBCs of leukemia.

Thymus extracts are useful to enhance the thymus gland function and thus the immune system.

Autoimmune urine and autoimmune blood therapies enhance the body's defense systems against foreign substances including cancer proteins in much the same way that allergy shots do against pollen allergies.

Carbamide (urea) is in keeping with the autoimmune urine therapy. Carbamide is particularly effective for LIVER CANCER.

Beta-carotene taken with vitamin E can be taken at as much as 600,000 IU vitamin A equivalent! This will be of significant benefit in cancer therapy programs, especially CARCINOMAS. The vitamin A thus provided will also help the thymus gland produce antibodies and make laetrile more effective.

Selenium is a trace mineral that has been investigated very intensively as a cancer preventative and as therapeutic nutrition. 1,000–3,000 mcg/day is considered to be the proper therapy dose. The medical school at the University of Arizona (JAMA December 1996) showed that selenium given at 250 mcg per day will reduce your risk of esophageal cancer by 71 percent, prostate cancer by 69 percent, colon and rectal cancer by 64 percent, and lung cancer by 48 percent. The same study showed that if you give 250 mcg of selenium to a cancer patient, it can double their expected life span. In an earlier study, the Unversity of California at San Diego showed that 250 mcg of selenium every day will reduce the risk of breast cancer by 50 to 80 percent depending on the type of cancer. Plant derived colloidal selenium is 98 percent absorbable.

Shark cartilage and shark liver oil contain substances (angiostatin and endostatin) that stop the formation of capillaries that feed new metastatic growths of cancer. Although shark cartilage has been used by the Chinese for 5,000 years to treat cancer, the orthodox oncologists have pooh poohed this practice as quackery. Harvard Medical School and Yale Medical School have done 25 years of solid research on the effects of shark cartilage on the rate of cancer metastisis and have proved that angiostatin and endostatin do in fact retard the growth of capillaries that are necessary for the support of cancer growth. If you already have metastisis, the shark cartilage will shrink the metastisis and reduce pain. If the metastatic growth is smaller than a grape it may disappear altogether. You don't need to wait for the genetically engineered angiostatin or endostatin to appear on your doctor's prescription pad; if you have cancer start using shark cartilage at 70 grams per day. If you think this is expensive, wait til the genetically engineered angiostatin and endostatin hit the market!

Chemotherapy in "micro-doses" in conjunction with alternative therapies or chemotherapy into the arterial blood supply of the cancer infested tissue or organ can substantially reduce the negative side effects of chemotherapy.

Intravenous infusions with total nutrition, especially in the early phases of alternative therapy, are very useful in providing your body with much needed raw material for rebuilding normal tissue as well as replenishing the ravaged immune system. This total nutrition should include vitamins, minerals, amino acids, and essential fatty acids as well as electrolytes. It is well established that cancer patients have poor digestion and absorption. This poor absorption is probably from the long-term effects of food allergies on the gut producing celiac type changes.

CANDIDIASIS (chronic fatigue syndrome) is an infection caused by Candida albicans, a ubiquitous, normally harmless yeast (saprophyte) of your skin, mouth, vagina, and intestine. Under certain circumstances of reduced immune status this organism becomes a parasite and therefore pathological (disease creating) when its competitors—the normal bacteria of the gut—are killed by long term use of antibiotics, allowing them to proliferate unchecked. Hypochlorhydria, the reduced production of stomach acid (usually the result of salt restriction), allows the Candida albicans to move into the stomach—an unusual location. Stress will cause the reduction of stomach acid after stress reaches the point of decompensation. Food allergies change the lining of the gut in a manner very similar to celiac disease which causes an increased nutrient concentration in the gut—this hyperfertilized environment is very attractive to C. albicans. The overgrowth of the organism eventually spills over into the blood stream and, thus, infests the body proper.

Prevention includes being aware of your intestines and knowing your digestive and absorptive abilities and patterns. Do pulse tests for food allergies, avoid long term use of antibiotics, and as you grow older take betaine HCl and pancreatic enzymes before meals to offset the normal decrease in production of stomach acid. Be sure to take these digestive aids if you are under stress; deal aggressively with any disease that lowers your immune capacity!

The diagnosis of candidiasis may be made from symptoms. However, if you want a sure diagnosis, get a blood test for antibodies against Candida albicans or a skin test (very similar to a TB tine test). A positive test is a sure diagnosis. A negative test may or may not be revealing. Anergy is a state in which the immune system is so exhausted that it can't even react to a diagnostic test!!!

Symptoms of candidiasis include forgetfulness, irritability, fatigue, nausea, flu-like joint and muscle pain, and a high emotional state. Gastrointestinal symptoms may or may not be present (i.e. diarrhea, dyspepsia, gas, etc.). Most of the patients we see have been on oral Nystatin for some length of time with little or no positive effect. No wonder, since Nystatin is not absorbed into the body properly and therefore only controls the C. albicans in the gut.

Treatment for candidiasis includes treating food allergies, hypoglycemia, chemical sensitivities and any concurrent infection (i.e. herpes, EBV, CMV, etc.), and correcting indigestion. Hydrogen peroxide and enriched aloe vera juice may be taken orally at 1 oz. b.i.d. upon arising and retiring (we like H_2O_2 that is mixed with aloe vera which makes it palatable and makes it easy to take). Also, there is no danger in this diluted form. Hydrogen peroxide 10cc in a DMSO 10cc and 5 percent dextrose solution; 500cc should be administered IV to kill the systemic infestation. It takes 10–12 infusions to get the desired effect.

Germanium orally and IM is a good adjunctive therapy as it helps get oxygen into the cells. Remember Candida albicans is anaerobic and doesn't like oxygen.

Replantation of Lactobacillus acidophilus, a friendly resident of the gut and a primary competitor to Candida albicans, is a useful part of any treatment program. Use the retention enemas with 4 oz. of warm water containing 10 billion organisms (empty twenty 500,000 organism capsules into the water). A retention douche of 3 oz. for ten minutes weekly is suggested. The external genital area in both male and female may be washed with 3 percent hydrogen peroxide solution. Sixteen ounces of 3 percent hydrogen peroxide can safely be added to bath water. Autoimmune urine and blood therapies can be very useful in stimulating specific antibody production.

CANKER SORES (cold sores, fever blisters, aphthous stoma-stomatitis) can be precipitated by stress, consumption of certain foods as in food allergies (do the pulse test), and certain deficiencies. The canker sore is differentiated from herpes in that it only occurs on the movable oral mucosa of the lips and cheeks.

Treatment should include avoidance of allergens, zinc at 50 mg t.i.d., lysine at 1,500 mg/day, vitamin E at 800–1,200 IU/day, B-complex at 50 mg each t.i.d., and vitamin A at 300,000 IU/day as beta carotene.

CARBUNCLES (multiple boils): see boils

CARDIAC ARRHYTHMIA (irregular heart beat) is a common complaint of persons with food allergies and hypoglycemia, assuming organic heart disease has been ruled out. The classic for this syndrome is the "Chinese restaurant syndrome" which is caused by sensitivity to MSG. Many a patient with sudden irregular heartbeat and palpitations has called the ambulance thinking they had a "heart attack." By the time the ambulance arrived, they no longer had symptoms. A history of eating out, especially at a Chinese restaurant, is the give away.

Deficiencies that cause cardiac arrhythmia include B1 (i.e. beriberi), B3 (i.e. pellagra), B6, chromium, selenium (i.e. Keshan Disease, cystic fibrosis), magnesium, potassium, carnitine, and CO Q10.

Treatment of cardiac arrythmia includes avoidance of known allergens (MSG, sugar, etc.), autoimmune urine and blood therapies, chromium at 50–100 mcg t.i.d., B-complex at 50 mg t.i.d., selenium at 100–300 mcg t.i.d., magnesium at 1,000 mg/day, potassium at 500 mg t.i.d., plant derived colloidal minerals, carnitine, and CO Q10 per label.

CARDIOMYOPATHY (Keshan Disease, muscular dystrophy of heart) is recognized by the WHO as a selenium deficiency disease. This is the type of heart disease that makes individuals a candidate for heart transplant in the eyes of the "orthodox" physician. It is typical that $1/month in selenium supplement would prevent this disease and the "need" for a $250,000 procedure that carries a 20 percent mortality rate. This disease is also found in cystic fibrosis patients (one of the telltale signals that genetics has nothing to do with cystic fibrosis). Cardiomyopathy is known as "mulberry heart disease" in pigs and "white muscle disease" in cattle, sheep, and horses. It is interesting that veterinarians have eliminated this disease in animals with selenium injections and oral supplementation of diets. Again this is an example where it just might be better to go to your vet.

The diagnosis of cardiomyopathy is made from an ECG (electrocardiogram) and a x-ray or CAT scan in an "orthodox" cardiologist's office. The earliest signs are S-T and T wave changes. At this point, diet correction (avoid margarine and fried foods) and selenium supplementation will reverse this if the diagnosis is correct. The neglect of this will result in severe fatigue and sufficient heart muscle changes for the cardiologist to be able to "justify" a heart transplant.

The treatment of early cardiomyopathy includes selenium at 350 mcg t.i.d. or 1,000 mcg IM, plant derived colloidal selenium, vitamin E at 1,200 IU/day, and essential fatty acids at 5 gm t.i.d. I have personally seen individuals who have survived quite well with only selenium supplementation. They still have mild S-T or T wave changes but they have been working out in the rice fields as a field hand for 25 years after their diagnosis and treatment with selenium.

CARPAL TUNNEL SYNDROME (slipped tendon, perosis, angel wing) is caused by compression of the median nerve in between the tendons of the forearm muscles by a shrinking of the circular wrist ligament that holds everything together. This compressed nerve causes radiating pain in the palm of the hand and wrist, especially when the underside of the wrist is forcefully tapped with an index finger or a reflex hammer. Carpal tunnel syndrome is caused by a deficiency of arsenic, manganese, and choline.

Treatment includes B6 at 75 mg t.i.d., zinc at 50 mg t.i.d., plant derived colloidal arsenic, manganese, and choline. All of these nutrients are found in Dr. Wallach's Pig Arthritis Formula. Compare this with the "orthodox" therapy of wrist surgery!

CARSICKNESS (motion sickness, sea sickness, air sickness, or motion sickness) is common in some individuals when repetitive angular and linear movement occur at the same time. Fixing the gaze on a single geographic point can help in seasickness when the patient is on deck but is a fruitless exercise in other forms of motion sickness. Symptoms include "green at the gills" feeling including vertigo, nausea, and vomiting.

Prevention of motion sickness includes the use of scopolamine transdermal patches (can be worn behind the ear) or Dramamine (both medications can be purchased at the pharmacy without a prescription). Herbs that are useful for motion sickness include ginger.

CATARACTS are caused by changes in the eye lens, which makes them opaque and unable to transmit light to the retina of the eye. Cataracts are easily diagnosed with the ophthalmoscope in a darkened examining room. Severe mature cataracts are snow white and opaque like mothballs and are easily seen with the unaided eye through the pupil of the eye. Cataracts are the most common cause of blindness in older people and should be dealt with aggressively and without delay.

Treatment of cataracts includes avoiding fried foods and margarine, the base line vitamin/mineral supplement plus vitamin E at 2,000 IU/day, vitamin C to bowel tolerance, B1, B2, B3, B5, and B6 at 50 mg b.i.d., inositol at 150 mg/day, selenium at 250 mcg/day, zinc at 25 mg t.i.d., bioflavonoids at 300 mg, glycine at 200 mg, l-glutamine at 200 mg, l-arginine at 300 mg/day, l-cysteine at 400 mg/day, and glutathione at 40 mg/day. If diabetes or hypoglycemia is present, chromium and vanadium at 250 mcg t.i.d. should be added.

CATARRH (croup, whooping cough) is the mucus associated with a wide variety of nasal, throat, tracheal, and bronchial infections and/or irritations.

Treatment includes the use of steam at bedtime to break up the catarrh (mucus) and allow peaceful sleep. If this does not work and sleep is an urgent need, the use of drying agents such as Contac should be considered. Homeopathy can work quite well if a complete case is collected as there are many variables to be considered. Herbs that can be effective include vervain or wild hyssop (Verbena officinalis), cucumber (Cucumis sativa), wild cherry (Prunis serotina) and thyme (Thymus vulgaris).

CELIAC DISEASE (gluten enteropathy, nontropical sprue) is perhaps the most underrated disease in America today. Celiac disease is characterized by a loss of villi (finger-like projections) from the wall of the small intestines and a scaring of the supporting tissue, which effectively reduces the absorptive surface by as much as 85 percent. Classically celiac disease is caused by a wheat gluten sensitivity, thus the need for "gluten free diets." If this change were limited to wheat only, it would be of small consequence because it is easily recognized. Complicating matters is the fact that cow's milk albumen and soy protein can cause these same physical changes in the gut including loss of villi and scaring of supportive tissue of the small intestine progressing to the point where by age 45–50 years, 90 percent of the intestine can be damaged resulting in a significant reduction of absorptive surface. The result is poor assimilation of nutrients which are the raw materials for tissue repair, growth, and maintenance of all tissues and the immune system.

Celiac disease is, therefore, the basic cause of many diseases including diabetes (i.e. malabsorption of chromium and vanadium), cancer (i.e. malabsorption of zinc, vitamin A, and selenium), and muscular dystrophy and cystic fibrosis (i.e. malabsorption of selenium in the pregnant mother resulting in damage to the fetus).

Diagnosis and treatment of celiac disease includes using the pulse test for allergies (i.e. whole wheat is great unless your allergic to it!!!) especially wheat, cow's milk, and soy products and eliminating and/or rotating the offending allergen. Macrobiotic diets "work" not because there's brown rice, but because of the elimination of wheat gluten and milk products. It takes 90 days to repair the injured gut which means there is great hope if you take the effort to see if, in fact, you are sensitive to wheat, cow's milk, or soy.

CEREBRAL PALSY is a congenital birth defect which affects the cerebellum, the fine motor coordinator of the body. The cause is a preconception deficiency of zinc, copper, and B6 (perhaps celiac disease was the base cause of copper/zinc malabsorption in the mother). There is no treatment since the damage occurred to the fetus during the formation of the brain and you can't put the genie back in the bottle.

CEREBROVASCULAR DISEASE (senile dementia) is more common in the United States than anywhere else. The "hardening" of the middle cerebral artery (the main blood supply to the brain) results in poor oxygen supply to the brain, which causes loss of memory and typical "senile" changes. As with arteriosclerosis, the "hardening" of the arteries is caused by smooth muscle scaring, followed by calcification and fatty cholesterol deposits. The risk factors include elevated blood cholesterol which is a building block of vitamin D. Vitamin D is angiotoxic (toxic to blood vessels) causing scaring of arterial smooth muscle and subsequent calcification. Magnesium deficiency also results in "malignant calcification" of cerebral arteries.

Prevention includes comfortable collars and ties so "eddies" are not created in the carotid arteries, which contributes to the deposition of cholesterol. Reduce the amount of vitamin D intake to a maximum of 400 IU/day (this is a real toughie when you consider animal fat, cholesterol, milk, butter, various prepared cereals and snack bars, supplements, and sunshine). Optimal levels of all nutrients including magnesium can also prevent "malignant calcification."

Treatment of cerebrovascular disease includes EDTA chelation therapy to help remove plaque, hydrogen peroxide IV to increase oxygen, vitamin C to bowel tolerance, avoid alcohol, vitamin E at 800–1,200 IU/day, essential fatty acids at 5 mg t.i.d., selenium at 1,000 mcg/day, centrophenoxine at 1,000–2,000 mg/day, hydergine at 4.5–9.0 mg/day, vasopressin (DIAPID) at 12–16 units/day, Lucidril at 4.4–8.0 gm/day, piracetam at 1.6 gm t.i.d. and choline at 9 gm/day concurrently, and lecithin at 4 gm b.i.d.

CERVICAL DYSPLASIA is considered a "precancerous" change in the surface cells of the uterine cervix. The "orthodox" approach, cryotherapy, is primarily a "counter-irritant" procedure. In other words, create enough acute (new) damage so that the influx of WBCs and antibodies also help heal chronic changes as a "side benefit." It is known that cervical dysplasia is, in fact, a manifestation of a chronic zinc and vitamin A deficiency. Diagnosis is made from a PAP smear and/or biopsy.

Treatment of cervical dysplasia is accomplished by painting the affected surface with Lugol's Solution (an iodine preparation) and oral supplementation of beta carotene at an equivalent of 300,000 IU of vitamin A per day and oral zinc at 50 mg t.i.d. Don't forget the base line nutritional supplement here.

CHALAZION is the result of plugged "meibomian" glands in the eyelid. A chalazion is easily confused with a "sty" in the early stages. However, after a few days the swelling and pain disappear leaving a slow growing pea sized "mass" in the lid.

Treatment of chalazions include vitamin A at 300,000 IU per day as beta carotene, zinc at 50 mg t.i.d., and warm poultices of 3 percent boric acid on the closed lid, and an herb called eye bright. Boric acid ophthalmic ointment may be obtained from the pharmacy without prescription.

CHEILOSIS (angular stomatitis) is the result of vitamin B2 or riboflavin deficiency. The deficiency shows up as cracks in the corners of the mouth, nasolabial folds, and "geographic" tongue.

Treatment of cheilosis includes identification of food allergies and supplementation with B2 at 75 mg t.i.d.

CHICKEN POX (Varicella, Herpes zoster-shingles) is an acute viral disease in children and a chronic, painful disease in adults (i.e. shingles). Epidemics occur in children in winter and early spring. Day care children are almost guaranteed to contract chicken pox in their first year of day care. For those that are into vaccination, a post exposure vaccine is available for up to 72 hours post exposure. Clear vesicles surrounded by a small red zone characterize chicken pox. These lesions occur primarily on the upper torso.

Treatment of chicken pox in children is primarily symptomatic and includes Caladryl lotion topically, oatmeal baths, colloidal silver, and vitamin E oil applied directly to each vesicle or papule. Regardless of therapy, chicken pox will last from seven to twenty days.

CHIGGERS (mites) are small arthropods (eight-legged critters) that burrow into the skin and cause a severe pruritis (itching). These little creatures can be repelled while walking in the woods or meadows by placing pet "flea collars" around your ankles, waist, and wrists. The use of poultry dusting powder containing pyrethrums can be used in socks or belt line.

Treatment of chiggers once they establish themselves is limited to covering each burrow opening with clear nail polish, which literally smothers them.

CHILLS (fever) are associated with the flu and other viral infections. The patient will be sweating, shaking, trembling, and unable to feel warm, even when bundled up with blankets.

Treatment for chills includes wearing warmups with a hooded sweatshirt to cover the neck and head, massage, homeopathy, acupuncture, and herbs to include willow (Salix alba).

CHILBLAINS (hypothermia) are the lowering of body and/or limb temperature to subnormal levels for some length of time resulting in near frostbite. Severe numbness and loss of function may occur. Colds and flu may follow this challenge to the immune system. Prevention includes proper dress for the weather.

Treatment includes rapid warming in warm water and/or warm enemas, and electric blankets if available (underneath as well as on top).

CHOLESTEROL (elevated) is considered a risk factor for cardiovascular disease. Elevation of cholesterol above 270 mg per 100 ml of blood is a sign of increasing risk for cardiovascular disease, diabetes, and liver disease (including gallstones). There are numerous causes of elevated cholesterol including low fiber diets, elevated vitamin D intake, deficiency of EFA and chromium and vanadium, diets high in refined sugar and flour, liver malfunction, and poor exercise habits. CAUTION: Low cholesterol below 200 can be equally or more dangerous than elevated cholesterol!

Treatment for elevated cholesterol includes regular exercise, base line supplement program, one to two heaping tablespoons of oat bran or protein fiber (soy powder) in an eight oz. glass of juice, vitamin C to bowel tolerance, essential fatty acids at 5 gm t.i.d., niacin at 450 mg b.i.d. as time release tablets, calcium and magnesium at 2,000 mg and 1,000 mg per day, chromium at 250 mcg., vanadium 250 mcg, selenium at 300 mcg., and herbs to include evening primrose (Oenothera biennis). A good liver flush can be very useful.

CHOREA is characterized by uncontrolled jerky or crampy type movements that may be regular in frequency. The onset of chorea is subtle and may be limited to mood changes, faltering or hesitant speech, then progressing to uncontrolled facial movements and grimaces, "prancing" gait, torticollis (marked twist in the neck), and difficulty in swallowing. Chorea is considered to be a genetic disease by the "orthodox" doctors, however, this is highly unlikely as the onset classically occurs between the ages of 30 to 55 years (we have seen chorea in preteens and teenagers). There is organic disease of the brain with degeneration of the frontal cerebral cortex as well as deeper portions of the brain. The "orthodox" treatment for chorea is limited to sedation and tranquilization.

We recommend the base line supplement program, essential fatty acids at 5 gm t.i.d., B-complex at 100 mg b.i.d. each, vitamin E at 800–12,000 IU/day, selenium at 500 mg/day, lecithin at 2,500 mg t.i.d., and choline at 500 mg/day. Avoid fried foods, margarine, sugar natural and processed, and caffiene. Pulse testing for food allergies and hair analysis to monitor absorption is essential.

CHRONIC FATIGUE (candidiasis, EBV, HBLV, CMV, food allergies and hypoglycemia) by its very name (syndrome rather than a disease) lets you know that this is a complex of symptoms with multiple causal factors. To our knowledge all patients with Chronic Fatigue Syndrome have two or more of the causal factors associated with their "disease." Symptoms include moodiness, highly emotional state, aches, pains, depression, gastrointestinal symptoms (i.e. "belch, burp, and bloat"), intense fatigue, drowsiness, and muscular weakness. Blood tests for antibodies against Candida albicans, EBV, HBLV, and CMV are available for specific diagnosis; there is also a skin test for candidiasis.

Treatment for Chronic Fatigue Syndrome should include IV hydrogen peroxide in a solution of DMSO and 5 percent dextrose, IV nutrition, IM germanium, base line nutritional supplement program, and hydrogen peroxide (20 drops per oz. in aloe juice) 1 oz. b.i.d. Do the pulse test for food allergies and do a six-hour GTT for hypoglycemia. Eliminate caffeine, eliminate refined sugar, and avoid any food allergens. Treat hypoglycemia with chromium at 75 to 200 mg t.i.d. Employ autoimmune urine and blood therapies. Detoxify with liver flushes and colonics (especially for the first two weeks of therapy) to cope with toxins generated by organism die-off. For chronic fatigue related to viral infection, Isoprinosin at 500 mg t.i.d. and Ribavirin at 250–1,200 mg per day are suggested. Reflexology, massage, and naturopathic or chiropractic manipulation are great adjunctive therapies.

CLAUDICATION (intermittent) is a cramping of leg muscles following exercise as a result of poor blood supply. The reduced blood supply to the legs is almost always due to arteriosclerosis of the femoral and popliteal arteries. Typically, after a few moments rest, the patient can start walking again.

The diagnosis of intermittent claudication can be made from symptoms alone. The symptomatic findings can be supported by taking the "pedal" pulses (at the instep of the foot). These pulses should be strong and equal—very frequently one or both are weak or absent.

Treatment of intermittent claudication includes the base line nutritional supplements, IV EDTA chelation therapy, IV hydrogen peroxide, vitamin C to bowel tolerance, vitamin E at 800–1,200 IU per day, chromium at 75–200 mcg t.i.d., selenium at 100–500 mcg t.i.d., B6 at 100 mg b.i.d., hydrotherapy, reflexology, massage and light exercise (i.e. walking, swimming, etc.), and herbs including ginseng (Panax spp.) and cayenne pepper (Capsicum minimum).

CLIMACTERIC (menopause) is the cessation of ovarian function and the stopping of the menstrual cycle. Menopause is a natural event in a woman's life and usually occurs between the ages of 45–55 years. Menopause may be artificially induced by ovariectomy or hysterectomy. When the process is normal and thus takes a gradual course, the adrenals and liver increase their output of female hormones (primarily estrogen) and make up the difference from the lost ovarian function. "Hot flashes" and night sweats are common symptoms when insufficient estrogen is being produced by the adrenals or liver. Other symptoms include sweating, nervousness, fatigue, depression, insomnia, tingling, volatile emotions, crying jags, dry vaginal tract, and urinary frequency and incontinence. Osteoporosis is a common result of improperly managed menopause.

Treatment for menopause is probably an improper term as normal events don't need "treatment" but rather "support" or "management" on occasion to help smooth the transition. Estrogen supplements should not be used as they increase the breast and uterine cancer induction risk. Eat two eggs every day, red meat once each day, and the liver flush at least once per month. Use the base line supplement program, plus calcium and magnesium at 2,000 mg and 1,000 mg per day and herbs to include Lady's mantle (Alchemilla vulgaris), motherwort (Leo nurus cardiaca), and St. John's wort (Hypericum perforatum) and Betaine HCl and pancreatic enzymes at 75–200 mg t.i.d. 15 minutes before meals.

"CLUSTER HEADACHES" (histamine headache) are related to allergic reactions and may occur by themselves or be associated with other diseases and syndromes including Chronic Fatigue Syndrome and hypoglycemia. The symptom of one-sided headaches that come on suddenly, cause debilitating pain and that come and go in severity is diagnostic. Pulse testing and rotation elimination diets with the use of a "diet diary" for keeping track of symptoms (in this case, the "cluster headache") can be helpful. In addition to foods, there are many inhalant allergens including cigarette smoke, perfume, house dust, etc. that can precipitate a "cluster headache."

Treatment includes the use of the base line supplement program, vitamin C to bowel tolerance, bioflavonoids at 150 mg t.i.d., autoimmune urine and blood therapy and avoidance of environmental allergens, and avoidance or rotation of food allergens.

COLDS (nasal catarrh, coryza) are caused by more than 100 different viruses, this is why no vaccine has been made available. Symptoms last for 7–14 days regardless of therapy. The incubation is very short (1–3 days) compared to most viral infections (10–21 days) with a sudden appearance of symptoms which include tingling in the nose and throat, scratchy throat, nasal mucus, coughing, headache, and laryngitis. Elevated temperature or fever is variable depending on the particular virus that is causing the "cold."

Treatment of the "common cold" should include vitamin C to bowel tolerance, bioflavonoids at 150 mg t.i.d., garlic, gelatin capsules t.i.d., base line supplement program, chicken rice soup (proven by Harvard to be the best cold therapy) for protein (to replace that lost in the mucus— yes, mucus is protein similar to egg white) and electrolytes (especially potassium). Also have bed rest and avoid chills. Homeopathic remedies and herbs to include oldman's beard (Usnea barbata), bigleaf linden (Tilia platyphyllos), dogrose (Rosa canina), European elder (Sambucus nigra), European Holly (Ilex aquifolium), hemp acrimony (Eupatorium cannabinum), purple coneflower (Echinacea angustifolia), Queen-of-the-meadow (Filipendula ulmaria), sea buckthorn (Hippophae rhamnoides), white willow (Salix alba), wormwood (Artemisia absinthium), yellowbark cinchona or Peruvian bark (Cinchona succiruba), feverfew (Chrysanthemum parthenium), bachelor's buttons (Pyrethrum parthenium), sweet balm (Melissa officinalis), and cayenne pepper (Capsicum minimum) can be helpful.

COLIC (severe belly pain) can be initiated by a variety of causes including food allergies, hypochlorhydria (low stomach acid), and gas bubbles from fermentation, to more serious causes such as kidney or gallstones or blocked bowel. In this section, we will limit the discussion to food allergies, hypochlorhydria, and fermentation since they are all three related. Food allergies cause "celiac" like changes in the gut resulting in malabsorption. Bowel organisms "ferment" the unabsorbed nutrients causing "bubbles" which cause sufficiently sharp pain from distension to create colic. This is especially true in babies. In adults, stress and/or food allergies and salt restriction can cause hypochlorhydria allowing organisms to move into the normally sterile stomach and ferment food crating the "belch, burp, and bloat" syndrome or "colic."

The treatment for colic in adults includes the base line supplement program, betaine hydrochloride and pancreatic enzymes at 75–200 mg each t.i.d. 15 minutes before meals, and pulse testing to determine presence of food allergies. In babies, pulse testing and diet diaries to determine offending foods, pancreatic enzymes at 75–200 mg t.i.d. before meals (enzymes may be constipating), one to two drops of flaxseed oil after each meal, and B6 at 10 mg b.i.d. In older children and adults, herbs including dill (Peucedanum graveolens) and peppermint tea may be of value.

COLITIS is an inflammation of the colon, which can be caused by stress, food allergies, bacterial or viral infections, or low fiber diets, etc. Symptoms vary from cramping and diarrhea to constipation alternating with diarrhea, bloody mucus, ulcerative colitis, and diverticulitis.

Treatment includes cathartics or antidiarrheals as necessary, high fiber meals (i.e. potato, well-cooked oat bran, multi-grain breads), and avoidance of raw carrots, peanuts, and corn for the first week of therapy. Use pulse test to determine if food allergies are involved. If food allergies are present, use a rotation diet and autoimmune urine and blood therapy. Drink a minimum of eight glasses of water each day and eat four to six cups full of green leafy vegetables (i.e. spinach, cabbage, etc.) preferably steamed or cooked. Take oral hydrogen peroxide 25 drops of 35 percent in 1 oz aloe vera juice b.i.d. and aloe powder (Aloe vera) at 65–300 mg per day. Avoid fried food, margarine, and caffiene.

CONGESTED LUNGS (with bronchitis) can be treated with homeopathy, acupuncture, hydrotherapy to include a steam sauna, massage, and herbs including penny royal (Mentha pulegium) as concentrated tea. Treat with magnesium, manganese, and the essential fatty acids at 9 grams per day. Remember the baseline nutritional program. Avoid dairy products, fried foods, margarine, and sugar natural and processed.

CONGESTIVE HEART FAILURE can be caused by lung disease, anemia, low blood protein, high blood pressure, nutritional deficiencies including B1, iron, copper, and selenium. There is usually a rapid irregular heartbeat and edema (swelling from tissue water) in the legs and/or belly cavity ("dropsy"). Two natural medications stand out in their efficacy (these herbs are even used by the "orthodox" doctors): 1) Lily of the valley (Convallaria megalis), and 2) foxglove (Digitalis purpura). These two herbs can be taken as whole leaf preparations or fluid extracts. **Note: Foxglove is potentially dangerous so you should**

get commercially prepared sources and advice on doses!

English hawthorne (Crataegus oxyacantha) is a useful herb for regulating heart rhythm and treating dropsy of congestive heart failure. This herb may not be strong enough in severe or advanced cases. The precipitating cause of the congestive heart failure should be identified and dealt with aggressively.

CONJUNCTIVITIS is an inflammation of the membrane that forms in the inner surface of the eyelids and covers the white of the eye. Dust, allergens (i.e. pollens), and foreign bodies including eyelashes and microorganisms (bacteria and viruses) can all initiate conjunctivitis.

Treatment of conjunctivitis includes using artificial tears, commercial eye washes (hydrogen peroxide eye drops) and/or boric acid ophthalmic ointment as appropriate. Pulling the upper lid over the lower lid by grasping the eyelash, lifting out, then down induces tear flow to wash eye and flush foreign bodies.

CONSTIPATION is not only uncomfortable but is also a significant risk factor for cancer. If you are not having two to three bowel movements per day, you are constipated! Very frequently exercise such as walking and eight glasses of water per day will solve simple constipation. Very frequently food allergies will initiate constipation; do the pulse test to determine if this might be a factor. Milk products, including cheese, have a constipating affect on certain individuals.

Treatment of constipation includes eight to ten glasses of water per day, fiber/protein at 1 tbsp. in 8 oz. of juice b.i.d., rotation/elimination diet, autoimmune urine therapy for allergies, four to six cups of vegetables per day, exercise for 30 minutes per day, homeopathy and herbs including castor oil (Rincinus communis), olive oil (Olea europaea), blackroot (Leptondra virginica), American mandrake (Podophyllum peltatum), alder buckthorn (Rhamnus frangula), cascara sagrada (Rhamnus purshiana), flaxseed or oil (Linum usitatissimum), senna (Cassia angustifolia), and psyllium (Plantago psyllium).

CONTRACEPTION is historically a touchy subject. For knowledge of contraception and abortion herbs midwives were deemed to be "witches" and burned at the stake! Today, because of population problems, AIDS, and teen pregnancies, contraception cannot be ignored if we are to survive. Some governments—like that in China—have imposed "one child" limits on their citizens, give free contraceptives to anyone who asks for them, and most are offering a form of "sex education." Sex outside of marriage is "Russian roulette," anal sex is putting a loaded gun to your mouth and pulling the trigger!

Contraception is divided into abstinence, barriers, hormones (this is the least desirable from the standpoint of side effects), IUDs (intrauterine devices—be careful here—remember the Dalcon Shield!!!), and surgery (vasectomy or tying the fallopian tubes). The "rhythm" method cannot be considered a safe form of contraception outside of marriage because of the AIDS risk. Few couples have the consistent self-control necessary to prevent pregnancies.

CONVULSIONS (seizures, fits) are uncontrolled body movements set off by an electrical malfunction of the brain. High "fevers" of 104.0–105.0 F are often a cause of convulsions in children. Epilepsy is a form of convulsion that is easily diagnosed by abnormal brain waves seen on an EEG (electroencephalogram). Unfortunately, the "orthodox" neurologist doesn't think "allergy" or fat/cholesterol deficiency when a hysterical mother brings a child to his office with a history of one or more convulsions. The "orthodox" approach to treating convulsions is Dilantin and/or phenobarbital.

Treatment of non-temperature induced convulsions should include a pulse test to determine if allergies are a factor. If it is determined that allergies are associated with the convulsions, the patient may avoid the foods or chemicals or rotate foods on a five-day "rotation" diet. A high fat, high cholesterol diet is indicated. Supplements of value include calcium and magnesium at 2,000 and 1,000 mg respectively, B6 at 100 mg b.i.d., chromium at 75–100 mcg t.i.d., and herbs to include peony (Paeonia officinalia), catnip (Nepeta cataria), and skullcap (Scutellaria lateriflora). Chiropractic care and acupuncture can be of great value here.

COR PULMONALE is classically thought of as an enlargement of the right ventricle of the heart as a result of severe and chronic lung disease (i.e. asthma, cystic fibrosis, bronchiectasis). There is usually a rapid pulse, palpitations and edema of head, neck, and lungs (the latter can be fatal). Sometimes there is angina. "Clubbing" of the finger and toenails and cyanotic (blue from lack of oxygen) nail beds are frequently seen when the lung disease is chronic. X-ray will easily diagnose this problem.

Treatment of cor pulmonale includes resolving the precipitating lung disease and oxygen, IV hydrogen peroxide, and selenium at 500–1,000 mcg per day for adults. Remember the baseline supplement program.

COUGHS (catarrh, asthma, chest complaints) are very bothersome and distracting to everyone around the patient. Coughs can be caused by minor irritations of the throat including allergies (i.e. milk), viral infections, and chemical irritations. If a fever is present don't rule out milk allergies as milk allergies will cause a rise in temperature—use the pulse test.

Treatment should include avoidance of any allergen or irritant, autoimmune urine therapy (if allergic), steam vaporizers at night for sleep, and herbs to include anise (Pimpinella anismum), English plantain (Plantago lanceolata), licorice (Glycyrrhiza glabra), mullein (Verbascum densilorum), thyme (Thymus vulgaris), onion (Allium cepa), sweet chestnut (Castanea vesca), and comfrey (Symphytum officinale).

"CRABS" (pubic lice) are transmitted primarily by sexual contact. The "crab" (Phthirus pubis) causes a great deal of pubic and anal itching. They are relatively large yet difficult to see. Very close inspection with good lighting is required to find these insects. Very frequently dark "specks" of droppings of the lice can be found in white underwear.

Treatment should include specially formulated shampoos containing 1 percent gamma benzene hexachloride and direct removal of any visually noted "crabs."

"CRADLE CAP" (seborrheic dermatitis of infants) can occur as early as one month of age in babies. Cradle cap appears as a greasy thick crust on the scalp and behind the ears and face.

Treatment of cradle cap includes shampooing regularly to loosen the greasy scale, B6 at 10–25 mg per day, and zinc at 15–25 mg per day. Food allergies can contribute to this problem—do a pulse test.

CROHN'S DISEASE (regional enteritis) is a chronic infiltration or invasion of defensive WBCs and "macropohages" (special scavenger cells) into the terminal ileum (last portion of small intestine that joins with the colon). Several theories are currently in vogue as to the cause of Crohn's Disease including infection with T.B-like organisms (similar to Johne's Disease in camels!!!). Of interest here is the high incidence of Crohn's Disease in Minnesota compared with all other areas of the United States. A second and perhaps more realistic cause is a food allergy (i.e. wheat, milk), do a pulse test, and practice rigorous avoidance program of any identified allergens—this will prevent acute (sudden) attacks and actually result in reversal of the Crohn's changes to normal. Compare this with cortisone and surgery that the "orthodox" medics would have you choose!!!

Treatment of Crohn's Disease includes a high fiber diet. Use the pulse test to make sure you're not allergic to the type of fiber you use to supplement your diet. Take folic acid at 5–10 mg t.i.d., vitamin A at 300,000 IU/day as beta carotene, B12 at 1,000 mcg/day (best by injection in this disease), and vitamin C to bowel tolerance if it can be tolerated.

Calcium and magnesium at 2,000 and 1,000 mg per day, selenium at 300 mcg t.i.d., chromium at 75 mcg t.i.d., and zinc at 50 mg t.i.d. as well as the basic supplemental plan.

CUTS (lacerations) are caused by paper, glass, metal, knives, and tools. Most cuts, except deep facial wounds, can be dealt with at home without stitches (sutures). Superficial cuts from kitchen knives, glass, and metal can be cleaned with soap and water. The edges of the wound are then brought together with butterfly bandages or wound steri-strips. Actually there will be less scar formation with this method than with sutures.

Cuts contaminated with dirt (resulting from falls on gravel, concrete, wood, or soil) need to be washed with soap and water to remove gross dirt and debris. The second step for contaminated wounds is to flush well with 3 percent hydrogen peroxide to "bubble" out the microscopic dirt that harbor microorganisms. The wound edges can then be brought together with butterfly bandages or wound strips. A drainage site should be provided to allow free exit to any possible infection. Bleeding from cuts can usually be stopped with pressure bandages unless an artery is cut. A cut artery will "spurt" blood each time the heart contracts. Small arteries can usually be controlled by pressure with a sterile sponge (gauze square). Bleeding from a large artery in the arm or leg may require a tourniquet to control until you get professional help.

CYSTIC FIBROSIS (mucoviscidosis) is the "crime" of the century second only to diabetes. And it's second only because diabetes affects millions and CF "only affects thousands each year." In that CF is 100 percent preventable and 100 percent curable in the early stages in laboratory animals and can be far better managed in chronic cases than it is currently managed by "orthodox" medicine, it's the leading crime. Cystic fibrosis is an important fatal disease of humans. CF was originally thought to be limited to white populations of central European origin. Today, CF has been diagnosed in all peoples of the earth.

CF is thought to be genetically transmitted by the "orthodox" pediatricians, yet "they" have failed to prove their theory despite multimillions of dollars spent in research. Classically, the diagnosis is made when any two of four criteria are present, yet most "orthodox" pediatricians will not diagnose CF without a positive "sweat test" (elevated level of sodium, chloride, and potassium in the sweat—greater than 65 mEq/L).

The "sweat test" has been elevated by dogma to "the diagnostic test" for CF, yet there are at least 17 known diseases and syndromes other than CF that can give a positive sweat test, leading at least one group of investigators to refer to CF as a syndrome rather than a disease.

Initially described in 1933, CF was first thought to be the result of a vitamin A deficiency in children dying with celiac disease. In 1938, the term "cystic fibrosis" was coined because the pathologist mistakenly thought the changes in the pancreas were true cysts (fluid filled spaces lined with normal tissue). It is well known today that the "cysts" of CF are, in fact, a dilation of the pancreatic functional unit (acini) with atrophy (shrinking) of the lining tissue.

In 1952, the fact that congenital CF occurred in a significant number of CF patients was established. The foundation of the genetic theory of CF transmission is based on the frequent congenital appearance and two very poor papers, one published in 1913 which claimed that two children with diarrhea had an "inborn error in fat metabolism" and one in 1965 that did an epidemiological study of a group of 232 Australian families with CF. Despite six sets of twins, the study failed to shed clear light on the proposed genetic theory. These papers were so poor they would not get past the letter opener at any "orthodox" medical journal today. I have spent an inordinate amount of time on CF in DDDL because this syndrome again demonstrates very clearly that if any medical specialty will be eliminated by a discovery, that discovery will never be given to the public by the "orthodox" doctors!!!

In 1978, I made the first universally accepted diagnosis of CF in a laboratory animal (rhesus monkeys). The diagnosis was based on characteristic CF changes in the pancreas and liver in baby monkeys. These were confirmed by CF experts from Johns Hopkins School of Medicine, Emory University, and the University of Chicago! Experts from NIH and the CF Foundation were overjoyed—that is until they learned that I could reproduce the CF changes with a congenital selenium deficiency in almost any animal species. With this revelation, I was fired with 24 hours notice and "blackballed" from research. Just to show you how ruthless medical doctors are, I was fired ten days after my first wife died of cancer.

It has been learned recently that the positive "sweat test" is the result of an essential fatty acid deficiency that causes a secondary deficiency of "prostaglandin" (very short lived hormones) that control the sodium, chlorides, and potassium levels of the sweat!!! Remember the talk by the distinguished anthropologist, Dr. Jonathon Leaky, Sr. who said "the more facts you have, the better the truth you have."

The prevention of CF has been accomplished in pet, farm, and laboratory animals by the veterinary profession by assuring adequate levels of selenium and essential fatty acid nutriture to the preconception, pregnant, and nursing mother. This is not as easy as it sounds because of malabsorption problems (i.e. celiac diseases and Crohn's Disease) in a percentage of women! All things being normal, a complete baseline supplement program that provided 250 mcg selenium per day and 9 gm of EFA per day prior to and during pregnancy would be adequate to prevent CF.

Treatment of CF is very basic. Treat the infant as early as possible with selenium IM at 10–25 mcg per day. Plant derived colloidal minerals may be used orally thereafter. Provide EFA at three percent of the total daily calories. Most importantly YOU MUST DETERMINE IF THE INFANT IS ALLERGIC TO WHEAT, COW'S MILK, OR SOY! If you do not correct the malabsorption problem, treatment will only be minimally effective. In the case of older CF patients, IV essential fatty acids and IM selenium provide excellent management, possibly leading to a normal life expectancy of 75 years. Compare this approach to the heart and lung transplant offered by the "orthodox" pediatricians! If the proper treatment is carried out early, the "typical CF lung disease" may not develop. The lungs of CF patients are normal at birth and only develop bronchiectasis after chronic essential fatty acid and copper deficiencies have taken their toll. Don't forget the base line nutritional supplementation here!

Ma Lan and I went to China in 1988 to study Keshan Disease, a known selenium deficiency disease of Chinese children. We studied 1,700 autopsies and found 595 cases or 35 percent had pancreatic CF. An amazing discovery to be sure when "orthodox" medicine says CF is supposed to be "genetic disease of children of middle European extract"! I'm sure some creative proponents of the genetic theory will no doubt claim that a very virile English missionary impregnated 125,000 Chinese girls and, unfortunately, he was "carrying the gene for CF." Believe me, they'd rather postulate that outrageous theory than give up all that money for "genetic" research.

CYSTITIS (bladder infection) is a common urinary bladder infection in women. Low immune status, improper hygiene habits following bowel movements, pantyhose that are too tight, and frequent sexual activity (the reason for the term—"honeymoon disease") are common causes. The symptoms include frequency, urgency, and burning on urination. The diagnosis can frequently be made from symptoms alone, however, a urine "dipstick" test will show a positive nitrate test indicating bacterial infection. The test will be positive for a large number of WBCs in the specimen. Blood may be present in severe infections. Note: blood may also be present during the menstrual period so if the nitrate is negative and no WBCs are present, disregard. In older individuals, cystic calculi (bladder stones) may be considered as part of the cause of cystitis, especially in males.

Treatment of cystitis consists of acidifying the urine by consuming one to two quarts of unsweetened cranberry juice per day for the first day then reducing the intake to one quart per day as needed. Herbs are very useful and include bearberry (Arctostaphylos uvaursi), birch (Betula pendula, B. pubescens), juniper (Juniperus communis), lovage (Levisticum officinale), prickly restharrow (Ononis spinosa), and rupture wort (Herniaria glabra).

DANDRUFF is caused by a change in the surface cells of the scalp which results in a "scaling" or "flaking." This change is caused by one or more nutritional deficiencies. Dandruff may or may not be accompanied by itching.

Treatment of dandruff includes washing the hair in vinegar to remove all of the loose scales. Oral supplementation with EFA at 5 gm t.i.d., PABA at 100 mg/day, vitamin E at 800–1,200 IU/day, B6 at 50 mg t.i.d., 300,000 IU vitamin A as beta carotene and zinc at 50 mg t.i.d., and plant derived colloidal minerals are recommended.

DEMENTIA (memory loss, as in senile) is a common symptom yet not a true result of aging. Nutritional deficiencies (magnesium, vitamin B1, cholesterol), arteriosclerosis, and alcoholism are the common causes of dementia. Symptoms include loss of recent memory, inability to do simple thinking tasks such as math or spelling, losing things, forgetting names, etc. The use of memory enhancing drugs such as hydergine and piracetam will provide excellent prevention of dementia when used to augment good nutrition and supplement program. Don't forget the base line supplement program and plant derived colloidal minerals. Check patient for food allergies and hypoglycemia and take appropriate action if either are positive.

Treatment of dementia includes IV chelation with EDTA, B1 at 100 mg t.i.d., B6 at 50 mg t.i.d., B3 at 450 mg q.i.d. (time release), folic acid at 3–5 mg/day, choline at 500–1,000 mg/day, lecithin at 2,500 mg b.i.d., vitamin E at 800–1,200 IU/day, vitamin C to bowel tolerance, copper at 2–3 mg/day, magnesium at 1,000 mg/day, zinc at 50 mg t.i.d., hydergine at 9 mg/day, vasopressin (Diapid) at 12–16 units/day, centrophenoxine (Lucidril) at 4.4–8.0 gm/day, Piracetam at 2.4–4.8 mg/day, and betaine

HCl and pancreatic enzymes at 75–200 mg t.i.d. 15–20 minutes before meals. Useful herbs include ginko (Ginko biloba).

DEPRESSION (manic depression) is a common problem in the human population throughout the world—so common that some pharmaceutical companies specialize solely in antidepressant drugs. It should be no surprise, however, that very few of the supposedly "expert" psychiatrists ever consider hypoglycemia and food allergies when they do an intake history on a patient who complains of depression. Before you run off and spend $75–$150 per session with a "shrink," do a "pulse test" and a six-hour GTT on yourself. If you're really depressed, you will have to get a family member to help you run these tests to completion. Look for "allergic shiners" at the peak of depression. Spontaneous crying, thoughts of suicide, and hopelessness are common. Depression may be cyclic as in PMS (premenstrual syndrome). Food allergies, hypoglycemia, and PMS account for 90 percent of the diagnosed "depression" today.

Treatment of depression should include dealing with the food allergies (i.e. avoidance, rotation diets) and hypoglycemia (i.e. hypoglycemia diet). In addition to the base line supplement program, also use chromium/vanadium supplementation at 50–200 mcg t.i.d, iron at 15 mg/day, B6, B2, B1 at 50 mg t.i.d., B12 at 1,000 mcg/day, vitamin C to bowel tolerance, calcium and magnesium at 2,000 mg and 1,000 mg/day, potassium at 250 mg q.i.d., essential fatty acids at 5 gm t.i.d., and dl-phenylalanine, l-trypto-phane, and l-tyrosine at 2 gm t.i.d. each. Plant derived colloidal minerals with lithium can be useful. Avoid all sugar, natural and processed (read labels—it's in everything that comes out of a package, bottle, or box); avoid caffiene and fried foods.

DERMATITIS (atopic, eczema, herpetiformis) is a common form of skin disease but, unfortunately is treated incorrectly by the "orthodox" dermatologists who typically use cortisone or prednisone creams. Ninety-seven percent of these patients have food allergies to wheat gluten; an almost equal number are sensitive to cow's milk. The scary thing is that the symptoms you see on the skin are also happening in the lining of your small intestine. The lesions on your skin are a cosmetic problem; the lesions on your intestine area a serious life-threatening absorption problem which, in the end, will deplete your immune system of essential nutrients and result in a variety of serious illnesses including diabetes, cancer, arthritis, and birth defects.

Atopic dermatitis is characterized by patchy areas of crusty, weeping lesions frequently located on the lips, ears, neck, hands, and joints.

Atopic dermatitis is very frequently associated with asthma . Both together in the same patient is referred to as "atopy" or an "atopic patient."

Eczema is essentially the same lesion as atopic dermatitis but less localized.

Herpetiformis type dermatitis is characterized by clusters of itchy blisters that look like a Herpes eruption. Hair loss, or alopecia, is a commonly associated problem with any of the above dermatitis and a concurrent essential fatty acid deficiency.

Treatment of all three of the above manifestations of dermatitis should include a gluten free and cow's milk free diet. It is also prudent to do a pulse test on frequently consumed foods to determine if they are also affecting you. The supplementation of EFA at 5 gm q.i.d., PABA at 200 mg q.i.d., and betaine HCl and digestive enzymes at 75–200 mg each t.i.d. before meals should be added on top of the base line supplement program. Have patience; it will take 60–90 days to heal the intestinal lesions to the point where you can absorb nutrients efficiently. Vitamin A at 300,000 IU/day as beta-carotene and zinc at 50 mg t.i.d. and colloidal minerals are also recommended.

DIABETES is the number one shame of the "orthodox" doctors in the 20th century. Diabetes is easy to prevent, easy to cure and treat (in laboratory animals and probably in humans) so you can avoid all of the terrible side effects (i.e. blindness, hypertension, amputations, early death, etc.). Since 1958, it has been known that supplemental chromium will prevent and treat diabetes as well as hypoglycemia. Just ask any health food storeowner or N.D.! Walter Mertz (the director of the U.S.D.A. field services) published the facts associated with chromium and diabetes in the Federation Proceeding. Here is the ultimate case of a whole specialty of medicine which could be wiped out by universal chromium supplementation. Nevertheless these facts are kept secret and away from the public for purely economic reasons. Additionally, in 1985, the medical school at the University of Vancouver, BC, Canada stated that "vanadium will replace insulin for adult onset diabetics."

Chromium/vanadium and the diabetes story should be on the front page of the newspaper in the same bold print as VE DAY instead of announcing things like artificial heart pumps that will temporarily save one life for $250,000!

The diagnosis of diabetes is very easy to make and it should be considered in any disease where there is a chronic weight loss or weight gain. Frequent urination and chronic thirst are warning signs that should be explored. A six-hour GTT will show a steep rise of blood glucose at

30–60 minutes to over 275 mg % and may keep rising to over 350 and stay elevated after 4–6 hours. The urine should be tested for sugar with the "dipstick" test every time the blood is tested for sugar. A positive diabetic will always include a positive urine sugar during the six-hour GTT. A morning fasting urine sugar test is useless for the initial diagnosis of diabetes. Blood of the diabetic is also typical in that the lipids and cholesterol are elevated as well as the sugar.

Treatment of diabetes should include chromium and vanadium at 250 mcg/day in the initial stages to prevent "insulin shock" (sudden dropping of blood sugar because of a relative insulin overdose). Keep checking urine blood sugar before and after meals, and as the blood sugar level drops you can adjust your insulin or pill medication just like you have been taught. You will also need to deal with food allergies that cause celiac-type intestinal lesions (i.e. wheat gluten, cow's milk, soy, etc.) and supplement with betaine HCl and digestive enzymes at 75–200 mg t.i.d. before meals. Have patience; the intestinal lesions take 60–90 days to heal.

Treatment of diabetes should also include zinc at 50 mg t.i.d., B-complex at 50 mg t.i.d. (be sure to include niacin which is part of the GTF "glucose tolerance factor"), essential fatty acids at 5 gm t.i.d., B12 at 1,000 mcg/day, bioflavonoids including quercetin at 150 mg/day, copper at 2–3 mg/day, lecithin at 2,500 mg t.i.d., and glutathione at 100 mg/day.

High fiber, high complex carbohydrate diets are recommended. No natural or processed sugar and carbohydrates should be consumed. Eat meat, eggs, and poultry three to six times per day to stabilize blood sugar in the beginning stages of the therapy. Every time you eat processed carbohydrate (i.e. sugar, honey, alcohol, mashed potatoes, etc.), you will loose 300 percent more chromium in your urine than when you consume complex carbohydrates! Herbs are useful in treating diabetes and may include licorice (Glycyrrhiza glabra), jaborandi (Pilocarpus jaborandi), yarrow (Achillea Millefolium), Canadian fleabane (Erigeron canadense), and Jerusalem artichoke. Plant derived colloidal minerals are fantastic for diabetics!

DIAPER RASH is all too frequent in babies and toddlers, not only because of infrequent changes but also because of food allergies (i.e. wheat, cow's milk, soy, corn, etc.). Do a pulse test on babies as you introduce them to new foods (be sure to test the old ones, too). Use avoidance or rotation diet systems, B6 at 5–25 mg t.i.d., zinc at 5–15 mg b.i.d., and vitamin E oil and/or aloe vera topically.

DIARRHEA (dysentery) can be caused by simply eating too much of a good thing (i.e. fruit, juices, etc.), food allergies (i.e. celiac disease, strawberries, fish, etc.), soap ingestion from improperly rinsed dishes, or can indicate a more serious problem such as parasites, food poisoning, or even cancer. Knowledge of your own body and how it reacts is important here, as you will have to sort things out. Did you go to an apple farm yesterday and eat a peck of apples? Have you had diarrhea since your trip to Mexico? What medications are you on? Have you been losing weight and have diarrhea off and on for six months? If the latter, you may consider "irritable bowel syndrome" or the more serious, cancer. At any rate you should consider a "lower GI" or a colonoscopic exam.

Treatment for simple diarrhea can include commercial products such as Pepto Bismol or Kaopectate, charcoal capsules, fiber, and herbs including American blackberry (Rubus villosus), barley (Hordeum distichon), clove root (Geumur-banum), whortleberry (Vaccinium myrtillus), black currant (Ribes nigrum), hounds tongue (Cynoglossum officinale), Lady's mantle (Alchemilla vulgaris), and tormentil blood root (Potentilla erecta). Be sure to consume lots of fluids (i.e. soup, herbal tea, hot water with lemon, etc.) and all 90 essential nutrients to replace nutrients lost through diarrhea.

DIETING (weight loss) is a common practice in the western world because "thin is in." There are some basic habits that will help the weight loss effort and help keep the weight off:

1. First, avoid caffeine as it causes a drop in blood sugar 30–90 minutes after consumption and thus creates "hunger pangs," cravings, the "munchies," and binge eating behavior.

2. Drink eight to 10 glasses of water each day. As many trips to the icebox are caused by thirst rather than hunger, and a restricted diet doesn't decrease your need for water. Restricted diets do reduce your water intake from food as much as 40 percent, though.

3. Diagnose any health problems you may have such as addictive food allergies (pulse test), hypoglycemia (six-hour GTT), pica and cribbing (mineral deficiencies), or hypothyroidism (basal body temperature) that might contribute to a weight problem.

4. Don't skip meals. Eat a breakfast like a queen (or king), lunch like a princess (or prince), and dinner like a pauper. Stay on a meal schedule. If you are going out to eat, don't skip a meal but rather have one of those high fiber/low cal drinks or food bars for lunch to assure a limited calorie intake—then enjoy your dinner date!!! Remember, in the long run it's the basic habits that will help you

lose weight and keep it off. Don't forget the 90 essential nutrients. Supplementing with minerals eliminates cravings (pica and cribbing behavior).

5. Dr. Wallach's "Salad Fork Trick" is useful for people who "eat only salads, but still gain weight." DO NOT PUT SALAD DRESSING ONTO YOUR SALAD. Put the salad dressing in a small dish or shot glass. Dip your salad fork vertically (no scooping) into the salad dressing. This technique will reduce your calories from salad dressing from 1,000 calories per salad to 50 calories per salad, yet give you the salad dressing taste.

6. Exercise, if done in moderation and on a schedule, will help you lose weight and not make you overly hungry for a snack. Eat a piece of fruit or have some nuts after exercise. Don't wait three hours until your next meal to eat or drink. The plant derived colloidal minerals are excellent after-event refreshers.

7. Before meal fibers (i.e. carrots) taken with eight ounces of water 30 minutes before meals will help curb appetite.

8. Don't forget the base line supplements. Remember restricted diets restrict nutrients and result in pica and cribbing. Plant derived colloidal minerals are fantastic here!

9. Essential fatty acids in the form of flaxseed oil at 5 gm t.i.d. will help regulate and normalize fat metabolism.

10. Thyroid (US Armour) will help if your basal body temperature is low (below 97.6 F). Too much thyroid will cause increase in basal pulse rate and make you speedy and unable to sleep. Start out with 1/2 grain per day and cut back or add to as needed.

11. Use a good weight loss support product that contains pyruvate (fuel for the Krebs Cycle, the body's most basic metabolic process), chromium picolinate (allows carbohydrate and fats to be burned), and chitosan (a saturated fat binder) before each meal.

12. DO NOT EAT AFTER 7 P.M. Frequently, more than half of your daily calorie intake will occur after 7 P.M. Drink water if you get hungry.

13. If you do all of the above, you will be slim, slim, slim!

DIURETIC: use broom-corn (Sorghum vulgare), horse tail, coffee, tea, unsweetened cranberry juice.

DIURETIC & LAXATIVE: use asparagus (Asparagus officinalis), cascara sagrada, and dandilion root.

DIURETIC & CATHARTIC: use broom (Cystisus scoparius).

DIVERTICULITIS is an inflammation of the small pea sized sacs in the outerwall of the colon. This inflammation is the result of a low fiber diet over a long period of time which allows tiny concretions to build up to a size that does not allow them to exit into the colon. These concretions irritate the colon wall to the point of causing painful spasm. Prevention includes high fiber diet (i.e. oat bran, 4–6 cups of vegetables per day, etc.). Certain foods, including corn, peanuts, and raw carrots can result in severe spasms. Rarely is blood detected in the stool with uncomplicated diverticulitis. Diverticulitis is easily diagnosed with a lower GI series.

Treatment of diverticulitis includes colonics two to three times per week, high fiber diet, eight glasses of water per day, and regular exercise. Avoid fried foods, margarine, and caffiene. Don't forget the 90 essential nutrients.

DOUCHE: This is a useful feminine hygiene practice, especially if one has a history of discharges or infection. Retention douches are particularly effective. This is accomplished best in a bathtub with the feet up on the sides to aid in retaining the fluid for 10–15 minutes. Use 4–8 oz. of diluted vinegar (4 oz/pint of warm distilled water, 1 1/2 percent hydrogen peroxide (4–8 oz.), bayberry myrtle (Myrica cerifera—one oz. powdered bark to one pint water—warm to body temperature), and numerous commercial products. Plain unsweetened yogurt or Lactobicillus acidophilus capsules emptied into warm water (10–20 per 4 oz.) may be used to replant L. acidophilus to normalize vaginal flora after vaginitis and/or antibiotic therapy.

DROPSY (water belly, abdominal edema) is a common occurrence in chronic kidney, liver, or heart disease and cancer. Low protein diets will also result in "dropsy." "Dropsy" is fluid accumulating in the belly cavity because the protein content of the blood is so low that fluid can't be held in the blood vessels (an osmotic gradient); poor circulation because of liver or heart disease is also a common cause.

Treatment of dropsy should include an improvement of the protein level of the blood, IV amino acids and the basic health of the liver, kidneys and heart and diuresis. Herbs are particularly useful and may include foxglove (Digitalis purpurea)—BE CAREFUL HERE, THIS PLANT IS POTENTIALLY DANGEROUS—lily-of-the-valley (Convallaria magalis), English hawthorne (Crataegus oxycanthus), Canadian fleabane (Erigeron canadense), kidney bean (Phaseolus vulgaris), Scotch broom (Cystisus scoparius), parsley (Petroselinum crispum), prickly restharrow (Ononis Spinosa), and nettle (Urtica urens).

DRY SKIN (cracked cuticles, hang nails, cracked index finger and thumb) is a common malady in the western world. In itself, it is a cosmetic problem. It is a signal of a potentially more serious problem—essential fatty acid deficiency that can result in cardiovascular disease (i.e.—thrombosis, stroke, heart attack, etc.). Superficial creams will temporarily deal with the superficial problem, but the more ominous results of the body's deficiency of essential fatty acids can be sudden and deadly!!! DSM/EFA or "dry skin means essential fatty acids"!!! If you are supplementing with more than 50,000–100,000 units of vitamin A over a long period of time, dry skin may signal the early stages of vitamin A overdose.

Treatment of dry skin includes flaxseed oil orally at 5 gm t.i.d., B6 at 50 mg t.i.d., zinc at 50 mg t.i.d., vitamin E at 800–1,200 IU/day. If you are not already supplementing vitamin A in excess, use vitamin A at 300,000 units/day as beta-carotene for 30 days then reduce to 20,000 units per day.

DUMPING SYNDROME is the sudden "dumping" of stomach contents into the small intestine all at once, thus overloading the natural intestinal buffer system. The resulting acid condition in the intestine prevents proper functioning of pancreatic enzymes, which require an alkaline environment. Dumping syndrome is a common side effect of stomach surgery. Anemia and osteoporosis are common secondary diseases of the dumping syndrome.

Treatment of the dumping syndrome should include any of the classic "bitters" (i.e. gentian, Gentiana lutea), folic acid at 3–5 mg/day, pectin at 1/2 oz. in water before meals, and high animal protein diets. Eat six to eight small meals per day and you should lay down for a half hour after meals. Don't forget the base line supplements here!

DYSENTERY (diarrhea) is characterized by a watery projectile diarrhea that creates cramping, urgency, and exhaustion from loss of electrolytes. Causes of dysentery range widely from "too rich" a diet (usually too much party food—such as wine, lobster, creamy desserts, etc.), improperly stored food that results in bacterial overgrowth, food poisoning (i.e. E. coli, Staphlococcus, Salmonella, food allergies, celiac disease), etc. Prevention of dysentery requires attention to details of food storage, hygiene, self-discipline, and preparation.

If you have a busy schedule that can't be altered, you will have to resort to commercial products such as Pepto Bismol or Kaopectate. Fortunately, they have tablets that you can quietly carry with you on your errands. Weak black tea, rice water, lime (calcium carbonate) water, chicken broth, or bouillon to replace electrolytes are indicated. Another good source for fluids and electrolytes are the athletic "thirst quenchers." Herbs such as Irish moss (Chondrus crispus) and common ivy (Hedera helix) are of great benefit in quieting the runaway colon.

DYSLEXIA (learning disorder, hyperactivity) is a complex syndrome rather than a specific disease. To be sure, there are some dyslexic children who have true organic or biochemical brain injury (I.e.—fetal alcohol syndrome) who will require intense "special" education and training programs. It is a sad testimony to American "orthodox" medicine that as many as 80 percent of these "dyslexic" kids are really suffering from food allergies and/or sugar sensitivity. For them sugar acts as a drug and produces a "pharmacological effect" just like "speed." These food sensitivities create learning disabilities that "mimic" organic and chemical disease and too many salvageable kids are put on drugs (i.e. Ritalin), shunted off into "special" education programs or worse yet, given up on as "lost" by frightened, frustrated families. Food allergies and sensitivities should be seriously investigated and dealt with (i.e. pulse test, elimination diets, and diet diaries) if these children are to have a fair shot at a normal life.

I speak with a great deal of experience with this problem as my youngest son was deemed to be a "learning disabled" child. "Zero brain waves" would be a better description; at age six he couldn't print his first name or count to ten. To make a long story short, he was cured in two weeks by eliminating sugar, milk, wheat, and corn from his diet. His teachers were convinced that I had exchanged him with his "normal" twin. They couldn't believe such a turn around with just a dietary program! To condemn a "dyslexic" child without investigating food allergies and sensitivities is equal to finding an innocent man "guilty" of murder and sentenced to life in prison—what a waste and what a tragedy.

Treatment and prevention are closely intertwined. Digestive enzymes and betaine HCl are essential to prevent progression of the problem as well as aid in onset of symptoms. The "Feingold Diet" is a good place to start, however, it, in itself, is not a "shield" to be totally relied upon. There are many foods and food additives not excluded by the Feingold program that will set off some kids like skyrockets. We had one dyslexic child patient that did everything the Feingold Diet required except eliminate honey. We found him on top of a 40-foot dome! Rotation diets, allergy elimination diets, and autoimmune urine therapy should be aggressively pursued. The rewards are beyond your wildest expectations. The entire family needs to eat the same way as the dyslexic child if you want this to work. You can't be guzzling Pepsi and expect them to drink distilled water.

DYSMENORRHEA (menstrual pain) is a common event in western women, so common that it is frequently considered part of PMS. Sometimes the discomfort of dysmenorrhea is intense enough to be debilitating. There are a number of excellent commercial products that will dampen the pain but not deal with the basic problem—an abnormal prostaglandin metabolism.

Treatment includes B3 and B6 at 50–100 mg t.i.d., calcium and magnesium at 2,000 and 1,000 mg/day, vitamin E at 800–1,200 IU/day, and essential fatty acids at 5 gm t.i.d. Don't forget the base line nutritional supplements and avoid caffeine. Herbs such as blue cohosh (Caulophyllum thalictroides) and black cohosh (Cimicifuga racemosa) are the ideal natural approach to pain of dysmenorrhea.

DYSPEPSIA (poor digestion, indigestion) is characterized by "belching, burping, and bloating" and "acid stomach." The reason for "burp, belch, and bloat" is that your stomach's "acid" is not acid enough and is burped up with bacterially generated gas. Dyspepsia is probably the most common "disease" in the western world and is certainly the most costly from the amount of money spent on "relief." Even more costly is the secondary results of chronic dyspepsia: food allergies, osteoporosis, anemia, debilitated immune system, degenerative disease. Prevention includes reduced stress levels, exercise, healthful diet habits, and reasonable food volumes. An unforgiving event as we age is a decrease in stomach acid production, the main cause of dyspepsia in seniors. Prevention in this case includes the regular use of digestive aids.

Treatment of dyspepsia includes supplementation of 75–200 mg betaine HCl and pancreatic enzymes t.i.d. 15–30 minutes before each meal. "Antacids" are a good "temporary fix" in an emergency, but regular use will eventually damage you by reducing the nutrients you absorb. Herbal preventions and remedies include papaya (Carica papaya), common barberry (Berberis vulgaris), and bitters such as gentian (Gentiana lutea). In some cases, a glass of wine or several oz. of vinegar before meals will be helpful.

EARACHE (ear infections) like tonsillitis, sinusitis, and bronchitis are related in cause, prevention and cure. Allergies to cow's milk is the most frequent common denominator. So well does it mimic strep throat (including pain and fever) that most "orthodox" doctors will prescribe penicillin syrup for affected children over the phone!!! The "orthodox" EENT will want to surgically place "tubes" in the ears of infants and toddlers to treat "chronic earaches." Simple avoidance of cow's milk and cow's milk products will prevent chronic "earaches" and tonsillitis.

Treatment of milk allergy "earaches" and tonsillitis includes avoidance of milk and milk products and avoidance of sugar. Fever and discomfort are treated with demulcents and antipyretics (i.e. willow, Salix alba), and hydrogen peroxide eardrops and/or mullein oil drops (Verbascum thapsus). Treat as with any allergy including autoimmune urine therapy. True "strep throat" requires the use of penicillin.

ECCHYMOSIS (easy bruising) is very common, especially in women and children on low fiber, low fruit, and low vegetable diets (i.e. fast foods, lots of coffee, tea, and soft drinks).

Treatment includes alfalfa tablets at 4–6 b.i.d., vitamin C to bowel tolerance, vitamin K at 15 mg/day, vitamin E at 800–1,200 IU/day, and 4–6 cups of green vegetables each day. Avoid fried foods, margarine, sugar, and caffiene.

ECZEMA (atopic dermatitis, psoriasis) is a dry patchy scale on localized skin areas (i.e. ears, nose, joints, breasts, etc.). Eczema is usually the result of food allergies, especially cow's milk, wheat, and soy. Do pulse tests and elimination diets to determine the culprits. This is not only a cosmetic problem as the same damage is occurring in the intestinal lining which can lead to malabsorption, lowered immune status, and chronic degenerative diseases.

Treatment includes avoidance of offending foods, betaine HCl and pancreatic enzymes at 75–200 mg t.i.d. before meals, folic acid at 3–5 mg/day, essential fatty acids at 5 mg t.i.d., vitamin A at 300,000 IU/day as beta-carotene, zinc at 50 mg t.i.d., vitamin C at bowel tolerance, and vitamin E at 800–1200 IU/day; topical herbs include aloe vera (Aloe spp.), wild strawberry (Fragaria vesca), araroba (andira araroba) and Labrador tea (Ledum latifolium), comfrey (Symphytum officinale), English walnut (Juglans regia), European snakeroot (Aristolochia clematitis), flaxseed or linseed oil (Linum usitatisimum), German chamomile (Matricaria chamomilla), great burdock (Arctium lappa), high mallow (Malvia sylvestris), hounds tongue (Cynoglossum officinale), marigold (Calendula officinalis), oak (Quercus robur), and pansy (Viola tricolor).

EJACULATION (premature) is a common problem in today's busy world. Premature ejaculation is usually equated as "poor performance" on the part of the male. Premature ejaculation can easily be prevented and cured if both the "guy" and "doll" understand the basic cause. Again "orthodox" sexologists would have you believe that there is a "mental block" or some "deep seated guilt trip" that you have to deal with—anything to keep you coming again (pardon the pun). The true basics of premature ejaculation, which happens to all men given the classic circumstances, include a mental state of high expectation, infrequency of sex, and too much friction. The "orthodox" approach to therapy is to "think of draining your car's oil" so you're not thinking of sex! How absurd! How can you participate in the sex act and not be aware of sex? Who would want to?

Treatment and prevention of premature ejaculation are interrelated. The most important part of the treatment is to be very open about you and your "doll's" bodies. Spend a lot of time together naked, take showers together, read in bed together naked on top of the covers, have sex in any room (obviously you have to make sure the kids are somewhere else), give each other massages (both naked) until the sight of each other's naked body is no big deal.

Step number two is to have frequent sex. This definitely requires effort by both the "guy" and the "doll." Frequent sex means two to three times per night three to four nights per week. This is easier than it sounds when both are cooperating. The "doll" can't expect the "guy" to give a marathon performance once each week when she's in a high demand state but has been fending the "guy" off all week because she is into shopping with the girls or taking the kids to ballet, aerobics, movies, and grandma's. For the "guy's" part, he can't expect the "doll" to be receptive regularly if he isn't "romantic" (i.e. kindness, flowers, dancing, gifts, compliments, wine, perfume, shower, shave, after-shave—you know, just like when you were courting). The "wham, bam, thank you, ma'am" approach just isn't attractive to the "dolls."

The third aspect of preventing and curing premature ejaculation is lubrication. The "guy" must make sure that the "doll" is properly lubricated. This can be accomplished in many ways, including the "doll's" natural lubrication that results from emotional and sexual excitement and sexual stimulation. If the "doll" is a slow responder, the "guy" can liberally cover his penis with a water soluble gel (i.e. K-Y Jelly) as well as apply some to the vaginal opening. Slowly insert the penis into the vagina and just "let it soak." After awhile, the "doll" relaxes and the "guy" can move around a little without premature ejaculation. This is one process that there are no short cuts for. (Who would want any?!?)

Herbs, ginseng (Panax spp.), Dr. Wallach's Stud Horse Formula, and herb combinations (Zumba) are excellent tonifying agents for increasing the "guy's" potency. A prescription drug, Viagra, is available to help maintain an erection. It is expensive, however, and does have side effects.

ELECTRIC SHOCK can be fatal, even with the 110 electric outlets in the home. Toddlers sticking bobby pins or keys into the outlet can have a fatal shock; radios or appliances falling into the bathtub can be fatal to adults as can electrical repairs without turning off the breakers. Electricity kills by disrupting the electrical signals of the heart's regulating mechanism which causes the heart to "fibrillate" (quiver rather than beat normally) and the breathing muscles to become paralyzed.

Treatment of electric shock includes shutting off the source of electricity or breaking the electrical contact with the patient and reestablishing the basic functions of life with CPR (cardio pulmonary resuscitation) and oxygen. HAVE SOMEONE CALL 911 FOR EMERGENCY HELP!

EMESIS (vomiting) is a distressing event that may indicate overeating, cancer, excessive alcohol consumption, poisoning, food poisoning, food allergies, and infection (i.e. flu, EBV, Candida, etc.). In infants, vomiting with lethargy (unresponsive) and fever can be an ominous signal indicating meningitis. You may wish to cause vomiting when a child (or adult, for that matter) consumes a noncorrosive poison (i.e. rat poisons, toxic plants, household chemicals, etc.). "Coffee grounds" vomiting indicates large amounts of blood from a bleeding ulcer and/or stomach cancer and is a critical sign as death from uncontrolled bleeding can occur. Seek emergency help here. Early pregnancy often times will be heralded by nausea and vomiting ("morning sickness").

Treatment of vomiting can be simply to not eat for several hours, suck ice, drink small amounts of peppermint tea, and drink small amounts of chicken or beef bouillon. Drinking small volumes of athletic fluid/ electrolyte replacers is of value because significant amounts of potassium are lost through vomiting. If stomach irritation is severe don't be bashful about taking Pepto Bismol or Kaopectate—preferably the liquid to coat the stomach.

To cause vomiting in case of noncorrosive poisoning including drug ingestion, you can use the syrup of ipecac from your home "pharmacy" at 1 tsp. for children and 2 tbsp. for adults. Have the patient take in a large amount of water (one quart for an adult and as much as one pint for a child), and repeat the dose in 15 minutes if necessary.

ENDOMETRIOSIS is the abnormal implantation of the nonmalignant uterine lining cells in the body cavity. The endometrial cells are still sensitive to estrogen and therefore swell during high estrogen parts of the female cycle. Normally the uterine lining detaches from the uterus each month resulting in a mix of blood and tissue tags known as a "period." Normally the endometrial cells and blood flow out of the uterus through the vaginal tract out of the body. Any obstruction or damming of the normal vaginal flow pattern of the endometrial tissue and blood results in a retro-flow into the adominal cavity, where the endometrial cells find nurishment from the serosal surface of the bladder, colon, uterus, ovaries, etc. Tampons and sex during the "period" are the most common causes of endometriosis.

Treatment should include refraining from using tampons and refraining from having sex during the period. All 90 essential nutrients, including the use of wild Mexican yam (natural progesterone source) and herbs such as blue cohosh, black cohosh, and donqui will minimize the clinical discomfort. The use of Luperon (prescription posterior pituitary hormone) can shrink the maverick endometrial tissue to the size of a pea so it can be easily removed with endoscopic surgery. Luperon produces temporary menopausal symptoms that reverse after withdrawal.

ENURESIS (bedwetting) in children is another one of those outrageous syndromes botched by the "orthodox" pediatrician or, worse yet, the psychiatrist!! The "orthodox" view of enuresis is that it is "genetic," associated with "passive-aggressive" behavior, "dependency," "sleepwalking," "anti-social behavior," and "speech disorders."

Enuresis is, in fact, the result of food allergies (i.e. sugar, milk, etc.) and/or severe reactive hypoglycemia (chromium/vanadium deficiency). Calcium/magnesium deficiencies complicate the food allergies and hypoglycemia. All the behavioral symptoms associated with enuresis are pretty typical of "hyperactivity" which again is caused by the food allergies and/or the hypoglycemia, combined with unnatural interest in fire and cruel behavior. Bedwetting is a potentially serious sign of future violent behavior, especially if the child likes to play with fire and is cruel to little animals and little children—the "bad seed" syndrome. Employ the pulse test and a six-hour GTT to get a complete picture of the cause.

Treatment of enuresis includes eliminating the offending foods for food allergies, and eliminating sugar natural and processed including sweet juices, i.e. grape and apple from bedtime treats. Use digestive aids (i.e. betaine HCl and pancreatic enzymes) at 75–200 mg t.i.d. 15–20 minutes before meals, calcium and magnesium at 2,000 mg and 1,000 mg, and don't forget the base line supplement program for the 90 essential nutrients and the plant derived colloidal minerals.

EPILEPSY (fits, convulsions) is classically categorized by severity. 1) "petite mal," or small seizure, is often times a blank stare or dizziness that comes over the patient for but a brief moment, and 2) "grand mal," or large seizures, are spectacular convulsive attacks where the patient becomes stiff, falls over and begins to gnash his teeth and "flop" or "jerk" around the floor. The "grand mal" seizure can be fatal if the patient vomits and inhales the vomitus or hits his head; tongue biting commonly occurs.

Treatment of epilepsy by the "orthodox" doctor will include the use of phenytoin at 5–10 mg/kg in children and 300–500 mg in adults, phenobarbital at 5–10 mg/kg in children and 2–5 mg/kg in adults, and premidone at 10–20 mg/kg in children and 0.75–1.5 gm in adults (may need to increase slowly). These allopathic drugs will stop symptomatic convulsions. They do have dramatic and potentially dangerous side effects such as uncontrolled eye movements, weakness and stumbling, arthritis and osteoporosis, skin rashes and/or dermatitis, anemia, learning disabilities and hyperactivity. Vitamin B6 alone will frequently "cure" epilepsy at 50–100 mg t.i.d.. Long-term administration can cause some numbness and tingling in the face or hands. Adding Calcium magnesium at 2,000 and 1,000 mg/day, folic acid at 15–25 mg/day and B12 at 1,000 mcg/day IM can also be curative. Manganese at 50 mg/day, zinc at 50 mg t.i.d., essential fatty acids at 5 gm t.i.d., choline at 4 gm/day, taurine at 500 mg t.i.d., and dimethyl glycine at 100 mg b.i.d. are also indicated. High fat, high cholesterol diets are often helpful in resolving acquired seizure disorders not related to trauma.

EXOPHTHALMOS (bug eyes) is a prominent protrusion of the eyes from any of several causes including hyperthyroidism, tumor (especially if only one eye is affected), or glaucoma.

Treatment is specifically related to the cause. Blood test or axillary test for thyroid function, a glaucoma pressure exam and consideration of brain tumor (orbital or eye) is indicated.

EYE REDNESS (sties, pink eye) can be caused by dust, pollen allergies, bright sunshine, overwork, irritants (i.e. cigarette smoke), staying up late, infection, foreign body, etc.

Treatment of the eyes should be taken seriously. Infection can be treated with ophthalmic ointments with either boric acid or neomycin from your home "pharmacy." Commercial eye drops such as Visine work very well for simple irritation. Pulling the upper eyelid outward and over the lower lid will cause enough tear flow to wash out small foreign bodies such as eyelashes and dust. Herbs can be used for eye washes including eyebright (Euphrasia rostkoviana), fennel (Foeniculum vulgare),

German chamomile (Matricaria chamomilla), oak (Quercus robur), pasque flower (Pulsatilla vulgaris), and cornflower (Centaurea cyanus).

FAILURE TO THRIVE is a term used to describe an infant that falls below expected growth rates. Celiac disease and/or other food allergies and cystic fibrosis should be considered as the most common cause. Plant derived colloidal minerals are of great value here as most of these children are severely depleted in trace minerals and rare earths.

FARTING (bowel gas) is usually caused by digested but poorly absorbed food reaching the colon and being fermented by bowel organisms. Some foods such as beans, garlic, and onions are legendary for their production of bowel gas. Food sensitivities to wheat, wheat gluten, and dairy can cause celiac disease type changes in the small intestine, which results in malabsorption. The unabsorbed proteins reach the colon and are the source of sulfur that smells like rotten eggs.

Treatment for pathological amounts of unpleasant bowel gas includes the avoidance of offending foods and betaine HCl and pancreatic enzymes at 75–200 mg t.i.d. 15–20 minutes before meals where food allergies have caused celiac disease type changes in the small intestine.

FATIGUE (chronic fatigue syndrome, Candidiasis, Epstein-Barr Virus, cytomegalovirus, human herpes 6 virus, human B lymphotrophic virus, food allergies, hypoglycemia, diabetes, anemia, malnutrition) is the disease of the 80s. See specific disease description.

Treatment should be specific as described in appropriate section, and in addition, herbs may be of value including American ginseng (Panax quinquefolius), lavender (Lavandula augustifolia), rosemary (Rosmarinus officinalis), sweet flag (Acorus calamus), and pasque flower (Anemone pulsatilla). Avoid all sugar natural and processed, avoid soft drinks, and avoid fried foods, margarines, and caffiene. Take all 90 essential nutrients as a daily supplement to ensure that there are no nutritional deficiencies.

FERTILITY (problems) that are not related to physical blockage of egg or sperm transport systems are usually the result of some form of malnutrition, either overt (i.e. diet fads) or secondary to food allergies and/or malabsorption. One also must be sure that the woman is cycling and ovulating properly (i.e. slim women with less than 20 percent body fat do not ovulate regularly). Infertility usually means that the condition can be reversed whereas sterility usually means permanent nonreversible conditions. Do hair analysis and pulse test.

My oldest daughter and her husband had desperately been trying to have a child for 12 years and tried all the in vitro techniques with no results. She was brought to tears when she was told that she was "hopelessly sterile." I finally was able to get her to supplement with all 90 nutrients while she waited for adoption paper work to be processed. In just three months she was pregnant! It is amazing what a little nutrition will do.

Treatment of this form of infertility includes the base line nutritional supplement. Pay special attention to selenium deficiency in male infertility, betaine HCl and pancreatic enzymes at 75–200 mg t.i.d. before meals, correction of quality animal protein intake to a minimum of 100 gm/day (the RDA is only 40 gm/day), and essential fatty acids at 5 gm t.i.d.

FEVER or elevated temperature (normal is 98.6°F) is part of the body's defense mechanism. Many enzymes, antibodies, and cell (WBCs) responses are more efficient in slightly elevated temperatures. Elevated temperature during the day is not bad per se but should be reduced at night to allow comfortable sleep. Infants with high fevers of 104°F or above may have convulsions, which must be prevented or reduced quickly by immersion in tepid water.

Treatment of fever can include a number of commercial products including aspirin, Tylenol, Nuprin, etc. Ice packs on the forehead, running cool water over the wrists, cool baths, and herbs to include feverfew (Chrysanthemum parthenium), meadow-sweet (Filipendula ulmaria), sea buckthorn (Hippophae rhamnoides), European holly (Ilex aquifolium), white willow (Salix alba), mugwort (Artemisia vulgaris), and cinchona bark (Cinchona succirubra) can be used. Obviously, all of the above are symptomatic treatments. The basic disease process (i.e. cold, flu, pneumonia, cancer, etc.) must also be dealt with forthrightly with fluids (chicken soup), herbal tea, and tomato juice.

FIBROIDS are a runaway production of fibrous connective tissue and smooth muscle cells of the wall of the uterus. There are no agreed upon nutritional preventions or nutritional deficiencies that cause uterine fibroids. Looking at the tissue, however, there are certain similarities between fibroid tissue and the early changes of arteriosclerosis in the walls of muscular arteries and fibrocystic breast disease, giving some clues as to best approach uterine fibroids naturally. We know that magnesium deficiency is the cause of "malignant calcification" (arteriosclerosis) in the walls of muscular and elastic arteries. We know that eliminating caffiene and the supplementation of vitamin E and selenium enhance the healing process of fibrocystic breast disease.

Treatment of uterine fibroids should include avoidance of fried foods, margarine, and caffiene, as well as supplementation with all 90 essential nutrients. Crank up the magnesium level to 1,000 mg per day, vitamin E level to 2,000 i.u., and the selenium level to 500 mcg per day. If satisfactory results are not achieved in four to six months, one can consider the use of Luperon (posterior pituitary hormone sold originally to dry up milk supply). The fibroids will shrink suffiently to remove them with endoscopic surgery without the need for a hysterectomy. The side effects of Luperon treatment include temporary induced menopause that reverses after withdrawal of the drug.

FIBROCYSTIC BREAST DISEASE is cosmetically unpleasant and often painful during peak estrogen production. Cysts may vary in size from pea size to grapes and occasionally larger. Prevention and treatment are the same course of action.

Treatment of fibrocystic breast disease includes avoiding methyl xanthines (i.e. caffeine, coffee, black tea, ice tea, carbonated soft drinks with caffeine, chocolate, sugar, etc.), avoiding margarines and fried foods (avoid trans fatty acids and free radicles), vitamin E at 800–1,200 IU/day, vitamin A at 300,000 IU/day as beta carotene, essential fatty acids at 5 gm t.i.d., iodine at 200 mcg/day, and selenium at 500 mcg/day.

FIBROMYALGIA (stiff lamb disease, white muscle disease, adult onset muscular dystrophy) is a disease that was eliminated from lambs, calves, and pigs in 1957. It is a multiple deficiency disease caused by a high intake of fried foods and vegetable oils (margarine, cooking oils, and salad dressing) and deficiencies of selenium, vitamin E, and sulfur amino acids (methionine, mysteine, cystene).

Treatment includes eliminating all vegetable oils and fried foods (be sure to supplement EFA at 9 grams per day since you are cutting back on oils) and supplementation with selenium at 300 mcg/day, vitamin E 1200 i.u/day, and an amino acid program that includes methionine, cysteine, and cystine. Use Dr. Wallach's Pig Arthritis Formula.

FINGERNAILS (white spots, ridges, brittle) are good barometers of absorption and nutritional status. Bluish fingernails indicate chronic lung conditions (i.e. not enough oxygen); white spots indicate zinc deficiency; ridges can indicate iron and/or calcium deficiency; brittle nails indicates sulfur amino acid and protein deficiencies. Don't forget the base line nutritional supplements with all 90 essential nutrients.

Treatment of fingernail problems should include collagen (Willamette Valley which is 100 percent Kosher beef, diabetic Jello, or Knox gelatin— this is especially important for those who have been vegetarians for any length of time), essential fatty acids at 5 gm t.i.d., and betaine HCl and pancreatic enzymes at 75–200 mg t.i.d. before meals.

FITS (see epilepsy) can be caused by a variety of problems including epilepsy, high fever in children, low fat low cholesterol diets and certain poisons. See epilepsy. You may wish to call your local poison center "hotline" for poisoning. Keep the telephone number taped on your telephone, especially if you have small children. In addition to the medications indicated for epilepsy, you may consider mullein tea (Verbascum thapsus).

FLATULENCE (bowel gas, colic, farting) is a signal that unabsorbed foods, especially proteins, are reaching the colon where they are fermented by colon organisms. Do the pulse test to see if any allergies are present that might cause celiac changes in the small intestine.

Treatment of flatulence includes digestive enzymes at 75–200 mg t.i.d. 15–20 minutes before meals, betaine HCl at 75—200 mg before each meal, avoidance and/or rotation of offending food allergens, and herbs including angelica (Angelica archangelica), anise (Pimpinella anisum), caraway (Carum carvi), dill (Anethum graveolens), fennel (Foeniculum vulgare), and black pepper (Piper nigrum).

FLU (influenza, grip) is a potentially fatal viral disease. Infants and elder citizens are susceptible to the most serious complications if they are poorly nourished, immune compromised, or have a serious respiratory ailment (i.e. emphysema, asthma, pneumonia, CF, etc.). Flu is characterized by prostration, fever, diarrhea, bronchitis, coughing, headache, pneumonia, muscle aches, joint aches, and chills (feel cold and shaky but sweating). Flu typically occurs as a winter epidemic. Vaccination is very questionable for several reasons: 1) there are numerous strains and serotypes of flu virus (perhaps thousands!) so a vaccine for one strain or serotype is a "crap shoot" at best; usually you will come up "snake eyes" and get vaccinated for the wrong strain, 2) carte blanche vaccination has been identified as the probable vehicle for a variety of human epidemics including the first wave of HIV, and 3) permanent damage to the brain and nervous system is possible as a result of autoimmune reactions to the vaccine itself. Treatment for the flu includes antiviral agents such as Ribavirin at 1–2 tablets q.i.d. and/or Isoprinosin at 1 capsule b.i.d.; Fluviatol is another good choice at 2 tablets q.i.d. (pregnant women should avoid these DNA and RNA inhibitors because they potentially can cause birth defects). You will also want to include some protection against secondary bacterial pneumonia (i.e. Staphylococcus or Pneumococcus) such as echinacea (Echinacea angustifolia) or golden seal (Hydrastis canadensis). Individuals with low immune status or severe respiratory disease may choose to take antibiotics rather than a pneumococcus vaccine which is usually used on seniors at risk for pneumonia. Fluids (i.e. juices, chicken/rice soup, vegetable soup, etc.) are essential to prevent dehydration and replace electrolytes lost through diarrhea or vomiting. Vitamin C to bowel tolerance (if you already have diarrhea, take 1,000 mg time release tablets hourly during your waking day), vitamin A at 300,000 IU/day as beta-carotene, bioflavonoids at 150–300 mg/day, zinc at 50 mg t.i.d., ACE (adrenal cortical extract sublingual or IV), herbs including wormwood (Artemisia absinthium), cinchona bark (Cinchona succirubra), eucalyptus (Eucalyptus globulus), hemp acrimony (Eupatorium cannabinum), meadowsweet (Filipendula ulmaria), sea buckthorn (Hippophae rhamnoides), European holly (Ilex aquifolium), dog rose (Rosa canina), white willow (Salix alba), European elder (Sambucus nigra), broad-leafed lime (Tilia platyphllos), and bearded usnea (Usnea barbata).

FOOD ALLERGIES (sensitivities) are a concern for everyone. The reason is that the celiac disease type changes they cause in your intestines will prevent the absorption of essential nutrients that are required to keep your immune system, as well as your various organs, maintained, repaired, and in tip top working order. Many of the maladies caused by food allergies are not a direct cause but rather an indirect cause by cutting off the flow of essential raw materials necessary for your body to repair itself. A list of symptoms of food allergies would perhaps fill ten pages of this book. Suffice it to be said that if you have any chronic disease (i.e. cancer, diabetes, arthritis, heart disease, etc.) and/or emotional problems (i.e. hypoglycemia, depression, neurosis, schizophrenia, hyperactivity, paranoia, etc.) you have food allergies and hypoglycemia! Allergic "shiners" and "geographic" tongue are red flags. Incompletely digested proteins (polypeptides) getting into your blood stream cause food allergies. This happens to the fetus through the placenta (i.e. cystic fibrosis, celiac disease, etc.), to the nursing baby through the breast milk, and to the rest of us when our digestive system is not working perfectly (i.e. stress, aging, salt restricted diets, etc.).

The diagnosis and identification of specific food allergens takes quite a bit of work on your part to identify, but it is worth the effort as it will add 10–20 years to your life and make an enormous improvement in your quality of life. The easiest way to identify food allergies in yourself is the Coca Pulse Test. To perform this test, you learn your base pulse rate, then eat a single food (i.e. milk only, wheat only, etc.) and check your pulse 15, 30, and 60 minutes after you eat the single food item. An elevation in pulse rate of more than ten beats over the baseline pulse is an indicator that you are allergic to that food. You must be serious and aggressive at this project because it takes time and effort. After you get cancer, it is a little late to realize that you spent more time working on your lawn's health than you did on your own!!! A second method of allergy diagnosis can be used in conjunction with the pulse test is the diet diary. This diary is especially useful when emotional symptoms and headache are associated with food allergies. First, you eat a single food (as you do with the pulse test) noting the time on a pad of paper. Then record emotional symptoms and/or headache with the time. The symptom will appear within minutes to a few hours of ingesting the offending food (this includes hyperactivity and dyslexia). Do a six-hour GTT as almost everyone with food allergies has hypoglycemia because the celiac changes in the intestine prevent the efficient absorption of chromium and vanadium.

Treatment of food allergies includes religious use of the base line nutritional supplements (be sure to use hypoallergenic supplements—no corn, wheat, soy, egg, or milk). Avoid vaccinations that have egg, blood, or beef origins. Use vitamin C to bowel tolerance levels, vitamin A at 300,000 IU/day as beta-carotene, bioflavonoids at 150–300 mg/day, zinc at 15 mg t.i.d., essential fatty acids at 5 gm t.i.d., selenium at 300 mcg b.i.d., chromium and vanadium at 200 mcg t.i.d., betaine HCl and pancreatic enzymes at 75–500 mg t.i.d. 15–20 minutes before meals, ACE sublingual or IV, five day rotation diets, avoid offending foods, and have patience! It takes up to 90 days to repair the intestinal injury. The good news is that repair will take place even if you're 100 years old. IV hydrogen peroxide speeds up the healing process.

FRACTURES (broken bones) can result from malnutrition (i.e. calcium/magnesium deficiency, improper calcium/phosphorus ratio, osteoporosis) and severe trauma (i.e. a blow during a fight, auto accident, fall, etc.). Good mineral status in your bones will prevent most types of "spontaneous" fractures, compression fractures, and fractures from simple falls. Diagnosis of a fracture can be made by seeing a digit or limb at an abnormal angle, noticing severe pain at a specific place on the bone, and use a vibrating tuning fork to touch the suspected fracture site because the vibrations will be painful if there is a fracture present. X-rays in an emergency room may be warranted to differentiate between a fracture and a sprain or strain.

The use of the base line nutritional supplements (Dr. Wallach's Pig Arthritis Formula) including calcium and magnesium at 2,000 mg and 1,000 mg per day, plant derived colloidal minerals and digestive aids (i.e.

betaine HCl and pancreatic enzymes at 75–200 mg t.i.d. before meals) is an almost sure guarantee against nontrauma fractures especially in post-menopause women. The use of comfrey (Symphytum officinale) orally and over the injury site will speed healing of fractures as well as reduce pain and swelling.

FRECKLES (liver spots, age spots, sun spots) are caused by melanin pigment in response to sunlight in fair skinned people. "Liver spots" or "age spots" in middle aged and older people are sometimes difficult to distinguish from freckles. Liver spots and age spots are caused by "ceroid lipofuchsin" pigment build up in the skin from peroxidation of fats in your body (i.e. trans fatty acids and free radical damage) and are a more ominous sign than freckles. Freckles may be prevented or reduced by the religious use of sun screens by fair skinned people.

Treatment of freckles and "liver spots" includes avoiding fried foods and margarine, the use of vitamin E at 800–1,200 IU/day, selenium at 200–500 mcg t.i.d., vitamin C to bowel tolerance, vitamin A at 300,000 IU/day as beta carotene, essential fatty acids at 5 gm t.i.d., and the herb English mandrake (Tamus communis) topically on the spots b.i.d.

GALLBLADDER DISEASE (gall stones) is generally caused by liver problems, especially with fat and cholesterol metabolism. Gallbladder "attacks" are caused by a cramping of the muscles in the gallbladder after a fatty meal or a temporary blockage of the bile duct by a gallstone. Gallstones are composed of almost 100 percent cholesterol and fat when they first form. On rare occaisions they become calcified after the passage of time. Prevention of gallbladder problems includes the faithful use of all 90 essential nutrients to assure optimal liver nutrition, glycyrrhizin (an extract of the licorice plant, Glycyrrhyza glabra), and the base line nutritional supplement including 5 gm of EFA t.i.d. Fried eggs are known to precipitate 93 percent of all gallbladder attacks, followed closely by fried onions, fried potatoes, and pork.

Treatment of gallbladder disease and gallstones includes the use of high fiber diets (i.e. make sure you are having 2–3 bowel movements per day), lecithin at 2,500 mg t.i.d., EFA at 5 gm t.i.d., vitamin E at 800–1,200 IU per day, vitamin C to bowel tolerance, selenium at 200 mcg t.i.d., and taurine at 500 mg t.i.d. A liver "flush" is a time tested home remedy. Herbs to use include acrimony (Agrimonia eupatoria), blessed thistle (Cnicus benedictus), vumitory (Fumaria officinalis), horehound (Marrubium vulgare), licorice (Glycyrrhiza glabra), peppermint (Mentha piperita), wormwood (Artemisia absinthium), artichoke (Cynara scolymus), sweet coltsfoot (Petasites hybridus), celandine (Chelidonium majus), chicory (Cichorium intybus), and dandelion (Taraxacum officinale).

GEOGRAPHIC TONGUE (benign migratory glossitis) like allergic "shiners" is a red flag that you are not absorbing B3, B2, B6, B5, B12, folic acid, or zinc (the cause is usually malabsorption from celiac disease-like changes in the small intestine). Geographic tongue is recognized by irregular denuded areas on the top surface and sides of the tongue. Do a series of pulse tests to determine what foods you may be allergic to. Geographic tongue is not painful and taste may or may not be affected.

Treatment of geographic tongue includes avoidance of any offending food allergens, zinc at 15 mg t.i.d., betaine HCl and pancreatic enzymes at 75–200 mg t.i.d. before meals, B-complex IM in the early stages of therapy, and be sure to get on the base line supplement program.

GINGIVITIS (periodontal disease, receding gums, loose teeth, facial and jaw osteoporosis) is the shame of the dental profession, second only to mercury amalgam fillings. Gingivitis is totally preventable with proper nutrition and can very frequently be reversed with nutrition. It is the contention of the "orthodox" dental profession that food caught between the teeth and between the gums and tooth is the root cause of gingivitis and they have duly raised the stock worth of the dental floss companies. In reality, the reason the gums recede and food gets packed into the gingival space between the gums and tooth is that the "alveolar" bone supporting the tooth root has dissolved from a calcium deficiency and/or a phosphorus excess (i.e. too much meat, too much phosphate-containing soft drinks, etc.). The alveolar bone is very thin and fragile so minute losses in bone density are reflected more severely in the face and jaw than, in say, the femur (thigh bone). The truth would get rid of an entire specialty of dentist (periodontists), so it is kept in the dental research literature. Think about it, dogs and cats don't floss and they don't get periodontal disease or receding gums unless we feed them table scraps. Complete dog and cat rations have been formulated to prevent this malady. Again the veterinary profession is treating their patients better than their human counterparts!

Treatment of gingivitis includes the correction of the calcium-phosphorus ratio in the diet (consider gingivitis and periodontitis as an osteoporosis of the face and jaw). The correct calcium/phosphorus ratio is 2 calcium/1 phosphorus (most American diets are 15–20 phosphorus/1 calcium) and it is impossible to achieve without supplementation of calcium and consciously reducing the phosphorus intake (i.e. give up soft drinks, reduce meat intake, etc.). Take calcium at 2,000 mg and magnesium at 1,000 mg t.i.d. with meals until teeth tighten up and gums calm down and are not so inflamed. Plant derived colloidal minerals make this aspect of prevention and treatment easy. This heavy supplementation of calcium will not cause kidney stones (kidney stones are the result of raging osteoporosis). Rinse the mouth with hydrogen peroxide tooth gel and mouth wash, take vitamin C to bowel tolerance, and colloidal silver and herbs may be used for mouthwash to relieve inflammation and pain. Herbs to use include arnica (Arnica Montana), bilberry (Vaccinium Myrtillus), German chamomile (Matricaria Chamomilla), high mallow (Malva Sylvestris), and tormentil bloodroot (Potentilla Erecta).

GLAUCOMA is caused by an increased pressure in the eye itself which causes a change in shape, obstructing the normal flow of fluid from the eye. Food allergies are among the most common causes of increases in eye pressure. Do the pulse test to determine if you are allergic to any foods. Another common cause of increased eye pressure is muscular dystrophy or fibromyalgia of the eye muscles.

Treatment of glaucoma by the "orthodox" doctor is limited to a prescription of pilocarpine 4 percent every 15 minutes, surgery, or cortisone. You must do pulse testing and eliminate foods you are sensitive to, betaine HCl at 75–200 mg t.i.d. before meals, vitamin C to bowel tolerance, rutin at 20–50 mg t.i.d., and the base line nutritional supplement. DO NOT REDUCE MEDICATION WITHOUT A TEST THAT SHOWS A REDUCTION IN EYE PRESSURE.

GLUTEN ENTEROPATHY: see celiac disease

GOITER (colloid goiter, hypothyroid) is caused by a simple deficiency of nutrients (i.e. iodine, copper, molybdenum, the amino acid tyrosine, etc.). Nitrates are goiterogenic (stimulate goiter formation); they are found in luncheon meats, hot dogs, sausages, and a variety of prepared meat products. Another source of goiterogens is the nitrates in fertilizers, which gets into well water. If you get your water from a farm well, have it tested for nitrates because they are carcinogenic as well as goiterogenic. Cabbage, broccoli, and Brussels sprouts are also goiterogenic. Goiter is easy to diagnosis because the nutrient deficient thyroid gland enlarges 50–100 times its normal size; it is located just below the larynx in the front of the neck.

Treatment of goiter includes the removal of all goitrogens from the diet (read labels to exclude nitrates), supplement iodine at 250 mcg/day, and thyroid USP at 2–5 grains each morning. Kelp is a good natural source of iodine. Don't forget the 90 essential nutrients.

GOUT (gouty arthritis) is caused by deposits of uric acid crystals in the joints and surrounding tissues. These joints, classically the great toe of each foot, are very tender and may become deformed in chronic or long-standing cases. Kidney disease and uric acid kidney stones may develop in chronic untreated cases. Elevated uric acid in the blood (above 7 mg/100 ml of serum) along with sudden onset of tender "gouty" joints is a red flag for gout.

Treatment for gout should include an avoidance of alcohol, organ meats, seafood, lentils, beans, peas, and fructose sources. Use folic acid at 20–50 mg/day, cherries, and unsweetened cherry juice, and herbs including gout weed (Aegopodium podagraria) and meadow saffron (Colchicium autumnale). The "orthodox" doctors use colchicine almost exclusively as the treatment of choice, but add prednisone for inflammation.

GROWING PAINS (Osgood-Slaughter disease) are common in American children today. All you have to do is go to the zoo and watch parents carrying around six and seven year old children on their hip or pushing them around in an "18-wheeler" stroller! Growing pains are totally unnecessary and are red flags for one or more nutritional deficiencies. Prevention of growing pains includes the base line nutritional supplement rich in calcium, magnesium, selenium, vitamin E, and vitamin C including Dr. Wallach's Pig Arthritis Formula at 1 tsp/ 20 pounds body weight for kids.

Treatment of growing pains includes calcium and magnesium at 2,000 mg and 1,000 mg per day, selenium at 50–200 mcg b.i.d., and betaine HCl and pancreatic enzymes at 75–200 mg t.i.d. before meals, and Dr. Wallach's Pig Arthritis Formula at one tsp per 20 pounds body weight.

GUMS (bleeding, sore, pyorrhea) see gingivitis. You may also wish to rinse mouth with colloidal silver or a tea from the root of the white pond lily (Nymphae odorata).

HAIR LOSS: see alopecia

HANGNAILS are caused by an essential fatty acid deficiency. Treatment of hangnails includes flaxseed oil at 5 gm t.i.d. and 100 percent Kosher beef gelatin at one half ounce powder or 6 to 12 capsules daily. You may also wish to put vitamin E oil or aloe vera directly on the hangnail to soften it and reduce the probability of further tearing or infection. Small scissors or fingernail clippers can be used to "surgically" remove the skin flap.

HAY FEVER (pollen allergies) is caused by plant pollen allergies and tends to be seasonal and coincides with plant cycles. Symptoms include headache, red itchy eyes, nasal congestion, and asthma.

Treatment of hay fever includes autoimmune urine therapy after the first attack each year, commercial antihistamine products (i.e. Allerest, Contac, etc.), vitamin C to bowel tolerance, bioflavonoids at 150 mg q.i.d., and rutin 50 mg t.i.d. or as needed. The faithful supplementation of all 90 essential nutrients (including plant derived colloidal minerals) often times will reduce or even eliminate clinical symptoms.

HEADACHES are caused by a wide variety of problems. Food allergies (the primary cause of migraines) and hypoglycemia are major causes of headaches. Sinus headaches are often caused by allergies to pollens and milk products. Headaches can also be cyclic in PMS. Do a complete series of pulse tests and a six-hour GTT.

Treatment for headaches comes in the form of a wide variety of commercial products (i.e. aspirin, Tylenol, Nuprin, Bufferin), chromium at 50–200 mcg t.i.d., and betaine HCl at 75–200 mg t.i.d.

Avoid offending foods including all sources of caffeine. Use autoimmune urine therapy, vitamin C to bowel tolerance, B3 at 450 mg time release q.i.d., B6 at 100 mg t.i.d. or as needed, choline at 150 mg/day, and flaxseed oil at 5 gm q.i.d. Avoid simple carbohydrates, use proteins and amino acids for snacks. Herbs including feverfew (Tanacetum parthenium), fleabane (Erigeron canadense), balm (Melissa officinalis), cowslip (Primula veris), lavender (Lavandula angustifolia), queen-of-the-meadow (Filipendula ulmaria), valarian (Valeriana officinalis), and white willow (Salix alba) can be helpful.

HEARING LOSS (deafness) may require a "hearing aid" to amplify or correct the problem. On the other hand, sometimes cleaning the wax out of one's ear with hydrogen peroxide eardrops or a commercial earwax solvent will do the trick. I used to have an office down the hall from a hearing aid retailer—this fellow was so honest, he would always send his clients down the hall so I could clean their ears before he would examine them for hearing loss and fit them for hearing aids; we saw many a miracle of hearing return!!!. In children, manganese and/or tin deficiency can cause reversible hearing loss. Do a pulse test for milk allergies (another common cause of deafness in kids).

HEART DISEASE (heart attack, cardiovascular disease): see cardiovascular disease, see arteriosclerosis. Prevention is the name of the game when it comes to heart disease. Good nutrition means moderation in all things with no fried foods. The base line nutritional supplements are a must. Pay special attention to EFA, avoid as much of the polyunsaturated fatty acids as you can (other than the essentials—i.e. flaxseed oil and/or salmon oil), and pay special attention to selenium (500 mcg/day) and vitamin E (800–1,200 IU/day). Exercise in moderation (i.e. a 30-minute walk each evening is enough) and avoid vitamin D as an adult. More than 400 IU/day results in calcification of coronary arteries—the target tissue for vitamin D poisoning! Keep a 30-minute oxygen tank in your house (a two-hour supply if you live in a rural area), learn CPR, have nitroglycerin capsules or transdermal nitroglycerin patches on hand, obtain an IV infusion set and several 500 ml bottles of lactated ringers to set up an IV should a heart attack occur. Don't relegate your survival to an EMT who might or might now get there on time. Learn as much about emergency heart care as you know about your home's electrical system. Remember: UNPREPAREDNESS KILLS!

Treatment once you have had a heart attack includes EDTA chelation (with H2O2 added). You may need as many as two chelations per day for 80 or more days to ensure full recovery for your heart. Be aggressive. Your "orthodox" cardiologist will not agree to this so you will have to arrange it yourself! Increase your selenium intake to 1,000 mcg/day and your vitamin E to 1,200 to 2,000 IU/day and take 5–10 alfalfa tablets with each meal in addition to the base line nutrition program. Take two ounces of an oxygen supplement in the morning when you awake and two ounces before retiring. Take betaine HCl and pancreatic enzymes at 75–200 mg t.i.d. before meals. REFER TO YOUR PHYSICIAN'S DESK REFERENCE BEFORE TAKING ANY MEDICATION YOUR "ORTHODOX" CARDIOLOGIST WANTS TO PRESCRIBE FOR YOU! Don't take any medication you do not fully understand! Remember 40 percent of all patients are in the hospital because of iatrogenic disease (doctor mistakes in medication or surgery). Get back into your walking and/or swimming program as soon as you can.

HEARTBURN (dyspepsia, reflux) is one of the more common diseases in the USA today. Stress, salt restricted diets, and aging cause a decrease in stomach acid production which allows bacteria to grow in the stomach. These opportunistic bacteria generate gas and acid that results in the "belch, burp, and bloat" syndrome. Prevention includes eating small meals, no fried foods, and drinking eight glasses of water each day to prevent constipation.

Treatment should include betaine HCl and pancreatic enzymes at 75–200 mg t.i.d. before each meal. For acute attacks of "heartburn," any of the commercial products advertised on TV (i.e. Rolaids) may be helpful. Herbs to try include peppermint (Mentha piperita) and angelica (Angelica archangelica).

HEMORRHOIDS (piles) are varicose veins in the rectum and anus that itch, bleed, become painful, and eventually blocked with clots (thrombosed). The cause of hemorrhoids is primarily a copper deficiency (a breakdown of elastic fibers in veins), low fiber diets, the resulting constipation, and lack of exercise. The increased pressure needed to force out a constipated bowel movement causes ballooning of the hemorrhoidal veins. Bright red blood on the toilet paper after a bowel movement is usually from an irritated hemorrhoid. You may be able to feel the large grape sized "balloon" in the hemorrhoidal vein. Prevention includes high supplementation with all 90 essential nutrients, eight to 10 glasses of water each day, highfiber diets, and exercise.

Treatment of hemorrhoids includes high fiber diets (you may need to add oat bran at two heaping tbsp. in eight oz. of juice or water before bed) to encourage two bowel movements per day, hydrotherapy (Jaccuzi jet directed at hemorrhoidal tissue) b.i.d. as long as necessary, commercial topical products (i.e. Preparation H, etc.), and topical washes and/or compresses of herbs including German chamomile (Matricaria chamomilla), silver weed (Potentilla anserina), smart weed (Polygonium hydropiper), witch hazel (Hamamelis virginiana), yarrow (Achillea millefollium), juniper berries (Juniperus communis), horse chestnut (Aesculus hippocastanum), and plantain (Plantago major). SURGERY IS RARELY, IF EVER, NECESSARY!

HEPATITIS by dictionary meaning means any inflammation of the liver. In daily use hepatitis refers to any of three viruses that attack the liver: 1) Hepatitis A is transmitted by fecal-oral contamination (i.e. contaminated food, oral sex, etc.), 2) Hepatitis B is primarily transmitted by blood contamination through dirty "community" needles, and causes a more severe disease and is potentially fatal, 3) Hepatitis C is a newly identified virus associated with blood transfusions that causes chronic liver disease and death. Hepatitis can appear as a minor flu-like disease to a fierce fatal liver disease depending on your immune system's ability to fight off the virus. In China, where there is an endemic hepatitis rate of 10 percent (that is 100 million cases a year!), the rate of liver cancer is very high. Prevention of hepatitis is fairly simple—follow good personal hygiene, wash your hands after using the toilet, and wash your hands before cooking and eating. DOCTORS AND NURSES, PLEASE **WASH YOUR HANDS BETWEEN PATIENTS**. By not washing their hands between patients doctors and nurses cause two million infections each year in hospitals alone. Do not do illegal drugs, do not use "community" needles, etc. Follow the above simple rules and you will reduce your risk of contracting hepatitis by 97 percent. When my wife and I went to China, we took "Handi-Wipes" and washed all plates, cups, and eating utensils (i.e. chopsticks, spoons, etc.) before using them, even in public restaurants—we didn't contract hepatitis. Diagnosis of hepatitis is difficult in the early stages but easy after a week or so. Loss of appetite, prostration, nausea and vomiting, and fever are the early flu-like signs; after 3–10 days the urine will turn dark and jaundice (yellow eyes and skin) will appear. The patient feels better at this point. Blood test show a marked elevation in the SGOT (AST) and SGPT (ALT) up ten times the normal values; the elevated enzymes gradually decrease as recovery takes place.

Treatment of hepatitis includes bed rest and plenty of fluids including chicken soup. Avoid sugar, fat, margarine, and fried foods, and avoid alcohol. Vitamin B12 at 1,000 mcg/day, folic acid at 5–10 mg/day, catechin at 1.5 gm/day, vitamin C to bowel tolerance, and herbs including licorice (Glycyrrhiza glabra), chicory (Chichorium intybus), and dandelion (Taraxacum officinale), germanium at 25–50 mg/day, selenium at 200–500 mcg/day, and an oxygen supplement at one ounce on awakening and retiring.

HERPES (simplex, cold sores, canker sores) is a virus that causes recurrent blisters and ulcers on the lips (Type I) and on the genitals (Type II). This disease never goes away completely (once infected, always infected). The best you can hope for is long term remission. Herpes lesions itch at the early stages and can be very painful and disfiguring. These viruses are transmitted by kissing and sexual contact. Avoid kissing and sexual activity when the lesions are active. Use condoms during an active stage of genital Herpes.

Treatment includes ultra violet light directly on lesion for 1–6 minutes per day, avoid high arginine foods (i.e. avoid chocolate, peanuts, nuts, seeds, grains), eat high lysine foods (i.e. meat, potatoes, milk, yeast, fish, chicken, beans, eggs), vitamin C to bowel tolerance, bioflavonoids at 200 mg t.i.d., zinc at 75 mg t.i.d., l-Lysine at 1–6 gm/day to effect, then 500 mg/day maintenance, Ribavirin at 250–500 mg/day (do not take during pregnancy), and Isoprinosin at 500–1,500 mg/day (do not take during pregnancy), and topical herb compress with walnut (Juglans nigra). There are many commercial products available for topical application.

HERPES ZOSTER (shingles) is the result of a resurfacing of a long-standing infection with the "chicken pox" virus. The resultant skin eruptions are extremely painful, sometimes requiring hospitalization. Extreme pain can be elicited by the touch of clothes or sheets. The path of the virus is along nerves so a regular pattern for the skin lesions is typical.

Treatment of choice for shingles is Isoprinosin at 500–1,500 mg/day, Ribavirin at 250–500 mg/day, vitamin B12 at 1,000 mcg/day, vitamin C to bowel tolerance, vitamin E at 800–1,200 IU/day, lysine at 5 grams/day, and zinc at 15 mg t.i.d.

HIATAL HERNIA is usually a congenital birth defect (not genetic) of the diaphragm. It can also be caused by crushing the chest or abdomen as in an auto accident. Gas, dyspepsia, reflux, and chest pain that mimics a "heart attack" are common symptoms. It is said that more than 40 percent of the USA population has asymptomatic hiatal hernia by actual x-ray survey!

Treatment of hiatal hernia usually is restricted to treating the gas and dyspepsia with digestive enzymes and betaine hydrochloride. Six to eight small meals each day are suggested as is sleeping with the head of your bed elevated which often times prevents night-esophageal reflux while you sleep. When there is a large defect in the diaphragm (paraesophageal hiatal hernia) surgical repair is recommended to prevent strangulation of portions of the stomach, intestine, or liver.

HICCOUGHS are distracting and bothersome though rarely fatal. Hiccoughs are the result of spasmodic contractions of the diaphragm, closely followed by a sudden closure of the glottis. Hiccough "attacks" may be started by swallowing hot or irritating substances that irritate the vagus, phrenic, and recurrent nerves controlling respiration. Chronic hiccoughs can be the result of the vagus nerve being squeezed by connective tissue in the skull (osteoporosis) as the nerve exits the skull (a type of peripheral neuropathy).

Treatment of hiccoughs includes holding your breath. High levels of blood carbon dioxide inhibit hiccoughs. Drink a large glass of water, orange juice, or lemon juice slowly. Pressure on the closed eyes with the heels of your hands and digital pressure applied to the phrenic nerves just behind the sternoclavicular joint (where your collarbone joins your sternum) can be of benefit. Chronic hiccoughs should be treated as osteoporosis.

HOARSENESS (laryngitis) can be caused by too much yelling as at a football game or from many of the cold and upper respiratory viruses. If hoarseness persists there could be more sinister things going on such as muscular dystrophy or fibromyalgia of the laryngeal muscles.

Treatment of hoarseness includes use of demulcents such as slippery elm (Ulmus fulva) in lemon and honey, chickweed (Stella media), and the "singer's plant" or hedge mustard (Sisymbrium officinale) as a liquid extract. Avoid fried food, margarine, and processed sugar, and be sure to faithfully supplement with all 90 essential nutrients.

HYPERACIDITY (stomach acid, gas): see dyspepsia. Treat with fennel tea (Foeniculum vulgare).

HYPERACTIVITY (hyperkinesis, ADD, ADHD, Tourette's syndrome) is a very disruptive speeded up activity level to the point the attention span is less than a minute. The repetitive activity that develops is distractive to others in a classroom or family setting. Very frequently the activities are self-destructive, injurious to others, and create a learning disability. Food allergies, food sensitivities (i.e. sugar, milk, etc.), and hypoglycemia cause 95 percent or better of the cases of hyperactivity and hyperkinesis. Pulse testing for allergies and a six-hour GTT are essential here if you truly wish to correct the problem. Be sure to include the base line nutritional program. In addition to the behavioral problems, and certainly more insidious, are the "celiac" disease type changes in the intestines resulting from the food allergies which cause severe malabsorption of nutrients. In turn, the resultant malnutrition causes further behavioral problems.

Treatment of hyperactivity and hyperkinesis requires absolute adherence to a rotation and avoidance diet based on the results of the allergy testing and six-hour GTT. Supplement with betaine HCl and pancreatic enzymes at 75–200 mg t.i.d. before meals, Feingold diet (i.e. avoid sugar natural and processed, additives, food colors, etc.), IM or IV B-complex at 50 mg each per day, and chromium and vanadium at 25–250 mcg per day.

HYPERTENSION (high blood pressure) represents an elevation of the blood pressure above 140/90 mm Hg (the upper limits of normal). Either the systolic or diastolic numbers alone or both may be elevated. High blood pressure is complex and may be caused by many diseases ranging from simple nervousness in the examining room, arteriosclerosis, kidney disease, a variety of endocrine gland disorders, and food allergies. The most common reason for high blood pressure is a calcium deficiency and as a result high blood pressure is usually found in people with arthritis, osteoporosis, kidney stones, muscle cramps, etc. Do pulse test to identify offending foods. Do a hair analysis to check for excessive heavy metals (i.e. lead, arsenic, cadmium, and mercury). Don't forget the baseline nutritional supplements. CALCIUM DEFICIENT DIETS ARE KNOWN TO BE A MAJOR CAUSE OF HYPERTENSION.

Symptoms of hypertension include dizziness, red face, headache, fatigue, nosebleeds, nervousness, memory loss, edema of the optic nerve disc, strokes, etc. While not a symptom, obesity is a serious predisposing factor to hypertension; obesity also indicates mineral deficiencies.

Treatment of hypertension includes calcium (particularly useful is the plant derived colloidal minerals which are 98 percent absorbable), high fiber diets, rotation/avoidance diets, low fat diet (no fried food or margarines), avoid sugar and refined flour, avoid more than 400 IU of vitamin D, avoid caffeinated coffee or tea, chelation with EDTA, infusions with hydrogen peroxide, flaxseed oil at 5 gm t.i.d., garlic, reduce red meat intake, consume 4–6 cups of vegetables per day, CO-Q 10 at 60 mg/day, eight glasses of water per day, lecithin at 2,500 mg t.i.d., herbs including European hawthorn (Crataegus oxyacantha), rauwolfia (Rauwolfia serpentina), and olive (Olea europaea). Weight loss can drop elevated blood pressure dramatically.

HYPOGLYCEMIA (low blood sugar, hyperinsulinemia, narcolepsy) is placed in quotation marks in the medical literature. The "orthodox" idea for treatment of "hypoglycemia" is to "eat a candy bar anytime you feel an attack coming on" (by the way, these quotes are from the 1988 AMA Family Encyclopedia of Medicine!). With such an archaic approach to the treatment of such a simple problem, how can we trust the "orthodox" medical community with something as complex as cancer!!! The cause of hypoglycemia is almost always food allergies that cause a malabsorption of chromium and vanadium as a result of celiac disease type changes in the intestine and/or a large intake of sugar (natural and processed) and refined flour which increases the dumping of chromium and vanadium in the urine as much as 300 percent. The old wives' tale "if you eat sugar from the sugar bowl, you will surely develop diabetes" is then quite true as untreated hypoglycemia will very frequently develop into diabetes. The symptoms of hypoglycemia are highly variable and may include emotional symptoms (i.e. hyperactivity, paranoia, schizophrenia, memory loss, irritability, hallucinations, depression, manic depression, bi-polar disease, dyslexia, crying, learning disabilities, ADD, ADHD, Tourette's syndrome, etc.), sleepiness, narcolepsy, fatigue, heart palpitations, sweating, inability to do cognitive tasks (i.e. inability to think out simple problems), explosive reactive anger, negative thinking, and catatonia and/or coma-like states.

The diagnosis of hypoglycemia requires a six-hour GTT. A FASTING

BLOOD SUGAR ALONE WILL NOT DIAGNOSE HYPOGLYCEMIA OR DIABETES IN 98 PERCENT OF THE CASES; THERE ARE NO SHORT CUTS TO THIS DIAGNOSIS!!! A finger prick is done in the morning while fasting and the fasting blood sugar level is recorded (normal is 75 mg % give or take 5 points). Then 100 gm of glucose (Glucola) is ingested and a finger prick blood glucose is taken 30 minutes after ingestion and the results recorded. A finger prick blood glucose is taken at 60 minutes after ingestion of the glucose and at hourly intervals thereafter for a total of eight finger sticks (easy to remember as you have eight fingers!). It is of extreme importance to have an observer present during the entire test, not because the test is dangerous, rather because behavioral changes are best recognized by someone else. Having the "patient" write their name, draw pictures, etc. can be very useful, especially in children where they may have a difficult time describing how they feel. These tests and observations should be done every 30 minutes during the six-hour test. A chart is then developed using the numbers gathered to assess the patient's glucose status. Hypoglycemia exists when the low during the test drops below the level of the starting fasting blood sugar level. Elevated blood sugar can produce behavioral changes as the blood sugar rises after a meal much in the same way that alcohol or drugs do (in fact, many hypoglycemics are falsely accused of being intoxicated!). Diabetes can be diagnosed when the total of the results of the fasting, at the 30 minute, one hour, and the second hour blood sugar test exceeds 600 mg % and there is sugar in the urine during the test.

Treatment of hypoglycemia includes high protein (preferably animal protein) diets (six to eight small meals per day) as even complex carbohydrates will increase the excretion rate of chromium and vanadium in the urine. Simple sugars increase the excretion rate of chromium and vanadium up to 300 percent of the normal rate! Chromium and vanadium are the "magic bullets" for treatment of hypoglycemia at 50–200 mcg t.i.d. with meals. THOSE INDIVIDUALS ON INSULIN SHOULD START CHROMIUM / VANADIUM THERAPY AT 25 mcg t.i.d. TO PREVENT A SUDDEN DIP IN BLOOD SUGAR. Also B-complex at 50 mg each t.i.d., avoid alcohol (alcohol is a simple carbohydrate), zinc at 25 mg t.i.d., and betaine HCl and pancreatic enzymes at 75–200 mg t.i.d. before meals. Resolve the associated food allergies by using digestive enzymes, betaine HCl, and avoidance and rotation diets.

HYPOTENSION (low blood pressure) can be caused by prescribed drugs (check your PDR), heart disease, kidney disease, low blood sugar, food allergies, dehydration, adrenal exhaustion, and hypothyroidism.

The causative disease process must be dealt with to properly resolve hypotension. Symptoms of hypotension include low energy, dizzy feeling when you stand up fast from a lying down or sitting position, fainting, blurred vision, palpitations, inability to solve simple problems, and slurring of speech.

Treatment of hypotension includes resolving the original problem, vitamin C to bowel tolerance, zinc at 15 mg t.i.d., ACE (adrenal cortical extract) sublingual, IM or IV, and thyroid at 1 to 3 grains in the morning. Too much will cause increase in heart rate and uncontrolled shaking of hands. Find the OD level by gradual "titration" then back off one grain. Eight glasses of water each day, acupuncture, homeopathy, reflexology, and herbs including ginseng (Panax ginseng, P.quinquefolius), rosemary (Rosmarinus officinalis), and spring adonis (Adonis vernalis) are helpful.

HYPOTHYROID (low thyroid, goiter): States that frequently do not produce goiter (thyroid gland enlargement) can produce obesity, fatigue, disinterest, low blood pressure, water retention (edema), etc. Diagnose with a basal body temperature test. Upon waking up, take your temperature by placing a thermometer under your armpit before getting up and stirring around. If your temperature is below 97.6°F, you have low thyroid. Don't forget your thyroid gland requires all 90 essential nutrients to function properly and produce thyroxin.

Treatment of hypothyroidism includes eliminating all goiterogenic substances such as nitrates, cabbage, etc. Supplement with U.S. Armour thyroid at 1 to 3 grains each morning. An excess will cause increase in heart rate and shaking of the extended arm. Increase dosage to OD then back off one grain. Kelp and iodine supplement at 250–500 mcg per day and herbs to include quercus marine (Fucus vesiculosis).

HYSTERIA (melancholia, panic attacks) is a symptomatic diagnosis. Hysteria can result from PMS, food allergies, drugs (prescribed and illegal), alcoholism, hypoglycemia, etc. Our "orthodox" medical colleagues created the "hysterectomy" operation to resolve hysteria because of the PMS association! Test for food allergies (pulse test, etc.), hypoglycemia (six-hour GTT), and keep a daily diary to document PMS. Use a PDR to check out any medication that you might be on.

Treatment of hysteria includes avoidance of offending foods that you might be allergic to (i.e. sugar, dairy, caffiene, etc.), rotation diets, EFA at 5 gm t.i.d. with meals, chromium and vanadium at 50–200 mcg t.i.d. with meals, lithium, betaine HCl and pancreatic enzymes at 75–200 mg t.i.d. before meals, acupuncture, homeopathy, and herbs including black hellebore (Hellebores niger), blue cohosh (Caulophyllum thalictroides), mistletoe (Viscum album), B3 at 450 mg t.i.d. (time release), and B6 at 150–300 mg t.i.d. Take this dose for thirty days then cut it to 25 mg t.i.d.

IMMUNE DEPRESSION (immune exhaustion) is caused by many chronic processes such as unrelenting stress, chronic allergies, and chronic infections which result in exhaustion of the immune system and an inability to protect yourself against foreign invaders such as EBV, Candidiasis, food allergies, arthritis, cancer, etc. Anergy refers to a state in which your immune system is so exhausted that you may not react to diagnostic tests even though you have an overwhelming disease (i.e. TB, Candidiasis, etc.). DRUGS SUCH AS CORTISONE, PREDNISONE, AND CHEMOTHERAPY CAUSE IMMUNE DEPRESSION—READ YOUR PDR.

Treatment of a depressed immune system includes vitamin C to bowel tolerance, zinc at 50 mg t.i.d., vitamin A at 300,000 IU/day as beta carotene, ACE (adrenal cortical extract) sublingual, IM or EV, germanium at 50 mg orally or IM daily, acupuncture, homeopathy, herbs to include ginseng (Panax ginseng), selenium at 300 mcg/day, and all 90 essential nutrients and plant derived colloidal minerals.

IMMUNIZATION (vaccination) is perhaps the greatest interface between government and freedom of choice in your own health care. Today the government says you will vaccinate your children or they will not be admitted to school. This is the same government who says that AIDS infected children should be in public schools. State governments have even gone to the extreme to say that if you don't vaccinate your children, you will be charged with child abuse and your children placed in a foster home. Many states are trying to eliminate the religious exemption for vaccination. WARNING: VACCINATION APPEARS TO BE A BATTLEFIELD TAKING SHAPE BETWEEN THE ORTHODOX MEDICAL ADVISORS AND OUR CONSTITUTIONAL RIGHTS TO FREEDOM OF CHOICE. Don't forget that many vaccination programs are suspected to be the carrier for many catastrophic diseases. Some experts even believe that HIV was originally spread through vaccination programs including hepatitis, flu, and smallpox vaccines.

IMMUNOTHERAPY is a play on words as the "orthodox" medical doctors practice it as their approach is chemotherapy and cortisone which actually depress the immune system. Immunotherapy should be designed to increase the immune system's ability to cope and adjust to all invaders. The need for immunotherapy includes cancer, arthritis, food allergies, multiple sclerosis, SLE, and ALS.

Treatment to provide immunotherapy includes avoiding fried foods, margarines, and sugar (natural and processed), sublingual allergens regimen for allergies, autoimmune urine therapy, avoidance of food allergens, rotation diets, vitamin C to bowel tolerance, vitamin A at 300,000 IU/day as beta-carotene, zinc at 15 mg t.i.d., germanium at 50 mg/day orally or IM, selenium at 300 mcg/day orally, IV or IM, acupuncture, and herbs to include ginseng (Panax ginseng).

IMPETIGO (ecthyma) is a form of dermatitis in children that may take the form of blisters filled with straw colored fluid or pus or skin ulcers. Impetigo primarily affects the exposed areas of skin such as the face, ears, arms, and legs. The "orthodox" doctors believe that impetigo is caused by a Streptococcus bacteria and treat it solely with antibiotics over a long period of time. It appears, though, that impetigo is more sinister than a simple infection. Instead, it is an early sign of immune depression which allows normal skin organisms to flourish at an unchecked rate and cause disease. Food allergies (i.e. sugar, milk, wheat, soy) are frequently the original source of the immune depression in children. On occasion contact dermatitis from detergents will be diagnosed as impetigo. Untreated impetigo can result in deep infections of the tissue beneath the skin and in the lymph nodes.

Treatment of impetigo includes topical washes with boric acid, colloidal silver and herbs such as comfrey (Symphytum officinale), echinacea (Echinacea angustifolia), and golden seal (Hydrastis canadensis), and topical or systemic penicillin may be necessary in cases where impetigo occurs on the face to prevent scaring. Take vitamin C to bowel tolerance, vitamin A 25,000–300,000 IU/day as beta-carotene, zinc at 25–30 mg t.i.d. Practice the avoidance of sugar, fried foods, and margarine, use a rotation diet for food allergies, and increase animal protein level of the diet (i.e. eggs, chicken, and fish).

IMPOTENCE (inability to have an erection) can be caused by a wide variety of problems including an unstimulating partner, psychological domination by your partner (i.e. domineering wife syndrome), guilt (i.e. having had an extramarital affair), medication side effects (i.e. calcium channel blockers, etc.), malnutrition of various sorts, hypothyroidism, low blood pressure, adrenal exhaustion, hypoglycemia, stress, post surgical damage (prostate surgery), etc. Solving any associated problems first will guarantee results.

Treatment of impotence should include relaxation, spending time with your mate, and setting up romantic situations. The interpretation of the word romantic is an individual thing: flowers excite some people and turn others off, alcohol excites some people and anesthetizes others.

Also, acupuncture, homeopathy, and herbs to include ginseng (Panax ginseng), nux vomica (Strychnos nux vomica), sarsapilla (Smilax officinalis), saw palmetto (Serenoa serrulata), Zumba, and oral testosterone (i.e. glandular food supplements and testosterone IM), can be of value. A prescription drug called Viagra may be of value to maintain an erection, but there are side effects.

Don't forget the base line nutrition program and include the plant derived colloidal minerals (most satisfied wives ask for it by the 55-gallon drum!). The techniques of Master and Johnson can be very useful and can be a "self-help" technique employed without the need for an expensive counselor: Step 1) nongenital pleasuring (i.e. massage, reflexology, etc.), Step 2) genital pleasuring (i.e. genital foreplay), and Step 3) nondemand lovemaking (i.e. neither the "guy" or the "doll" expects to be brought to a climax).

INCONTINENCE (inability to control bowels or bladder) can be caused by a wide variety of diseases (i.e. benign prostatic hyperplasia, MD, MS, cancer, ALS, stroke, etc.), injury (including surgery, obstetrical procedures), food allergies, and hypoglycemia. Correcting the underlying diseases or injury is a must if the desired results are to be achieved.

Treatment of incontinence should include Kegel's exercises (i.e. contracting the floor of the pelvis as if trying to stop a bowel movement) at about 250–500/day, essential fatty acids at 5 gm t.i.d., selenium at 500 mcg/day, vitamin E at 800–1,200 IU/day, betaine HCl and pancreatic enzymes at 75–200 mg t.i.d. before meals, and the avoidance and rotation diets with respect to offending food allergens. Also chromium and vanadium at 25–200 mcg/day, and herbs to include saw palmetto (Serenoa serrulata) and ginseng (Panax ginseng).

INFARCTION (cerebral-stroke, heart-heart attack) is the death of an area of tissue because the blood supply was stopped by a plug or "thrombi" (i.e. blood clot, clump of tumor cells, clump of bacterial cells). If vital areas of the heart or brain are affected, the "stroke" or "heart attack" will be fatal. If nonvital areas are affected, speech, vision, muscular function, and heart capacity are significantly affected until repair and/or compensation by surrounding tissue can take place. Prevention is always better than trying to "come from behind" and repair a "stroke" or "heart attack."

Treatment and repair of infarction should include hyperbaric oxygen, oral oxygen supplements (i.e. hydrogen peroxide, etc.), vitamin C to bowel tolerance, vitamin E at 800–1,200 IU/day, selenium at 500–1,000 mcg/day orally or IM, vitamin A at 300,000 IU/day as beta carotene, chelation with EDTA, hydrogen peroxide IV, betaine HCl and pancreatic enzymes at 200–500 mg t.i.d. 15 minutes before meals. Avoid fried foods, margarines, and sugar. If clumps of bacteria are involved (i.e. rheumatic fever) then antibiotics (penicillin or tetracycline) will be required to resolve the current problem and prevent further damage to heart valves and joints.

INFECTION (invasion of tissues by bacteria, viruses, fungus) is caused by two factors: 1) an infective "dose" of organisms, and 2) a low state of resistance by the host. The base line nutrient program will provide the necessary 90 essential "macro" and "micro" elements for maintenance and repair of the immune system. Be sure to do pulse tests to determine food allergies. Use common sense and reasonable precautions when in contact with individuals who have contagious diseases (i.e. measles, mumps, scarlet fever, meningitis, hepatitis, herpes simplex, herpes II, venereal disease, flu, infectious mononucleosis, lungworm, athlete's foot, EBV, HIV, etc.).

Treatment of infections should include the use of echinacea (Echinacea angustifolia), golden seal (Hydrastis canadensis), garlic (Allium sativum), vitamin C to bowel tolerance, vitamin A at 300,000 IU/day as beta-carotene, zinc at 15 mg t.i.d., selenium at 500–1,000 mcg/day, Isoprinosin at 100–300 mg/day, Ribavirin, H_2O_2 in an IV infusion over four hours; antibiotics and antifungal medications are sometimes necessary in lifesaving situations.

INFERTILITY (curable inability to have children) is usually caused by a nutritional deficiency of some nutrient. We have "cured" several hundred cases of infertility by simple supplementation of vitamins, minerals, trace minerals, and digestive aids. Food allergies may be involved by causing celiac disease type changes in the intestine and, thus, affecting absorption.

Treatment of infertility should include the base line nutritional program (include plant derived colloidal minerals). Resolve food allergies by avoidance and rotation diets. Eat high protein diets (up to 200 gm/day), EFA at 5 gm t.i.d., 1-arginine at 500 mg t.i.d., zinc at 15 gm t.i.d., selenium at 250 mcg/day, vitamin A at 100,000 IU/day for 30 days then drop to 25,000 IU/day, germanium at 50 mg/day, acupuncture, and herbs including ginseng (Panax ginseng), leek (Allium perrum), and garlic (Allium sativum).

INFLAMMATION can result from injury, arthritis, infection, cancer, burns, chemicals. Symptoms of inflammation include swelling, tenderness, discharges, edema, fever, allergies, etc. Treatment of inflammation include DMSO, proteolytic enzymes orally (i.e. chymotrypsin, pancreatic enzymes, bromelin, trypsin), vitamin C to bowel tolerance, vitamin E at 800–1,200 IU/day, zinc at 50 mg t.i.d., essential fatty acids at 5 gm t.i.d., bioflavonoids 150 mg/day, quercetin 100 mg/day, d-phenylalanine, l-tryptophane, and dl-valine each at 1.5 gm/day, acupuncture, herbs including camphor (Cinnamonum camphora), comfrey (Symphytum officinale), licorice root (Glyccerizin glabra), and feverfew (Chrysanthemum parthenium).

INDIGESTION (dyspepsia, belch, burp, and bloat) occurs as a natural course of aging, as a result of stress, salt restriction, and overeating. In the course of aging, the stomach begins to loose its ability to produce hydrochloric acid. This process begins at about age 35. Food allergies can contribute to this syndrome. The pulse test should be used to determine food allergies.

Treatment of indigestion should include Kaopectate or Pepto Bismol for acute diarrhea, betaine HCl and pancreatic enzymes at 75–200 mg t.i.d. before meals, mint tea as needed to calm stomach, English bitters (Gentiana lutea) before each meal, vitamin E at 800–1,200 IU/day, selenium at 500 mcg/day, calcium and magnesium at 2,000 and 1,000 mg/day, acupuncture, homeopathy, herbs such as balm (Melissa officinalis), bitter orange (Citrus aurantium), celandine (Chelidonium majus), fennel (Foeniculum vulgare), hops (Humulus lupulus), masterwort (Peucedanum ostruthium), peppermint (Mentha piperita), wormwood (Artemisia absinthium), yarrow (Achillea millefolium), and marshmallow (Althacea officinalis).

INSOMNIA (inability to sleep) can be caused by stress, excitement, and drugs including caffeine (i.e. coffee, cola soft drinks, chocolate, etc.). Use your PDR if you are on prescription drugs. Food allergies and hypoglycemia can cause insomnia and nightmares. Use the pulse test and six-hour GTT.

Treatment for insomnia includes avoidance of caffeine and offending food allergens, calcium (especially plant derived colloidal calcium), chromium and vanadium at 25–200 mcg t.i.d., acupuncture, homeopathy, dl-phenylalanine at 250 mg t.i.d., l-tryptophan at 1,000 mg t.i.d., inositol at 500 mg/day, niacinamide at 1,000 mg at bedtime, and herbs including valerian (Valeriana officinalis), passion flower (Passiflora incarnata), hops (Humulus lupulus), and California poppy (Eschscholzia California), and B3 (niacin) at 450 mg t.i.d. (time release). Don't forget the base line nutrition program.

IRRITABLE BOWEL SYNDROME will alternate between constipation and diarrhea. Food allergies are the most frequent cause of this very distressing syndrome. Small intestine damage includes celiac disease like changes, edema, ulceration, and catarrhal inflammation. The "orthodox" approach to treating irritable bowel syndrome is low fiber diets, cortisone, and Tagamet. The pulse test is an extremely useful test for determining the individual cause of irritable bowel syndrome.

Treatment of irritable bowel syndrome should include high fiber diets, 4–6 cups of fruit and vegetables per day, elimination of fried food, margarine, caffeine, sugar, and offending foods based on the pulse test (i.e. wheat, milk, soy), betaine HCl and pancreatic enzymes at 75–200 mg t.i.d. before meals, folic acid at 5–25 mg/day, gluten free diet, and eight to ten glasses of water each day. Don't forget the base line nutrition supplement program. Herbs including marshmallow (Althaea officinalis). A macrobiotic diet can be of great benefit here.

ITCHING (pruritis) can be caused by dry skin, contact with irritants, and contact and food allergies. Pulse test and challenge tests are used to determine allergens and irritants. Resolving the basic problem is essential to eliminating itching.

Treatment (symptomatic) of itching includes the use of topical applications of Caladryl, aloe vera (Aloe spp), salt rubs, dilute vinegar (50 percent), and washes with herbal compresses (see dermatitis). Oral treatment should include 5 gm EFA t.i.d., zinc 15 mg t.i.d., and vitamin A at 300,000 IU/day as beta-carotene. Don't forget the base line nutritional program.

JAUNDICE (icterus, yellow eyes) can be caused by blockage of the bile duct system in the liver (gallstones, tumor, hepatitis), and/or destruction of RBC's (Rh factor, blood parasites-malaria). Diagnosis is a critical problem when jaundice is present. Examining the "whites" of the eye (sclera) will reveal jaundice by the presence of a yellow coloration which is absent when the skin is yellow from a high beta carotene consumption. Blood tests will differentiate between obstruction (i.e. elevated bilirubin—above 2.0–2.5 mg %) and RBC destruction (i.e. unconjugated or indirect bilirubin are elevated).

Treatment of jaundice includes exposure to ultraviolet light to speed up elimination of bile pigments, liver flush (three days of an apple juice fast sipping through the day as needed followed by a cup of olive oil and a cup of lemon juice), vitamin C to bowel tolerance, vitamin A at 300,000 IU/day as beta-carotene, selenium at 500–1,000 mcg/day, vitamin E at 800–1,200 IU/day, and herbs including licorice (Glycyrrhiza glabra), agrimony (Agrimonia eupatoria), celadine (Chelidonium majus), and chionanthus (Chionanthus virginica).

JOINT PAIN can be caused by a variety of disease processes including arthritis, osteoporosis, rickets, gout, obesity, and various nutritional deficiencies (i.e. calcium, magnesium, manganese, sulfur, sulfur bearing amino acids, and copper) and food allergies/sensitivities.

Treatment of joint pain includes the correction of any overt or underlying disease (arthritis, osteoporosis), calcium and magnesium at 2,000 and 1,000 mg per day, cartilage at 5 gm t.i.d., gelatin (unsweetened) once per day, copper at 2–5 mg/day (a copper bracelet can be of great value), B6 at 100 mg t.i.d., mineral bath hydrotherapy and ultra violet light exposure at 1–6 minutes; symptomatic treatment of joint pain includes pain gels, DMSO, and acupuncture. Avoid soft drinks, fried food, margarine, and sugar. Take Dr. Wallach's Pig Arthritis Formula twice each day. Chiropractic can be of great value in treating and providing symptomatic relief of a variety of joint problems including subluxations of the spine, ribs, and pelvis.

KEGEL'S EXERCISE is a great way to condition the voluntary muscles of the pelvic floor in both males and females. This exercise is useful for prenatal conditioning of the pelvic muscles, vaginal muscles, and urethral muscles in both male and female for urinary incontinence and urgency. To perform the Kegel's exercise you tighten the muscles of the pelvic floor as if you were trying to stop a bowel movement. You can also add the variation of stopping your urine stream at will as often as you can. Try to do several hundred each day.

KERATOMALACIA (xerophthalmia) is recognized as a hazy "bluish" dry cornea (the domed clear bulge on the front of the eye) that becomes ulcerated. Symptoms include extreme dryness of the eyes with blinking in attempts to keep the eyes moist, conjunctivitis, and night blindness. Fat-like spots (Bitots spots) can be found on the "white" of the eyeball. Untreated keratomalacia can result in permanent blindness.

Treatment of keratomalacia includes vitamin A at 25,000 IU as beta carotine (kids) to 300,000 I (adults) per day as beta carotene, zinc at 5 to 15 mg t.i.d. and increase the animal protein to 120 gm day (i.e. chicken, fish, eggs, milk, lamb, pork, or beef). Don't forget the base line nutritional supplement program.

KERATOSIS is a "goose bump" like keratin build up in the openings of the hair follicles. These pinhead sized "plugs" are found in greatest numbers on the backs of the arms, thighs, and buttocks. The "orthodox" doctors claim that treatment is unnecessary, however, keratosis is, in fact, a symptom of a chronic vitamin A deficiency.

Treatment of keratosis includes vitamin A at 25,000 IU as beta-carotene (kids) to 300,000 IU (adults) per day as beta-carotene and zinc at 5 to 15 mg. t.i.d. Increase protein at 120 gms per day, and don't forget the base line nutrition program.

KERNICTERUS is the depositing of bile pigments into the brain of newborn children after an extended elevation of bilirubin (bile pigments produced from RBC breakdown). Symptoms mimic those of cerebral palsy (i.e. lethargy, poor feeding, vomiting, uncoordination, seizures, and death). Prevention and treatment of kernicterus includes frequent feeding of the infant to reduce absorption of bile pigments and exposure to blue and ultra violet light to photo-oxidize bilirubin. Note: a transient lactose intolerance is associated with light therapy in infants that results in diarrhea—this does not appear to have any permanent consequences.

KETOACIDOSIS (ketosis) results from a low glucose supply to the liver, which forces it to metabolize fat. The resulting by-products are "ketone bodies" (i.e. acetoacetic acid, B-hydroxyburytic acid, and acetone). Ketosis occurs in diabetes, alcoholism, hypoglycemia, and starvation. The breath will smell like acetone, nausea and vomiting will occur, along with air hunger, confusion or coma, extreme thirst, and weight loss. A positive urine "dipstick" for ketone bodies is an easy way to confirm your suspicions.

Treatment of ketosis includes resolving the basic disease process (i.e. diabetes, hypoglycemia, alcoholism, starvation, etc.), increasing the complex carbohydrate intake, chromium and vanadium at 50–200 mcg t.i.d., and the base line nutritional program.

KIDNEY DISEASE (kidney stones, "malignant calcification") can be caused by a variety of infections, toxins, and nutritional excesses (i.e. hypervitaminosis D) and deficiencies (i.e. deficiencies of vitamin A, magnesium, calcium, selenium, and zinc). Kidney disease can be secondary to cardiovascular disease or diabetes. Kidney stones, contrary to popular belief by the "orthodox" doctor, are caused by calcium and magnesium deficiencies which cause a depletion of calcium from your bones, which is the source of the calcium found in kidney stones. Prevention of kidney stones includes adequate levels of supplementary calcium and magnesium (impossible to get enough from your diet especially if you are a big consumer of phosphorus—meat and carbonated soft drinks). Deficiencies of magnesium results in "malignant calcification," a deposition of calcium in the small elastic and muscular arteries typically found in the kidney. Excess vitamin D (suntanning, fish oil, and supplementation) concurrently with calcium deficiency will accelerate the depletion and, thus, increase the risk of kidney stones. Also check for cadmium toxicity with a hair analysis.

Treatment of kidney disease and kidney stones should include supplementation of calcium and magnesium at 2,000 mg and 1,000 mg per day, reduction of your phosphorus intake, adequate vitamin A nutriture at 25,000–300,000 IU, vitamin A per day as beta-carotene, B6 at 50 mg t.i.d., lysine and glutamic acid, and herbs including dandelion (Taraxacum officinale), dwarf elder (Sambucus ebulus), goldenrod (Solidago virgaurea), Java tea (Orthosiphon stamineus), parsley (Petro Selinum crispum), horsetail (Equisetum spp.), mugwort (Artemisia vulgaris), and unsweetened cranberry juice. Chelation therapy with EDTA may help kidney disease that is secondary to cardiovascular disease and cadmium toxicity. An acute or sudden kidney stone blockage may require the pain relief of morphine as it can be excruciating. You may also wish to use prednisone for three days to reduce the inflammation in the ureter (the tube from the kidney to the bladder) so that you can pass the stones. Stones lodged in the kidney can be reduced to harmless powder by a machine known as a "lithotripter," an ultra sound machine that actually shatters the stones without surgery.

KORSAKOFF'S SYNDROME (recent memory loss, false Alzheimer's Disease) is characterized by an inability to record and store new memory. The patient can perform detailed tasks learned before onset but cannot learn the simplest of new tasks. This type of "amnesia" can result from a blow to the head or be the result of chronic alcoholism and vitamin B1 deficiency associated with an excess intake of simple carbohydrate and sugar. Confabulation or producing imaginary experiences for those that cannot be recalled is a consistent feature of Korsakoff's syndrome. If the disease is the result of a blow to the head, there is a good chance of a gradual recovery; if the brain tissue has been damaged by alcoholism (Wernecke-Korsakoff's Syndrome) or chronic vitamin B1 deficiency, the process may be difficult to treat.

Treatment of Korsakoff's syndrome includes IV chelation, hydrogen peroxide IV, vitamin B1 at 100 mg t.i.d., lecithin at 2,500 mg. t.i.d., avoidance of alcohol and sugar, chromium and vanadium at 50–200 mcg t.i.d., betaine HCl and pancreatic enzymes at 75–200 mg t.i.d. before meals, hydergine at 4.5–9 mg/day, vasopressin (Diapid) at 12–16 units per day as a nasal spray, centrophenoxine at 4.4–8.0 gm per day, and piracetam (Dinagen) at 1.6–4.8 gm per day. This is the drug treatment program used to restore Princess Di's bodyguard's memory.

KWASHIORKOR (protein starvation) is thought of as a disease of starving African children. It is classed as protein/calorie starvation and is characterized by a distended bloated belly, edema and "dropsy" because low blood protein levels can't hold water in the blood vessels so it simply "leaks" out. By now you will recognize that this happens to unschooled dieters, cancer patients, vegans and fruitarians who take in less than optimal amounts of complete proteins. Don't forget the base line nutritional supplementation.

Treatment of Kwashiorkor includes adequate intake of complete animal protein (i.e. greater than 120 gms per day), a calorie intake of 3,000 calories per day, selenium at 200 mcg per day and chromium and vanadium at 50–200 mcg t.i.d. Don't forget the 90 essential nutrients here.

LABOR (induce) can be made easier and assisted by herbs including blue cohosh (Caulophyllus thalictroides) and raspberry tea (Rubus idaeus). Corn ergot (Ustilago maydis) can be used to stop postpartum hemorrhage (orally or IM). Taking training classes (i.e. Lamaze) will help train the mother-to-be to relax during contractions (labor pains) and help train the "coach" to assist and how to recognize potential trouble. Home births are safer than hospital births and, in addition, the hospital rate of caesarian section is 35 percent. Vaginal births net the "orthodox" OB/GYN $800–$1,200; caesarian sections net them $2,500!

LACTATION (induce) can be induced or enhanced with herbs including milkweed (Asclepias galioides), caraway (Carum carvi), fenugreek (Trigonella foenum-graecum), and goat's rue (Galega officinalis).

LACTATION (reduce) can be reduced and breast pain of engorgement can be relieved by goldenrod (Solidago petradoria). Luperon, a posterior pituitary hormone can stop milk production; however, side effects include temporary menopausal symptoms.

LACTASE DEFICIENCY (cow's milk sensitivity) is a form of carbohydrate intolerance that results from a deficiency of the enzyme required to breakdown milk sugar (lactose) into glucose and galactose. Lactase deficiency is characterized by bloating and diarrhea with violent abdominal cramps following the ingestion of cow's milk and cow's milk products (cheese, yogurt, ice cream, etc.). Lactase deficiency occurs in 20 percent adults of Northwest European origin, at 75 percent in adults of all other ethnic groups, 90 percent of all Orientals, and 75 percent in blacks and American Indians. The ability to digest lactose is gradually lost between the ages of 10–20 years of age.

Treatment of lactose intolerance includes avoidance of lactose-containing foods, predigestion of lactose by adding lactase to milk-containing foods and the use of digestive enzyme supplements that contain lactase.

LARYNGITIS (loss of voice) can be caused by bacterial and/or viral infections, extreme overuse of the vocal cords (i.e. yelling at a football or hockey game) and muscular dystrophy or fibromyalgia of the laryngeal muscles. Very frequently, the temperature is not elevated and voice loss is the only symptom. "Strep" throat can be a cause that can be potentially dangerous and lead to rheumatic fever or meningitis if not dealt with properly. Hoarseness, voice change or complete loss of voice (aphonia), and tickling/raw throat are all symptoms.

Treatment of laryngitis can include penicillin or tetracyclines for "Strep" throat at 250 mg orally q 6 h for 10–12 days, voice rest, honey/lemon preparations and herbs including cajuput (Melaleuca leucadendron), sunflower (Helianthus annus), pine oils (Pinnus sylvestris), black caraway (Pimpinella saxifraga), garden sage (Salvia officinalis), high mallow (Malva sylvestris), wild ginger (Asarum europium), and eucalyptus (Eucalyptus globulus). Viral laryngitis may be treated with Isoprinosin at 500–1,500 mg per day or Ribavirin at 250–1,500 mg per day. (**Warning: pregnant women should avoid these drugs, as they are teratogenic—that is, they cause birth defects in lab animals**). Avoid fried food, margarine, and cooking oil, and supplement with all 90 essential nutrients.

LAXATIVE includes many OTC preparations such as Ex-Lax and Milk of Magnesia and herbs including senna (Cassia aqutifolia), flaxseed or flaxseed oil (Linum ustatissimum), alder buckthorn (Rhamnus fragula), cascara sagrada (Rhamnus purshiana), juniper (Juniperus communis), and manna ash (Fraxinus ornus).

LEAD POISONING (plumbism): Lead is required to convert RNA into DNA at the level of parts per billion. An excess of inorganic or metallic lead can cause a wide variety of symptoms and syndromes including learning disabilities, kidney disease, anemia, stunted bone growth, headaches, and gastrointestinal disease. Very often the eating of lead, lead paint, and caulking is the result of pica or a compulsive eating of unusual things because of mineral deficiencies. Sources of metallic lead include paint chips, window caulking, glaze from pottery, lead arsenate garden sprays, pollution from leaded fuels, inhalation of smoke from burning batteries, and large lead insulated wire. Diagnosis of lead poisoning can be made from a hair analysis in chronic cases or blood and urine in sudden onset acute cases.

Treatment of lead poisoning includes vitamin C to bowel tolerance, IV chelation with calcium EDTA at 10–25 infusions, and/or oral D-penicillamine. Don't forget the base line nutritional supplement program containing plant derived colloidal minerals because the IV chelation process is not selective and will tend to deplete body stores of essential minerals (selenium is of particular value).

LEARNING DISORDERS (dyslexia, hyperactivity, autism): see ADD, ADHD, autism, dyslexia, food allergies, hypoglycemia, hyperactivity, and lead poisoning.

LEGIONNAIRES' DISEASE is caused by an infection with Legionella pneumophila. The disease is characterized by pneumonia, high fever, slow heart, rate, dry cough, chills, pleuritis, and diarrhea. Legionnaires' disease is a relatively new disease, only being discovered in 1976. URI (upper respitory infection) is significantly absent in this disease. Untreated Legionnaires' disease will be fatal in 80 percent of the cases. Diagnosis requires growing the organism on charcoal-yeast extract from sputum. Immunosuppressed patients such as chemotherapy treated cancer patients, transplant patients, and AIDS patients are most susceptible.

Treatment of Legionnaires' disease is specific with erythromycin at 500 mg to 1 gm orally or IV q 6 H every 6 hours for three weeks.

LENTIGO-MALIGNA MELANOMA (melanoma, skin cancer) originates from the Hutchinson's freckle on sun exposed areas on the face, neck, arms, and torso. These skin cancers appear as large flat, tan, or brown lesions with darker black or brown spots dotted on its surface. These are slow growing cancers requiring about ten years to invade the dermis or deep skin layers.

Treatment of L-M melanoma can include excision biopsy. Frequently these tumors are on the face and a caustic cream may be more desirable than surgery. Take vitamin C to bowel tolerance, vitamin A at 300,000 IU/day as beta-carotene, selenium at 1,000 mcg per day, and use a #40 sunscreen to prevent new cancers. Avoid fried food and margarine. Don't forget the base line nutritional supplement program.

LEPTOSPIROSIS (Weil's Disease, infectious jaundice) is an infectious disease caused by Leptospira spp, a spirochete bacteria carried by dogs, rats, and various species of wild animals. Individuals are infected by urine contaminated water and cuts while skinning or butchering infected animals. Symptoms include anemia, jaundice, proteinuria, hematuria, and, on occasion, aseptic meningitis. Fever and chills are consistent symptoms. Blood tests for antibodies or urine cultures are necessary for diagnosis.

Treatment with antibiotics is most effective if instituted within four days of onset. Tetracycline at 500 mg q.i.d. is effective.

LEUKEMIA (blood cancer) is a cancer of the blood forming tissues of the bone marrow. No exact cause is proven but viruses, radiation, electromagnetic fields from power lines, and chemicals such as benzene are implicated. Leukemia produces a defect in the maturation process of WBCs resulting in large numbers of immature WBCs in the circulating blood. Diagnosis is made from a blood test, which shows anemia, low platelets, increased lymphoblasts (immature WBC), and an elevated total WBC count. Symptoms include weakness, joint pain, anemia, enlarged lymph nodes, and enlarged spleen.

Treatment includes Laetrile, hydrogen peroxide, DMSO (matures the immature cells in the circulation) IV, shark liver extract, hydrazine sulfate, cesium chloride, polyerga, germanium, carbamide, and, as needed, micro-dose chemotherapy, amino acids IV, vitamin C to bowel tolerance, selenium at 500–1,000 mcg per day, and vitamin A at 300,000 IU as beta carotene. Avoid fried foods and margarine.

LEUKORRHEA (vaginal discharge) is a nonspecific vaginal discharge containing mucus, WBCs and, on occasion, is tinged with blood. Leukorrhea can be caused by Candida albicans, Hemophilus vaginalis, Streptococcus spp., Staphylococcus spp. (the bacteria that will cause toxic shock syndrome when vaginal tampons are used incorrectly), or Neisseria gonorrhoea. Culture (growth of bacteria) and/or looking at the discharge under the microscope is required for specific diagnosis.

Treatment of leukorrhea should include specific treatment for the causative organism, i.e., vaginal application of triple sulfonamide creams, oxytetracycline vaginal suppositories, and vaginal douches with vinegar 30 ml/pint of water. Gonorrhea will require systemic antibiotics as well. Please note that any venereal disease must be reported to the Public Health Department.

LICE (pediculosis) can infest the head (Pediculus humanus capitis), body (P.h. corporis), and pubic area (Phthirius pubis). Eggs (nits) are white oval shaped seed-like objects attached to the base of the hairs; adult lice can be seen scuttling through the hair on the surface of the skin. Itching and irritated skin are the most common symptoms. Diagnosis is dependent on finding the adult lice or "nits" in the hair and scalp.

Treatment of lice includes the use of Labordor tea (Ledum latifolium) or field larkspur (Delphinium consolida) as a hair wash. Use of a special fine toothed comb to "harvest" the "nits" is recommended. Treatment should be done daily for fourteen days to break the life cycle of the lice. For stubborn cases, you may wish to use 1 percent gamma benzene hexachloride daily for two days as a shampoo and reapplied in ten days. Avoid prolonged use of the insecticide as it can cause genital skin irritation, especially in males.

LIFE EXPECTANCY (life span) or the longevity potential for man is 120–140 years, yet the average life span based on insurance actuary tables is only 72 for American males and 78 for American females. This leaves a 40–50 year differential that we can work towards with hopeful expectations. The Mormons and Seventh Day Adventists live to 82 on the average by avoiding caffiene, alcohol, fried foods, and drugs. That's a gain of 6.5 years. The use of water filtration systems in the home, the use of air filters and conditioners for the home and work place as well as employing the base line nutrition program can add 10 to 20 to 40 healthful years to your life. The use of digestive aids (i.e. betaine HCl and pancreatic enzymes) will add an additional ten years to your life. Together, these measures add a total of 20 to 50 years when you actively and aggressively seek a healthful life.

The Hunza secret of longevity (average of 100 years with a top end of 140 to 160 years) is the daily consumption of an optimal supply of grains, vegetables, fruits, and nuts that are rich in plant derived colloidal minerals.

Exercise alone without attention to food allergies, digestive aids, base line nutritional supplement program, colloidal minerals, and avoiding pollutants will only shorten your life and make what life you do have very sweaty.

Take responsibility for your own health and you will add 20 to 50 more years of life. Remember that 40 percent of all patients in the hospital are there because of iatrogenic disease (doctor created). This statistic doesn't account for the number who died outside of the hospital because of mistakes in prescriptions, mistakes in diagnosis, and mistakes in procedures.

LIVER DISEASE (cirrhosis, nonviral hepatitis) can be diagnosed by blood test showing elevation in SGOT, SGPT, GGT, alkaline phosphatase, and bilirubin. Elevated ketones in the urine are clues to liver disease as well as faulty carbohydrate metabolism. Jaundice and problems with delayed clotting times and a swollen tender liver (under the ribs at the right upper quadrant), dry itchy skin (a result of problems with essential fatty acid metabolism), anemia (iron storage and B-12/folic acid) deficiencies, weight loss, and ketosis are all symptoms of liver disease.

Also see gallbladder disease.

Treatment of liver disease includes IV or oral chelation with complete IV supplementation including amino acids and interlipids, vitamin C to bowel tolerance, vitamin A at 10,000 to 300,000 IU per day as beta carotene, B-complex at 100 mg each t.i.d., selenium at 500–1,000 mcg per day, B12 at 1,000 mcg per day, folic acid at 15–25 mg per day, essential fatty acids (both salmon oil and flaxseed oil) at 1 gm t.i.d., and herbs including tamarac (Larix americana), parsley (Carum petroselinum), hemp acrimony (Eupatorium cannabium), and milk thistle (Silybum marianum). Don't forget the base line nutrition program and colloidal minerals and avoid fried foods and margarine.

LOCKJAW (tetanus) is caused by the toxin (waste product) of Clostridium tetani, which is a normal anaerobic inhabitant of animal manure. Puncture wounds contaminated by this organism cause the production of tetanus toxin which paralyzes the voluntary muscles including the jaw muscles (masseter) which gives the disease its name "lockjaw." Prevention of the infection is the best of the alternatives. Squeeze the puncture wound to make it bleed out the toxin. Small puncture wounds of the foot or hands may require opening to allow cleaning with soap and water. Follow this cleaning with disinfection with 3 percent hydrogen peroxide. Take cramp bark tea (Viburnum opulus) in tablespoon doses as needed. These very minimal procedures prevent lockjaw virtually 100 percent of the time.

Treatment of lockjaw after it develops requires the use of tetanus neutralizing non-fixed toxin. Clean infected wound, disinfect wound with hydrogen peroxide, use penicillin at two million units IV q 6 h or tetracycline at 500 mg IV q6 h, sedation to control muscle spasms, and IV fluids and electrolytes until the patient can eat and drink on their own.

LUPUS ERYTHEMATOSUS (SLE) is considered a connective tissue disease of unknown causes. It is of interest that 90 percent of all cases of SLE are diagnosed in women in their 30s. The "orthodox" theory is that SLE is an "autoimmune" disease that causes the patient's own antibodies to attack themselves. The fact is the autoimmune defect occurs as a result of the disease and the presence of abnormal proteins rather than being the cause. Multiple mineral deficiencies of sulfur, copper, selenium, etc. are characteristically present. The classical symptoms of SLE usually begin suddenly with fever, fatigue, arthritis, and/or joint pain. Because of this, many SLE patients are misdiagnosed as having rheumatoid arthritis. Also present are a characteristic facial "butterfly" rash (typical of allergies), severe alopecia (hair loss), and papular skin lesions. Diagnosis of SLE includes recognition of a fever with the facial "butterfly" rash, poly arthritis, kidney disease, leukopenia (low WBCs), elevated blood globulins, and the presence of LE cells (these only occur in 70 percent of SLE and are normal WBCs that have engulfed a nucleus from a destroyed cell).

Do the pulse test to determine allergies (i.e. wheat, cow's milk, and soy are the most common). Treatment of SLE includes avoidance of offending food allergens, fried foods, and margarine and rotation of non allergic foods to prevent aquiring new allergies, chelation with total nutrition for 15–25 infusions, essential fatty acids (salmon oil and flaxseed oil) at 5 gm t.i.d., selenium at 500–1,000 mcg per day, and B-carnitine at 500 mg per day. Dr. Wallach's Pig Arthritis Formula is very useful for SLE.

LYME DISEASE (LD, Lyme arthritis) is a spirochete bacterial disease that is transmitted by ticks. The disease was first described in 1975 in Lyme, Connecticut, thus the name. Three to 32 days after being bitten by an infected tick a skin lesion known as an ECM (erythema chronicum migrans) will appear on the thigh, buttock, or arm pit. The lesion expands to a diameter of 50 cm and the lesion feels hot to the touch. There will be recurrent attacks of arthritis, fatigue, chills, fever, stiff neck, sore muscles, nausea, and vomiting. Heart disease in the form of cardiomegaly and AV-block occur in 8 percent of patients.

Diagnosis of Lyme disease requires a high degree of awareness of the disease. Lyme disease occurs most often in children who play out in the grass or deep woods, or those who have a dog that goes out into the woods and brings home the Ixodes dammini tick. The disease occurs in clumps along the northeastern coast of the U.S., Wisconsin, California, and Oregon. Patients may initially be misdiagnosed as having rheumatoid arthritis and WBCs are elevated at 25,000; special blood tests for antibodies are required for specific diagnosis.

Treatment of Lyme Disease requires the use of tetracycline at 250–500 mg q.i.d. for 20 days. IV antibiotics over a period of 30 days will ensure a 100 percent cure. In children where teeth would be permanently discolored by tetracyclines, penicillin can be used at 20 million u/day IV in divided doses.

LYMPHOMA (cancer of the lymph nodes): see cancer

MACULAR DEGENERATION (spots of the eye): spotty atrophy and free radical degeneration of the retina of the eye. A common cause of blindness in aging individuals, it is characterized by "snow" vision.

Treatment approach includes elimination of all fried foods and margarine, elimination of all sugar (natural and processed), supplement with all 90 essential nutrients (including selenium—500 mcg., vitamin E—1,200 iu., methionine), taurine 2–5 grams per day, and the 60 essential minerals in the plant derived colloidal form.

MALABSORPTION: see celiac disease, food allergies, and hypochlorhydria

MALIGNANCY (cancer): see cancer

MALNUTRITION can occur as an overt nutritional deficiency or secondary to extended use of medications that interfere with absorption of nutrients or malabsorption of nutrients as a result of celiac disease or hypo-chlorhydria. "Orthodox" doctors tend to think of malnutrition as protein/calorie deprivation and fail to recognize macro and micro nutrient deficiencies either singly or in complex multiples, especially in their early stages. "Orthodox" doctors also fail to recognize that celiac disease changes in the small intestine lining occur as a result of "subclinical" allergies to wheat, cow's milk albumen, and soy as well as other foods (i.e. rye, barley, beef, eggs, etc.).

In reality, adult onset diabetes and hypoglycemia are deficiencies of chromium and vanadium frequently created by malabsorption as a result of celiac type changes in the small intestine. Cystic fibrosis is, in reality, a deficiency of selenium and essential fatty acids of the embryo and newborn brought on by celiac disease type changes in the pregnant mother and continued in the breast fed and developing infant. Arthritis is, in fact, a deficiency of calcium complicated by excess phosphorus in the American diet, and cancer appears to be the result of a depressed immune system that has run out of essential nutrients, including selenium required to keep itself in constant repair. As wild as it seems, "malnutrition" as a result of "malabsorption" appears to be the common denominator of almost all degenerative disease. Liquid plant derived colloidal minerals are the most efficient way to get minerals into malnourished humans.

MANIA (manic depression, Bi-polar disease): see depression, food allergies, hypoglycemia

MEASLES (rubeola) is a highly contagious viral disease with a sudden onset, cough, nasal drainage, conjunctivitis, Koplik's spots (eruptions on the oral and labial mucosa), and a pimple like skin rash that starts on the head and neck and spreads to the body, arms, and legs. Elevated temperature to 104° F is common. Pneumonia and encephalitis are unusual and potentially fatal side effects. Measles today affect young teenagers and young adults and less often infants. The incubation of measles is 7–14 days with the diagnostic Koplik's spots appearing four days after the fever starts. Having had measles once gives life long immunity.

Treatment of measles should include topical OTC products to relieve itching (i.e. Caladryl), herbs including salves made of marigold (Calendula officinalis) and orally columbine (Aquilegia vulgaris), yarrow (Achillea millefolium), and pleurisy root (Asclepias tuberose).

MEASLES, GERMAN (rubella, three-day measles) is a contagious viral disease that produces mild symptoms in children including swollen lymph nodes of the head and neck. The incubation period is 14–21 days and overt symptoms may be absent in teenagers and adults. The typical skin rash occurs first on the face then spreads quickly to the body and limbs with a general body flush not unlike scarlet fever. Adults may have enlarged lymph nodes on the head and neck and adult males may complain of brief testicular pain. RUBELLA IS A DANGEROUS DISEASE IN PREGNANT WOMEN THAT CAN INDUCE SPONTANEOUS ABORTIONS AND BIRTH DEFECTS. VACCINES FOR GERMAN MEASLES CAN CAUSE SIMILAR BIRTH DEFECTS AS THE DISEASE SO ARE TO BE AVOIDED DURING PREGNANCY.

Treatment for rubella is the same symptomatic and supportive therapy as that used for the nine-day measles.

MELASMA (chloasma, "mask of pregnancy") is dark brown spots with distinct margins found on the face and forehead of pregnant women and women on birth control hormones. Sunlight darkens the pigment and these are sometimes called "sun spots." The spots may fade after childbirth. Susceptible individuals should use sunscreens while exposed to the sun. These spots are cosmetic in nature and appear to be of no consequence to health.

MEMORY LOSS (senile dementia, Korsakoff's syndrome, Alzheimer's) can be much more devastating than a physical disability. There are a variety of causes of memory loss and it is suggested that you look up each one separately including food allergies and hypoglycemia. You should do the pulse test to determine allergies or sensitivities to various foods and do a six-hour GTT to rule in or rule out hypoglycemia.

Treatment of memory loss should include avoidance of offending food allergens, sugar, fried food, and margarine, avoidance of alcohol, the taking of chromium and vanadium at 25–200 mcg t.i.d., selenium at 200–1,000 mcg per day, vitamin E at 800–1,200 IU per day, B-complex at 50 mg t.i.d., Diapid (vasopressin) at 12–16 U/day (this is a nasal spray), Lucidril (centrophenoxine) at 4.4–8.0 gm/day, Dinagen (piracetam) at

1.6–4.8 gm/day (should take choline with this product), and hydergine at 9–20 mg per day.

MENARCHE (menstruation, "period") is the regular monthly cycle of women that alternates ovulation (mid-cycle approximately at day 14) with "periods" (the 3–7 day discharge of blood and uterine lining) at the end of the cycle. "Periods" will frequently stop in women athletes and women who drop below 20 percent body fat. The stopping of a period is of no health consequence in and of itself but is a signal that you may be too thin for a normal cycle and ovulation. Painful "periods" or PMS are not uncommon and can be severe enough to force bed rest. These extreme symptoms are usually the result of calcium and/or EFA deficiencies.

Treatment of painful or excessive menses ("heavy flow") can include OTC products (i.e. Midol) and/or herbs such as snapdragon (Linaria vulgaris), Bethroot (Trillium erectum), black cohosh (Cimicifuga racemose), blue cohosh (Caulophyllum thalictroides), tamarac (Larix americana), alpine ragwort (Senecio fuchsii), Ladies mantle (Alche milla vulgaris), St. Johns wort (Hypericum perforatum), shepherd's purse (Capsella bursa-pastoris), white deadnettle (Lamium album) and yarrow (Achillea millefolium), essential fatty acids (salmon oil and flaxseed oil) at 5 gm t.i.d., vitamin E at 800–1,200 IU/day, selenium at 500–1,000 mcg per day, iron at 25–50 mg per day (especially for vegetarian women who do not eat red meat or liver regularly). Dr. Wallach's Pig Arthritis Formula supplies significant amounts of calcium and magnesium.

MENINGITIS (infection of the brain and spinal cord covering) can be caused by a variety of organisms including bacteria (i.e. Neisseria meningitides, Hemophilis influenzae, Streptococcus [Diplococcus] pneumoniae, Listeria monocytogenes), fungi, and hundreds of viruses. There is great danger in this disease in that infants with meningitis often only show a fever and lethargy and there is a "blood-brain barrier" that prevents most medications from getting into the inner surface of the meninges or into the space beneath the meninges and into the brain itself. Symptoms of meningitis vary considerably but usually include a sore throat, fever, headache, stiff neck, and vomiting. Children and adults may become critically ill in 6–24 hours after the first appearance of symptoms. If you suspect meningitis, this is one disease that requires rapid diagnosis and treatment GET PATIENT TO AN EMERGENCY ROOM IMMEDIATELY AND DEMAND IMMEDIATE HELP. Meningitis patients often die because they have waited 2–4 hours in an emergency waiting room.

Treatment of meningitis requires rapid diagnosis (spinal tap) and injection of antibiotics into the subdural space (under the meninges), total IV fluid and electrolyte support, and very frequently mechanical respirators. MENINGITIS IS NOT A SELF-HELP DISEASE.

MENINGOCELE (severe anencephila or spina bifida) is a severe birth defect that results in exposure of the brain or spinal cord and its coverings (meninges) because of improper formation of the skull or vertebrae. This birth defect is caused by a deficiency of folic acid, B12, or zinc and vitamin A during early pregnancy. These deficiencies may be the result of deficient diets and/or malabsorption syndromes in the pregnant mother. Severe cases may be debilitating or fatal. A large cluster of anencephila babies born to migrant workers occured in McAllen, Texas in the early 90s. This cluster is thought by public health authorities to be due to some chemical pollutant. It actually appears to be a folic acid and zinc deficiency in the winter diet of poor migrant workers living on corn tortillas.

Treatment of meningocele is limited to surgery. PREVENTION is the goal here! All women of child bearing age should be taking all 90 essential nutrients as a preconception, prenatal, and postnatal supplement.

MENKE'S KINKY HAIR SYNDROME is thought by the "orthodox" pediatrician to be a genetic disease, but it appears to be a malabsorption problem in early infancy (i.e. celiac disease) that results in a copper deficiency (along with other deficiencies). It has long been known in the veterinary field that a copper deficiency causes "kinky wool" disease. Retarded growth, anemia, progressive brain degeneration, sparse brittle hair, loss of hair color, arterial aneurysms, and scurvy-like bone disease (ostosis) are characteristic. Hair analysis will show very low copper levels and blood will show a low copper and low ceruloplasmin.

Treatment of Menke's syndrome includes dealing with the malabsorption problems (i.e. avoid wheat, cow's milk, and soy), supplement with digestive enzymes and betaine HCl, give copper IV at 200 ug/kg/day, and give copper orally at 1–2 mg per day after relief of symptoms.

MENOPAUSE: see climacteric

MERCURY POISONING can result from the ingestion or inhalation of any mercurial compound and off gassing of mercury vapors from mercury amalgam dental fillings. Symptoms include gastroenteritis, salivation, burning mouth pain, abdominal pain, nausea and vomiting, colitis, kidney disease, gingivitis, mental and emotional disturbances, and nerve deficits. Multiple sclerosis is thought by many dentists and alternative health advocates to be the result of mercury poisoning. Diagnosis of mercury poisoning is easily made with a hair analysis and history of a mercury source. The mental and emotional symptoms of mercury poisoning in "hatters" in Victorian England led to the coining of the saying "as mad as a hatter" (don't forget the "Mad Hatter" in *Alice in Wonderland*).

Treatment of mercury poisoning includes the removal of the source of mercury including removing mercury amalgam dental fillings, chelation with EDTA (to include complete IV nutrition), and sweating (sauna) as mercury is excreted in sweat.

The use of selenium containing colloidal minerals is very effective in removing mercury from the tissues. Selenium is almost a specific antidote to mercury poisoning.

METABOLIC THERAPY is the resolving or curing of disease processes by correcting the whole body metabolism through nutrition, herbs, homeopathy, acupuncture, manipulation, and hydrotherapy.

METHADONE is the drug used to facilitate opiate withdrawal. Classically methadone is given in just enough amounts to prevent the most severe withdrawal symptoms (usually 20 mg/day). The opiate (i.e. opium, morphine, etc.) withdrawal symptoms are self-limiting and not life threatening, although addicts in withdrawal often wish they were dead. The use of <u>double</u> the base line nutrition program for 30 days will enhance the patient's ability to get through the withdrawal. After 30 days drop to the base line nutritional supplement program and remain on it. Do pulse test to determine food sensitivities/allergies and do a six-hour GTT. Individuals addicted to drugs and/or alcohol very frequently have "addictive allergies" to food and sugar.

MIGRAINE HEADACHES are frequently heralded by flashes of light or tingling and occurs between the ages of 10–30 years of age and more often in women than men. Nausea, vomiting, diarrhea, digital cyanosis (blue color from lack of circulation and/or oxygen), irritability, and photophobia are common symptoms. "Orthodox" doctors tend to think that migraine headaches are the result of blood vessel problems. In reality, migraine attacks are the result of food allergies with the "target" tissue being the arteries, which constrict the elastic arteries in the brain and dilate the muscular scalp arteries. Do the pulse test to determine which foods you are allergic to.

Treatment and prevention are related to avoidance of food allergens which are identified by means of a diet diary and the pulse test, rotation diets, autoimmune urine therapy, betaine HCl and pancreatic enzymes at 75–200 mg t.i.d., vitamin C to bowel tolerance, bioflavonoids at 200 mg b.i.d., and the base line nutritional supplement program.

MISCARRIAGE (spontaneous abortion) is usually due to deficiencies of vitamins, trace minerals, and/or protein. In particular, vitamin A, zinc, folic acid, selenium, and complete proteins are essential to maintenance of pregnancy. Restricted diets (i.e. weight loss, incomplete vegetarian diets, incomplete rotation diets, etc.) and malabsorption syndromes (i.e. celiac disease type intestinal injury) are the most common reasons for the malnutrition that causes miscarriages and birth defects. Do the pulse test to identify offending food allergens.

Treatment for, and prevention of, miscarriages includes the base line nutrition program for six months before attempting conception and herbs including crampbark (Viburnum opulus), blue cohosh (Caulophyllum thalictroides), and alfalfa.

MITRAL VALVE PROLAPSE is a common progressive change in the left AV valve (mitral valve) and surrounding heart tissue. Most people are not aware that they have a problem. Some have nonanginal chest pain, palpitations, fatigue, and/or breathing problems. A late systolic "murmur" is sometimes detected when doing "squat" type exercises. If you are asymptomatic, your activities need not be restricted. Magnesium deficiency is a common cause of mitral valve prolapse.

Treatment of mitral valve prolapse should include selenium at 500–1,000 mcg/day, magnesium at 1,000 mg t.i.d., salmon oil at 1–5 gm t.i.d., and English hawthorne (Crataegus oxyacantha). Don't forget the base line nutrition program. If the prolapse is due to a magnesium deficiency you can expect a significant improvement within 30–60 days.

MONCKEBERG'S ARTERIOSCLEROSIS is a circular calcification of the media (middle muscular/elastic layer) of small arteries. This disease is caused by hypervitaminosis D (excess vitamin D). Symptoms include hypertension and angina.

Treatment of Monkeberg's arteriosclerosis should include IV EDTA chelation, oral chelation, vitamin C to bowel tolerance, selenium at 500–1,000 mcg per day, and the base line nutritional supplement program.

MONGOLISM (Down's syndrome) is a birth defect caused by a zinc deficiency in the earliest moments of conception (one third of the extra chromosome comes from the paternal parent). The "orthodox" doctors feel that mongolism is the result of a chromosomal defect that increases in risk as the maternal parent ages. It is said that women over 35 have 20 percent of the Down's syndrome babies, yet these women have only 6 percent of the babies born each year. Teenage mothers produce perhaps as many as 60 percent of the remaining Down's syndrome babies.

Newborn Down's syndrome babies are termed "floppy" babies as they are without muscular tone, placid, and rarely cry. Physical and mental maturation is retarded and the average IQ is 50. A small head with a domed forehead is characteristic. Also the bridge of the nose is flattened, the eyes are slanted and have pronounced oriental folds (epicanthal folds), and there are Brushfield's spots (gray salt-like grains around the outer edge of the iris) at birth. Brushfield's spots disappear in the first year of life.

Prevention of Down's syndrome includes the base line nutritional supplement program for 90 days prior to attempting conception. Test for food allergies with the pulse test to eliminate the malabsorption of zinc and other nutrients.

Treatment of Down's syndrome should include zinc at 15 mg t.i.d. and the base line nutritional supplement program. Do pulse test in Down's patients to determine the presence of food allergies and avoid offending foods. You can expect an increase in IQ of 15–20 points and an improvement in physical features as long as the program is followed. Withdrawal from the program results in loss of all the physical and IQ gains.

MORNING SICKNESS is a nausea that occurs in the first three months of pregnancy because of rising progesterone levels. Having a complex carbohydrate or protein snack upon awakening will relieve much of the nausea. Herbal tea such as dogwood (Cornus sericea) and mint (Mentha sativa), B6 and B-complex at 25 mg t.i.d., essential fatty acids at 1,000 mg t.i.d., and the base line nutritional supplement help this temporary condition.

MOSQUITOES can be eliminated from your dwelling by using screen windows and doors. Electric insect "zappers" can be placed approximately 15–25 yards from the back door, the idea being that the violet light will attract the mosquitoes away from the house as well as kill a large number. In addition to being an irritant, mosquitoes carry a number of serious human diseases including meningitis, encephalitis in North America, and malaria, yellow fever, meningitis, and encephalitis in South America. There are numerous OTC flying insect sprays, herbs like pennyroyal (Mentha pulegium) oil rubbed on the skin, and vitamins such as B1 at 500 mg/day will also repel mosquitoes.

MULTIPLE SCLEROSIS (MS) is a progressive disease of the central nervous system. MS is characterized by scattered zones of demyelination (loss of the fatty insulation layer on nerves). Symptoms begin between the ages of 20–40 years and usually start with tingling and/or numbness in the arms or legs (usually "stocking" and "glove" distribution). See mercury poisoning. Weakness, clumsiness, visual problems, balance problems and dizziness, and problems with bladder control follow in months or years. Knee and ankle reflexes are often increased or exaggerated. Intention tremor, nystagmus, and a "scanning" speech (known as Charcot's triad) are frequent problems. Spontaneous remissions for months or years are typical of the untreated disease in the early stages. The untreated disease can be rapidly fatal in one year. Stress is known to precipitate acute attacks. Diagnosis is based on history and neurological exam (the cerebrospinal fluid is abnormal in 80 percent of the patients— normal CSF doesn't rule out MS). Do pulse test to determine food allergens.

Treatment offered by the "orthodox" neurologists is limited to cortisone or prednisone. Unfortunately, this course of therapy is like giving aspirin to treat a brain tumor. It is known that avoidance of fried foods and margarine and a relatively high consumption of flaxseed oil or fish oil (cod liver oil or salmon oil) at 5 gm t.i.d. will increase your survival rate by 50 percent. The consumption of cholesterol (eggs and red meat)is of extreme importance as the myelin sheath that disappears in MS is made almost exclusively of cholesterol.

Treatment should include removal of mercury fillings, the use of CaEAP (a european drug used for M.S.) at 1 q.i.d., octocosanol at two capsules t.i.d., and rattle snake venom injections daily for a contenr irritant therapy, d-phenylalanine at 500 mg t.i.d., betaine HCl and pancreatic enzymes at 75–200 mg t.i.d., along with the avoidance of known food allergens and rotation diets to heal the small intestine, and avoid large doses of vitamin C supplementation. Eat green vegetables and juices as a natural source of vitamin C. This treatment regimen has also proved effective for ALS (Lou Gehrig's Disease).

MUMPS is a contagious viral disease that causes painful enlargement of the salivary glands, especially the parotids. The mumps virus is very aggressive. It is found in the saliva, six days before the patient feels ill, and is also found in the urine and blood. Symptoms include fever (up to 104° F), chills, the skin over the salivary glands becomes tender and shiny, and edema of the parotid salivary gland that causes noticeable swelling in front of and below the ear. Complications occur in 20 percent or so of adult males as a painful testicular infection. Testicular atrophy may follow the infection although hormone production and fertility are rarely affected.

Treatment of mumps is symptomatic including pain relief (i.e. codeine, Tylenol, aspirin, etc.), bed rest, liquid diet including chicken rice soup, sugarless Jello, sports fluid and electrolyte replacer, juices, and herbs for symptomatic treatment including mullein (Verbascum thapsus).

MUSCULAR DYSTROPHY (MD, fibromyalgia) is another crime against the people by the "orthodox" medical doctors for reasons of money. If the total truth was shared with the public, muscular dystrophy would be totally preventable but a whole medical specialty would be wiped out!!! As crazy as this seems, look at the veterinary industry where muscle is "king" (i.e. pork chops, beef steak, lamb chops, roasts, ground red meat, chicken, turkey, etc.). There muscular dystrophy has been wiped out!!! A farmer with 100 cows can expect 100 conceptions, 100 live births, 100 normal calves, and 100 calves raised to market or reproductive age. How can this be that animals are treated better than people???

Prevention is the name of the game with MD. The selenium levels in preconception women is important to the maintenance of pregnancy as well as the prevention of muscular dystrophy in all of its forms (i.e. Duchenne, Erb {scapulohumerall}, Leyden-Moebius {pelvi-femoral}, Landouzy-Dejerine {facio-scapulo-humeral}, Becker's {benign juvenile} and Gowers {hands and feet}), which are in reality artificial classifications of MD by the groups of muscles initially affected. Keshan disease (heart muscular dystrophy) which is also caused by selenium deficiency should be added to the list of muscular dystrophies. In the veterinary profession, muscular dystrophy ("White Muscle Disease") has been eliminated by the use of selenium in pregnant females and rapidly growing prepubic animals. In addition to overt deficiencies of selenium in the diet, the celiac disease type changes in the small intestine caused by food allergies is the common cause of tissue deficiencies of selenium. The symptoms of MD can start with weakness, scoliosis (curvature of the spine), and enlargement of certain muscle groups (i.e. calves, trapezius, etc.) to compensate for the loss of strength of synergistic muscle groups. A muscle biopsy is usually done by a neurologist to make the diagnosis of MD. If selenium and vitamin E were to be given IM or IV at the very first onset of symptoms, the disease will be arrested or maybe even "cured." The "orthodox" doctors resort to prednisone and surgery. Death is the inevitable end for those kids with MD if they are "treated in the "orthodox" method—it would be much healthier to go to a veterinarian for help.

Treatment of MD and/or Keshan disease includes the use of selenium orally (plant derived colloidal minerals), IV or IM at 50–1,000 mcg per day (based on weight), vitamin E IM at 80 mg per day, selenium orally at

250–1,000 mcg per day, vitamin E 800–1,200 orally, sulfur amino acids IV as a complete amino acid infusion and orally in the form of free amino acids and sugarless Jello, and EFA at 5 gm t.i.d. Avoid food allergens, excessive fats (no more than 20 percent of the calories each day as fat), fried food, and margarine. Give choline as soy lecithin at 10–20 gm per day. Avoid exercise for one month during initial treatment period (this is the opposite recommendation from the "orthodox" treatment) to avoid undue injury to already biochemically compromised muscle tissue.

MUSCLE CRAMPS (Charley horse) are a "mini" convulsion that is taking place in the muscle as a result of deficiencies of calcium, magnesium, potassium, selenium, and/or vitamin E. Muscle cramps may be as subtle as the twitch of an eyelid and muscle flutter in arms or legs (fasciculations) to and including the hard cramps of the toes, feet, calves, back, and neck muscles. Prevention includes the base line nutritional supplement program. Do pulse test to determine food allergies that might cause celiac disease type changes and the resultant malabsorption. Do a hair analysis to determine mineral status.

Treatment of muscle cramps can include liquid plant derived colloidal calcium, magnesium, and potassium, betaine HCl and pancreatic enzymes at 75–200 mg t.i.d. before meals. Dr. Wallach's Pig Arthritis Formula works like a charm here.

NASAL CATARRH (runny nose, stuffy nose) can be caused by a wide variety of upper respiratory viral infections. Treatment includes Contac at 1 q 12 h, cayenne pepper (Capsicum minimum), eucalyptus (Eucalyptus globulus), German chamomile (Matricaria chamomilla), and scotch pine (Pinus sylvestris). Avoid fried food, margarine, sugar, and dairy products.

NAUSEA can be caused by a wide variety of diseases and syndromes ranging from nutritional deficiencies, pregnancy, hepatitis, and food allergies to cancer. If nausea is a recurring problem, detailed investigation should be pursued.

Treatment of nausea can include Pepto Bismol, Kaopectate, and herbs to include artichoke (Cynara scolymus), avens (Geum urbanum), and peppermint (Mentha piperita).

NERVOUS HEART (rapid beat, tachycardia, or palpitations when nervous) tends to be common in senior citizens. Many of these cardiac symptoms are the result of B1 (Beri beri) deficiencies, anemia, and deficiencies of stomach acid. Do pulse test to determine if food allergies are a contributing factor.

Treatment of "nervous" heart conditions should include B1 at 100 mg t.i.d., iron at 45–100 mg, and an improved general diet. Don't forget the base line nutritional supplement program and herbs including English hawthorn (Crataegus oxyacantha), hops (Humulus lupulus), lavender (Lavandula angustifolia), motherwort (Leonurus cardiaca), and valerian (Valeriana officinalis), and also avoid offending food allergens and employ rotation diets.

NERVOUS TENSION (nervous headaches) are usually brought on by tension and overwork. There may be a precipitating factor such as caffiene overdose, hypoglycemia, and food allergies involved, so don't forget to do a pulse test. Treatment includes avoidance of sugar, caffeine, food allergens, avoidance and/or reduction of stress and tension, exercise, homeopathy, acupuncture, color therapy, subliminal relaxation tapes, and herbs including balm (Melissa officinalis), bitter orange (Citrus aurantium), sweet woodruff (Gallium odoraturm), wild celery (Apium graveolens), and lily-of-the valley (Convallaria magalis).

NEURALGIA (Tinitis, Trigeminal neuralgia, Bell's palsy, spinal stenosis, neuropathy) is an irritation or a pinching of a nerve which can be caused by many diseases ranging from trauma, nutritional deficiencies (i.e. osteoporosis, B12, folic acid, B1, B6, etc.), infections (i.e. herpes, shingles, etc.), alcoholism, diabetes, MS, etc. Treatment requires attention to any and all underlying conditions. Treatment of neuralgia should also include B-complex 50 t.i.d., B12 1,000 mcg per day, essential fatty acids as EPA at 5 gm t.i.d. and flaxseed oil at one tbsp. b.i.d., calcium and magnesium at 2,000 mg and 1,000 mg per day, Isoprinosin at 500–1,500 mg/day and Ribavirin at 250–1,500 mg/day for viral neuralgias (i.e. herpes and shingles), acupuncture and herbs including lavender (Lavandula angustifolia), oats (Avena satifa), rosemary (Rosmarinus officinalis), St. Johns wort (Hypericum perforatum), and white willow (Salix alba).

NIGHT BLINDNESS (xerophthalmia) is caused by a vitamin A deficiency which can be overt dietary deficiency, fat malabsorption syndrome (vitamin A is fat soluble), zinc deficiency which results in poor conversion of carotene to vitamin A by the liver, cystic fibrosis, celiac disease and various food allergies resulting in intestinal changes that prevent absorption of fat soluble vitamins (i.e. vitamin A, vitamin E, vitamin D and vitamin K), as well as a deficiency of essential fatty acids. Symptoms of night blindness include delayed adaption or complete failure of adaption to darkness. Treatment of night blindness is very specific with 25,000–300,000 IU of vitamin A per day as beta-carotene and zinc at 15–50 mg t.i.d.

NIGHT TERRORS (nightmares) are almost always caused by food allergies and hypoglycemia. The pulse test and the six-hour GTT are necessary to determine the exact cause of night terrors. Remember the low point of blood sugar levels occur at 4–4 1/2 hours after consumption of food (especially sugar foods and drinks) so night terrors will occur four hours after consumption of food (especially sugar foods and drinks). For that reason, night terrors will occur four hours after consumption of "bedtime snacks" (i.e. cookies and milk). Bedwetting in children often accompanies night terrors and are the direct result of food allergies (usually milk) and hypoglycemia (sugar bedtime snacks). Treatment of night terrors includes avoidance of offending food allergens, avoidance of sugar, chromium and vanadium at 25–200 mcg t.i.d., high animal protein diets, base line nutritional supplement program, and avoidance of caffeine.

NOSEBLEEDS (epistaxis) are usually the result of vitamin K and/or vitamin C deficiencies. "Orthodox" EENTs like to do "minor" surgery on noses to cauterize (i.e. burn) capillaries in the nasal membranes to stop the nosebleeds. Treatment for nosebleeds should include increased consumption of green leafy vegetables, reseeding the colon with Lactobacillus acidophilus (the bacteria will synthesize vitamin K), vitamin C to bowel tolerance, calcium and magnesium at 2,000 mg and 1,000 mg per day, vitamin E at 800–1,200 IU per day, alfalfa tablets at 5 t.i.d. with meals, and herbs including toad flax (Linaria vulgaris).

NUMBNESS (tingling both hands, Carpal Tunnel Syndrome) can be caused by neuralgia (diabetes, B12 deficiency), circulation problems, and carpal tunnel syndrome. On occasion food allergies can cause numbness and tingling and should be considered in your diagnostic process. Also, don't forget the possibility of MS. "Tinnel's sign" (tap wrist) with the finger to elicit pain for diagnosis of carpal tunnel syndrome.

"Orthodox" neurologists love to do carpal tunnel surgery for this problem. Treatment for numbness and tingling should include aggressive diagnosis and treatment of any underlying condition as well as manganese, choline, arsenic, B12 at 1000 mcg per day, B6 at 200–300 mg t.i.d., calcium and magnesium at 2,000 mg and 1,000 mg per day and zinc at 50 mg t.i.d., B12 at 1,000 mcg/day, and plant derived colloidal minerals.

OBESITY (overweight, see diet) is a problem to various degrees in all industrialized nations and, in particular, the United States. Obesity has various causes and combinations of causes and is not a simple problem. Rendered down to its simplest terms, obesity is consuming and storing more calories than you are using. Starvation only complicates the correction of the problem as a starving body will shut off calorie consumption as an energy conservation move. To avoid this body maneuver, be sure to consume at least 1,000 calories per day. This way, a gradual but permanent loss of pounds and inches will occur. Moderate exercise in the form of walking, tennis, golf, swimming, and/or low impact aerobics (i.e. Chi Gong) is adequate. Don't forget the base line nutritional supplements, as your need for nutritional supplementation becomes critical when you are on a calorie-restricted diet. Ninety percent of obese people over eat and binge because empty calorie diets result in "pica", a nibbling behavior caused by the body's search for trace minerals! Use colloidal minerals to supply these needed minerals. Test for food allergies with the pulse test and do a six-hour glucose tolerance test to determine if you have hypoglycemia or diabetes. Remember a single fasting blood glucose test will miss 99.9 percent of all hypoglycemics and 85 percent of all diabetics.

"Treatment" of obesity is, in fact, a change in life style and habits requiring a complete commitment, just like the one required to stop smoking. Avoid offending food allergens, avoid sugar in all forms (i.e. solids as well as liquids), avoid caffeine which lowers blood sugar and makes you hungry, avoid carbonated soft drinks which ALL are loaded with phosphates which will cause osteoporosis over the long haul especially when you are already on a restricted diet, and drink filtered —not distilled—water. Distilled water is "hungry" water and will demineralize your bones over a long period of usage. Drink 8–10 glasses of water each day. Forty percent of your water normally comes from food. It only makes sense if you restrict your food, you will also restrict water unless you make a conscious effort to drink enough. "Compulsive" trips to the refrigerator are most often subliminal searches for water, especially if they occur right after meals. Use special salts to flavor meals (potassium salt with kelp is excellent).

DO NOT SKIP MEALS. Make breakfast your largest most complete meal. Lunch should be a moderate meal with animal protein and dinner should be a light "soup and salad." Take salmon oil at 5 gm t.i.d. with meals, flaxseed oil at one tbsp. b.i.d., two heaping tbsp. of nutritional fiber in an eight ounce glass of water before bed, glucomannan at 1 gm in eight ounces of water one hour before meals, and betaine HCl and pancreatic enzymes at 75–200 mg t.i.d. 15 minutes before meals. Take thyroid starting at 1–3 grains. Too much will make you a little jittery and increase your heart rate as much as 10–20 beats/minute. Adjust your intake up or down in dosage as needed. If you get above six grains before you OD on thyroid, you have celiac disease type because of your intestine. Do pulse test and avoid allergens. Take herbal laxatives and/or herbal diuretic teas as necessary. Subliminal weight loss tapes can be very helpful (especially at the beginning). THIS PROGRAM IS VERY COMPLEX TO BEGIN WITH. CHANGE ALL OF THE FOOD IN YOUR HOUSE TO HELP YOU GET STARTED. AFTER YOU REACH YOUR WEIGHT GOALS, YOU CAN SIMPLIFY YOUR WEIGHT LOSS PROGRAM.

OBSTRUCTION OF AIRWAYS (choking) will be heralded by the "universal choking sign" of both hands clutched at the throat and a loss of the ability to speak. This happens very frequently in restaurants and is often referred to as a "restaurant coronary" as most observers think the patient is having a "heart attack." Prevention includes the stopping of talking while you are chewing and swallowing food (especially meat and firm raw vegetables such as carrots and beets). Treatment of choking includes: 1) putting your finger into the back of the throat and manually removing the obstruction, and 2) performing a Heimlich maneuver (standing behind the patient, lock your arms around them with hands locked just below the xiphoid cartilage and suddenly thrust/squeeze, for babies use hands only). If the obstruction is lodged and cannot be coughed out with the Heimlich maneuver, a tracheotomy must be performed as a lifesaving maneuver. The EMTs will not get there in time so you must act quickly. You must use whatever is available (i.e. pocket knife, steak knife, etc.). The location of the incision is half way between the base of the larynx (voice box) and the notch where the collar bones join the breast bone—it must be dead center and large enough to accommodate the empty barrel of a ball point pen which will provide enough airflow for survival. The EMTs will arrive about five minutes after you have completed your "surgery," however, the patient would have died if you waited for them. If the patient's heart has also stopped as a result of the choking, you will have to perform CPR after you have created the airway.

OLIGOSPERMIA (low sperm count) is usually the result of nutritional deficiencies and/or malabsorption syndromes. Do a pulse test to determine if food allergies and celiac type changes are a factor. Infertility is the usual "red flag" that raises the question of sperm count. Place one drop of a semen sample on a slide with a cover slip on top, observe at high power. The live sperm should be highly motile and appear as swirling waves like battalions of Chinese infantry.

Treatment for oligospermia includes avoidance of offending food allergens, fried foods and margarine, sugar and alcohol, double the base line nutritional supplementation for 30–60 days, acupuncture, and herbs including ginseng (Panax ginseng) and herbal combinations such as Zumba that contain 500 mcg of testosterone.

OMPHALOCELE (umbilical hernia) is a birth defect characterized by a grape to basketball sized skin sac in the "belly button" that is lined with peritoneum (membrane lining of the abdominal cavity). The sac may contain fat and/or intestinal loops that can be pushed back into the abdominal cavity. This is a common birth defect that is caused by maternal deficiencies (and, thus, fetal deficiencies) of vitamin A and/or zinc.

Treatment of umbilical hernia requires surgery to repair the belly wall defect if the "hernial ring" (defect in the belly wall) is larger than your finger tip. If the defect is approximately the diameter of your finger tip you can heal this one at home without surgery. The technique is to place a golf ball sized ball of virgin wool on the hernia and tape it firmly down to the level of the skin. Three times each day, remove the wool ball and be sure the fat is pushed back into the belly cavity with the finger tip, at the same time, rub the "hernial ring" in a rotary fashion for several minutes to irritate it. Over a period of weeks to months, the defect will fill in and completely heal without surgery. A sclerosing oil or compound can be injected into the edge of the digit caliber hernial ring to get good closure.

ORGANIC BRAIN SYNDROME (pellagra, alcoholism, dementia, depression, hyperkinesis, ADD, ADHD hypoglycemia, diabetes, PMS, paranoia, schizophrenia, and learning disabilities) is caused by a wide variety of nutritional deficiencies (i.e. niacin, B1, B12, folic acid, chromium, vanadium, lithium, etc.) and toxicities (i.e. alcoholism, lead poisoning, mercury poisoning-dental amalgam). Do a pulse test to determine if food allergies are a part of the syndromes and do a six-hour GTT to rule in or rule out diabetes or hypoglycemia. Remember a single fasting blood glucose will miss 99.9 percent of the hypoglycemia and 85 percent of the diabetes. Treatment of organic mental disorders requires serious dedication to identify the underlying problems and dealing with them.

Treatment should include avoidance of food allergens including sugar, dairy, and wheat, rotation diets, betaine HCl and pancreatic enzymes at 75–200 mg. t.i.d. 15 minutes before meals, B3 (niacin) at 450 mg t.i.d. as time release tablets, essential fatty acids as salmon and flaxseed oils at 5 grams each t.i.d., chromium and vanadium at 25–200 mcg t.i.d., and zinc at 50 mg t.i.d. Don't forget the base line nutritional supplement program for all 90 essential nutrients.

ORNITHOSIS (parrot fever) is an infectious disease caused by Chlamydia psittaci. Parrot fever is transmitted by inhaling the contaminated dust from feathers, cage bedding, or feces of infected birds (i.e. parrots, parakeets, lovebirds, canaries, or pigeons). Parrot fever is characterized by an "atypical pneumonia." Symptoms of "parrot fever" include fever, chills, weakness, loss of appetite, and dry coughing initially that develops into a productive cough. At first, "parrot fever" may be diagnosed as "flu" or confused with Legionnaires' disease or Q fever. Exposure to birds (especially sick ones) will offer a clue that Sherlock Holmes wouldn't miss. A blood test is required for specific diagnosis.

Treatment of "parrot fever" includes the use of tetracycline orally at 250–500 mg q.i.d. for 10–14 days, the cough should be controlled with codeine, and strict bed rest should be enforced as untreated and uncontrolled "parrot fever" can be fatal.

OSTEOARTHRITIS (degenerative arthritis): see arthritis. Dr. Wallach's Pig Arthritis Formula is the treatment of choice here. Thousands of happy arthritis patients can't be wrong.

OSTEITIS FIBROSA (nutritional secondary hyperparathyroidism) is also known as Paget's Disease. This is a bone disease that affects men more often than women (women get osteoporosis more frequently) and is characterized by a loss of hard bone which is replaced by fibrous connective tissue. The first signs of Paget's Disease occur in the dental arcade by separating the teeth and loss of teeth because of loss of jawbone. The weight bearing bones of the pelvis, femur, and tibia are next, very frequently there is a loss of stature as the bones undergo rearchitecturing, and kyphosis ("dowagers' hump"). The cause is thought to be unknown by the "orthodox" doctors. In animals the cause is a reversed calcium/ phosphorus dietary ratio intake in the presence of relatively large amounts of vitamin D; men tend to be out in the sun without their shirts more often than women. Diagnosis of Paget's Disease can be made by x-ray of the teeth in the earliest stages and x-ray of the weight bearing bones in the more advanced stages. The blood shows an elevated alkaline phosphatase (calcium and phosphorus are usually in the normal range) and an elevated parathyroid gland hormone. It is interesting to note that "orthodox" orthopedic doctors think of Paget's Disease as a viral infection.

Treatment of Paget's Disease should include a vigorous effort to correct the dietary calcium/phosphorus ratio, reduce or eliminate red meat intake, avoid phosphate containing soft drinks, avoid all phosphate containing supplements, reduce vitamin D intake and exposure (i.e.

hats, long sleeve shirts, etc.), increase calcium and magnesium intake to 2,000 mg and 1,000 mg per day, take betaine HCl and pancreatic enzymes at 75–200 mg t.i.d. 15 minutes before meals, and don't forget the base line nutritional supplement program—or to make it very simple—Dr. Wallach's Pig Arthritis Formula.

OSTEOPOROSIS is a decrease in bone that usually occurs in older individuals (more frequently in women). The big push by the "orthodox" doctors is for estrogen and fluoride supplementation, yet these two compounds alone do not solve the problem. In our personal experience osteoporosis is easy to prevent and cure with proper supplementation of stomach acid (HCl) and calcium. Do a pulse test to identify any food allergens that might be causing a celiac disease type change and malabsorption syndromes. The symptoms of osteoporosis are characterized by bone pain, joint pain, "dowagers" hump, and "spontaneous" fractures. Osteoporosis is the 12th most frequent cause of death in adults (following fractured hips, etc.).

Treatment of osteoporosis should include betaine HCl and pancreatic enzymes at 75–200 mg t.i.d. 15 minutes before meals, and calcium and magnesium at 2,000 mg and 1,000 mg per day or more for the first 30 days. Estrogen may be contraindicated because of the potential carcinogenic effect: it is known to cause breast and uterine cancer. Don't forget the plant derived colloidal minerals that include calcium, magnesium, and boron. To make it simple again, use Dr. Wallach's Pig Arthritis Formula.

OTITIS (earache, fluid behind the eardrum) is an inflammation of the inner parts of the ear. Otitis externa involves the outside of the eardrum and the ear canal. Otitis interna involves the inside of the eardrum and the eustachian tube. Otitis media involves the middle ear. The "orthodox" EENT approach is to give antibiotic eardrops and oral antibiotics in acute cases and to insert "tubes" into the eardrum to relieve pain in chronic cases. In reality, 95 percent of all otitis (earaches) is the result of a milk allergy. Do a pulse test before the eardrums are pierced and weakened unnecessarily. Milk allergies will cause a severe fever, painful earaches, and burst eardrums if not corrected. Treatment of otitis should include the use of hydrogen peroxide or mullein eardrops to help relieve local inflammation. Avoid cow's milk in all forms and be sure to take the base line nutritional supplement program. Aspirin or Tylenol may be necessary for pain relief. Antibiotics are only justified when a streptococcal sore throat or internal otitis is cultured positive for bacteria.

PAIN is caused by any abnormal process that changes the architecture of bone or soft tissue i.e. edema, distension, swelling, ulcers, etc. Repairing or correcting the disease process will usually eliminate the pain without the continued need for pain medication. Treatment for pain necessarily must include an aggressive correction of any underlying disease process. Treatment of pain may include TENS (electronic pain masking), codeine, Tylenol-3, aspirin with codeine, aspirin, Tylenol, DMSO, acupuncture, hydrotherapy, chiropractic, and herbs including aconite (Aconitum napellus), comfrey (Symphytum officinale), chicory (Cichorium intybus), and English mandrake (Tamus communis). Don't forget plant derived colloidal minerals here. Again, use Dr. Wallach's Pig Arthritis Formula to make it simple.

PALPITATIONS (irregular heartbeat) can be the result of organic heart disease. This is easily determined by an EKG or ECG. Other causes: food allergies (i.e. Chinese Restaurant Syndrome or allergy to MSG), nutritional deficiencies (i.e. B1, B3, selenium, magnesium, potassium, etc.), and/or hypoglycemia.

Treatment of palpitations should include EDTA chelation for cardiovascular disease, IV hydrogen peroxide, avoid caffeine, avoid offending food allergens, avoid sugar and processed foods in all forms, vitamin B1 at 100 mg t.i.d., B3 at 450 mg t.i.d. as time release tablets, vitamin C to bowel tolerance, selenium 250 mcg/day, and the base line nutritional supplementation program. Use herbs including English hawthorn (Crataegus oxyacantha), lily-of-the-valley (Convallaria mejalis), hops (Humulus lupulus), lavender (Lavandula angustifolia), mother wort (Leonurus cardiaca), valerian (Valeriana officinalis), and foxglove (Digitalis purpurea). See previous warnings about the dosage of foxglove!

PARASITES (worms, amoebiasis, malaria) include a variety of roundworms (i.e. ascaris, hookworms, pinworms, and whipworms), tapeworms, flukes, and microscopic one cell organisms (i.e. amoeba, flagellates, malaria). Symptoms of parasites include diarrhea, abdominal pain, weight loss, anal itching, weakness, anemia, failure to thrive, and B12 deficiency (tapeworm). Diagnosis of parasites includes a microscopic fecal exam for all intestinal parasites, except for pinworms, which require a Scotch tape test on the anal opening to find the eggs. Blood tests are required to identify malarial parasites.

Treatment for parasites includes garlic (Allium sativum), peach (Prunus persica), and black walnut (Juglans nigra). With heavy infestations, stronger medication is required. Pyrantel pamoate (roundworms),

Niclosamide (tapeworms) and Metronidazole (protozoa) should be employed.

PARKINSONISM (shaking palsy) is caused by a degeneration of the basal ganglia of the brain; symptoms are relentlessly progressive and include muscular rigidity, lack of purposeful movement, tremor, and "pill rolling" tremors of the thumb and index finger. The cause of true Parkinson's Disease is unknown, however, there are numerous medications that will cause Parkinsonism-like symptoms (i.e. phenothiazines, haloperidol, reserpine) as well as carbon monoxide poisoning, mercury from amalgam fillings, and excessive manganese in a community water supply.

Treatment of drug induced Parkinsonism should include the elimination of the offending drug. Note that the "orthodox" neurologist will usually recommend an additional drug to deal with the symptoms of the offending drug. Have mercury amalgam fillings replaced with composite, take octacosanol at 300 mcg t.i.d., leucine 10 gm/day, 1-methionine at 5 gm/day, EFA at 5 grams b.i.d., 1-tyrosine at 100 mg/day, dl-phenoalanine at 100 mg t.i.d., B1 at 200 mg t.i.d., B6 at 100 mg t.i.d., betaine HCl and pancreatic enzymes at 75–200 mg t.i.d. before meals, and the base line nutritional supplement program. The "orthodox" neurologist treats with 1-Dopa and carbidopa which aggravates and speeds up the progress of Parkinson's Disease in a significant number of cases and has no beneficial effect in more than 50 percent of the cases.

PEPTIC ULCERS (gastric ulcer, duodenal ulcer) are thought to be caused by stress, deficiency of "vitamin U" (a mythological vitamin), and/or dyspepsia. In reality they are caused by an infection of the stomach or duodenal lining with Helicobacter pylori. Symptoms of peptic ulcer include burning stomach pain, dyspepsia, and weight loss. "Coffee ground" stool or vomit indicates that the ulcer is bleeding and that the patient is in eminent danger of bleeding to death. GO TO A HOSPITAL IMMEDIATELY! Treatment of peptic ulcer should include alfalfa (Medicago sativa) which is thought to be the richest source of "vitamin U" at ten tablets t.i.d. with meals, cabbage juice (Brassica oleracea), flax (Linum usitatissimum), German chamomile (Matricaria chamomilla), and licorice (Glycyrrhiza glabra). A 98 percent chance of a cure can be affected with antibiotics and bismuth every day for four to six weeks.

PERIODONTAL DISEASE (receding gums, pyorrhea, gingivitis) is thought by "orthodox" dentist to be caused by food particles packing into the space between teeth and between teeth and gums. In reality, all forms of periodontal disease are the result of bone loss under the gums, which causes the gums to recede and allow food to pack into the space created. Again, this disease has been eliminated by the veterinary profession as a result of nutritional investigations for better health and production of pet and farm animals. I have not seen too many cows, horses, dogs, and cats (nor wolves, giraffe, or elephants for that matter) floss, brush their teeth, or use mouthwash with fluoride. The reason that this simple concept has not been shared with the public is money. Think about the toothpaste, toothbrush, and floss companies that get the approval of the American Dental Association. Does it not seem odd that these same companies give large grants to the dental schools? Sherlock Holmes, and maybe some union stewards, would call this one a "sweetheart deal!". This appears to be another case of letting the fox "guard" the chicken house.

Treatment of periodontal disease should include a correction of the dietary calcium/phosphorus ratio. Give up phosphate containing soft drinks, reduce red meat consumption, reduce phytate intake (raw vegetables), supplement calcium at 2,000 mg per day and magnesium at 1,000 mg per day, and remember the base line nutrition supplement program including plant derived colloidal minerals. Take vitamin A at 300,000 IU per day as beta-carotene, vitamin C to bowel tolerance, zinc at 15 mg t.i.d., and betaine HCl and pancreatic enzymes at 75–200 mg t.i.d. 15 minutes before meals. Avoid sugar, use herbal and hydrogen peroxide mouthwashes, and dental floss to keep gum pockets and teeth clean so rebuilding of bone can take place.

PHLEBITIS (varicose veins) is most common in the hemorrhoidal veins and veins of the legs. Constipation and static vertical position are the primary precipitating factors; however, a copper deficiency is the root cause. Copper is required as a cofactor for manufacturing strong elastic fibers in the walls of veins. Treatment of phlebitis should include consumption of eight glasses of water, two heaping tbsp. of nutritional fiber in a glass of water at bedtime, vitamin E at 800–1,200 IU/day, B-complex at 50 mg each t.i.d., vitamin C to bowel tolerance, copper at 2 mg per day (Dr. Wallach's Pig Arthritis Formula), EFA at 5 gm t.i.d., and herbs including arnica (Arnica montana), comfrey (Symphytum officinale), rue (Ruta graveolens), yellow sweet clover (Melilotus officinalis), and cascara sagrada (Rhamnus purshianus).

PICA (cribbing, cravings for dirt, paint, snack food, sugar, salt, etc.) is a symptom of one or more nutritional mineral deficiencies. Only mineral deficiencies cause this pica behavior. Adults often evidence pica when they crave ice, chips, salsa, chocolate, and soft drinks. Children evidence pica when they eat dirt and/or paint chips. The latter is extremely dangerous as many paints contain lead or cadmium. A hair analysis will be invaluable to determine the patient's mineral status. Do a pulse test to determine if a celiac disease type malabsorption problem exists.

Treatment for pica should focus on mineral supplementation and must include the base line nutritional program including plant derived colloidal minerals. EDTA chelation therapy may be necessary if hair analysis shows elevated levels of lead or cadmium.

PILES (hemorrhoids): see hemorrhoids

PILONIDAL CYST is a midline congenital defect (zinc or vitamin A, folic acid deficiency) in the sacral area. The "pit" often contains a tuft of hair. The tract is usually asymptomatic unless it becomes plugged and becomes a cyst. Treatment of the pilonidal cyst should include a poultice of plantain (Plantago major), comfrey (Symphytum officinale), or boric acid b.i.d. until cyst opens up. On rare occasions surgical opening of the cyst is required; local anesthesia and a scalpel blade are all that is required for this relatively minor surgery.

PIMPLES (acne): see acne

PREMENSTRUAL SYNDROME (PMS, hysteria) has a long history in "orthodox" medicine. Historically the treatment for PMS was hysterectomy (derived from hysteria) since removal of the ovaries and uterus "cured" all of the cyclical emotional symptoms leaving a precipitous menopause, which could be palliated with estrogen. It is now known that deficiencies of calcium and essential fatty acids in concert with the cyclical hormone patterns of the women produce the classical PMS picture of fragile emotions, irrational behavior, mania, depression, and debilitating pelvic "cramps."

Treatment of PMS includes 100 mg B6 q 4 d, EFA at 5 grams t.i.d., vitamin A at 300,000 IU per day as beta carotene during the last 14 days of the cycle, vitamin E at 800–1,200 IU/day, calcium (especially plant derived colloidal sources), and herbs including mistletoe (Viscum album), black cohosh (Cimicifuga racemosa), and blue cohosh (Caulophyllus thalictroides). Don't forget to supplement with the entire compliment of the 90 essential nutrients

POISON IVY causes a contact papular dermatitis that produces a severe itch. Treatment of poison ivy dermatitis includes topical application of vinegar, Caladryl, Aloe vera, poultices of Solomon's seal (Polygonatum multiflorum), golden seal (Hydrastis canadensis), and plantain (Plantago major).

POOR CIRCULATION can be caused by cardiovascular disease (arteriosclerosis, low thyroid, magnesium deficiency, and vitamin E deficiency). Symptoms include cold hands and feet and numb tingling fingers and toes.

Treatment of poor circulation includes EDTA chelation, the highest quality (with no contaminents) hydrogen peroxide IV (oxygen source) administered slowly, vitamin C to bowel tolerance, vitamin E at 800–1,200 IU/day, massage, hydrotherapy, acupuncture, and herbs including ginkgo (Ginkgo biloba), English hawthorn (Crataegus oxyacantha), horsetail (Equisetum arvense), lavender (Lavandula angustifolia), lily-of-the-valley (Convallaria majalis), rosemary (Rosmarinus officinalis), scotch pine (Pinus sylvestris), and cayenne pepper (Capsicum minimum).

POX: see chicken pox

POST PARTUM HEMORRHAGE is the result of an atonic uterus that failed to contract hard enough and long enough, allowing the open vessels to leak blood. On occasion a piece of afterbirth will remain attached to the uterine lining and is the source of the bleeding.

Treatment of post partum hemorrhage should include firm digital pressure on the fundus of the uterus to stimulate contraction, and the use of ergot (Claviceps purpurea) orally at 10–20 minims (a minim is an old apothecary term meaning approximately 1 drop) or by injection will add sufficient contraction power.

PREGNANCY LABOR (labor) can be enhanced by the use of herbs including raspberry (Rubus idaeus) and blue cohosh (Caulophyllum thalictroides).

PREGNANCY TOXEMIA (eclampsia) is the result of low protein, low salt diets entered into in an attempt to prevent excess weight gain in pregnancy. The first thoughts of restriction of weight gain occurred at the turn of the century when "orthodox" OB/GYN practitioners learned that low birth weight babies could be delivered faster and, thus, allow more calls in one day. Symptoms of preeclampsia include sudden weight gain (because of fluid accumulation as a result of low blood protein), high blood pressure, and albuminuria. Eclampsia includes the symptoms of preeclampsia plus convulsions and/or coma. Both preeclampsia and eclampsia characteristically occur after the 20th week of pregnancy. The current "orthodox" treatment is hospitalization, and watching until convulsions occur and then give barbiturates.

Treatment of preeclampsia should include a high animal protein meal plan (150 gm or more whereas the RDA is 40 gm), no restriction of salt, and B6 at 100 mg per day. Drop to 50 mg per day at parturition (birth) if you plan to breast feed as high levels of B6 will reduce production of breast milk. In addition to the base line nutritional supplement program for all 90 essential nutrients, patients should receive 10–12 glasses of water and/or juice per day, especially in the warm summer months.

PROSTATE HYPERPLASIA (benign prostate hyperplasia): see benign prostate hyperplasia

PSORIASIS is well known as a cosmetically disfiguring dermatitis (i.e. "the heartbreak of psoriasis"). Psoriasis is characterized by dry, well-demarcated silvery, scaling plaques of all sizes that appear primarily behind joints (i.e. elbows and knees) and on the scalp and behind the ears. Celiac disease type changes in the intestine lead to malabsorption of essential nutrients causing psoriasis. Do a pulse test to determine specific food allergens. Treatment of psoriasis should include avoidance of offending food allergens, rotation diets, folic acid at 15–25 mg per day, vitamin A at 300,000 IU per day as beta-carotene, lecithin at 2,500 mg t.i.d. with meals, EFA at 5 grams b.i.d., vitamin E at 800–1,200 IU per day, zinc at 15 mg t.i.d., copper at 2 mg per day, selenium at 500–1,000 mcg per day, and betaine HCl and pancreatic enzymes at 75–200 mg per day. Topical herbal washes are of palliative value as are topical pureed onions, topical pureed cucumbers, and topical vitamin A & D creams.

PYORRHEA (periodontal disease): see periodontal disease

Q FEVER is an acute rickettsial disease caused by Coxiella burnetii and characterized by sudden onset, fever, headache, weakness, and pneumonitis. Q fever has a worldwide distribution and is maintained as an endemic infection in domestic animals. Sheep, goats, and cattle are the primary reservoirs for human infections. The infection is spread to humans by bites from the infected tick, Dermacentor andersoni, and from consuming infected raw milk. Diagnosis is made from a positive blood test. Treatment of Q fever should include tetracycline orally at 250 mg q 4 h. Chloramphenicol may be used in small children to prevent discoloration of permanent teeth by tetracycline.

QUINSY (peritonsillar abscess) is an infection of the tonsil between the tonsil and the pharyngeal constrictor muscle. These infections are rare in children but common in young adults. The "orthodox" EENT will want to do a tonsillectomy. DON'T LET HIM DO IT! SAVE YOUR TONSILS! Treatment should include vitamin A at 300,000 IU per day as beta-carotene, zinc at 50 mg t.i.d., vitamin C to bowel tolerance, gargles with herbal washes, and penicillin G or V at 250 mg q 6 h for 12–14 days.

RABBIT FEVER (tularemia) is caused by the bacteria, Francisella tularensis. This disease is contracted by skinning and dressing infected rabbits or ground squirrels (87 percent). The disease initially appears as a local ulceration at the infection site, and secondarily goes systemic causing typhoid like disease with diarrhea and pneumonia. High fever and recurring chills with drenching sweat are characteristic. I have had tularemia and my grandfather died from it as a result of skinning infected wild rabbits. Diagnosis comes following a high level of suspicion (appropriate history of wild rabbit contact), and the ulcerated primary lesion at the infection site is enough to make the diagnosis. Sputum cultures are highly infectious and labs should be warned of your suspicions. Treatment of tularemia is with streptomycin IM at 500 mg q 12 h until temperature drops into the normal range, then give tetracycline orally at 250 mg q.i.d. for 10–12 days.

RABIES (hydrophobia) is a highly dangerous viral disease that is transmitted by the blood, tissue (transplanted corneas, livers, kidneys, or hearts), urine, or saliva of infected animals or people. We are all aware of the dangers of bites from rabies infected bats, foxes, skunks, and unvaccinated dogs but most of us are not aware that many cases of fatal rabies occur following tissue transplants. Rabies in humans is a progressive paralytic disease that is often misdiagnosed as stroke, which is why rabies infected tissues get transplanted.

Many Americans spend over a hundred dollars to visit the "orthodox" doctor when their child gets bitten by the pet hamster, because of fears of rabies. Think about it; the incubation period of rabies is fourteen days. If you have had the hamster for three weeks or more, rabies is an impossible diagnosis. A free phone call to your veterinarian would be informational and save you a lot of money.

High risk research personnel can get preventative vaccinations for rabies. Treatment of rabies should be instituted quickly if survival is to be anticipated. Treatment includes the well known "rabies shots" every day for ten days and respiratory and fluid support in a hospital setting.

RACHITIC ROSARY (rickets) is the "beading" of the junction between the ribs and the rib cartilage. This is exclusively a malady of small children who are kept indoors and are not getting an oral source of vitamin D. The rachitic "rosary" is easily palpated. Treatment of the rachitic "rosary" should include oral vitamin D at 400–1,000 IU per day and the base line nutritional supplement program including calcium and magnesium. After the abnormal bony changes become normal, the vitamin D dose should be dropped to 250–400 IU per day. Be sure the patient receives daily exposure to sun for at least 30 minutes.

RADIAL NERVE PALSY ("Saturday night palsy") is the result of compressing the radial nerve against the humerus. Draping the arm over the back of a hard-backed chair for an extended period, such as a drunken stupor or deep sleep, usually causes this. A wrist "drop" and weakness characterize radial nerve palsy in the ability to extend the wrist and fingers. Sometimes there is a loss of sensory function between the first and second fingers. Treatment of radial palsy should include B-complex 50 t.i.d., topical DMSO, acupuncture, massage and hydrotherapy.

RAYNAUD'S DISEASE is characterized by tingling and numbness in the fingers (and sometimes the nose and tongue) which is caused by spasms of small arteries. The "orthodox" approach to Raynaud's disease is to cut sympathetic nerves and give anesthetics and tranquilizers. Food allergies can be the precipitating factor in Raynaud's disease when arteries are the target tissue. Do a pulse test to determine if food allergens are a problem. Rule out "thoracic inlet syndrome" (nerves or arteries coming out of the thorax are squeezed by muscles or bones). Treatment of Raynaud's disease should include calcium and magnesium at 2,000 mg per day and 1,000 mg per day respectively. Avoid offending food allergens, avoid caffeine (i.e. coffee, tea, soft drinks, chocolate, etc.), vitamin E at 800–1,200 IU per day, essential fatty acids at 5 grams t.i.d., 1-tryptophane at 500 mg t.i.d., acupuncture, chiropractic, and herbs to increase circulation such as cayenne pepper (Capsicum minimum).

RECTAL ITCHING can be caused by Candidiasis, food allergies, hemorrhoids, crabs, fleas, and pinworms. Do a pulse test to rule in or rule out food allergies. Take the self-test, blood test, or skin test to determine infection with Candidia albicans. The diagnosis of pinworms requires the scotch tape test to identify the parasite eggs. The presence of fleas and/or hemorrhoids will require the use of a mirror for self examination of the anal folds. Treatment of rectal itching can be palliated with a variety of herbal washes (see hemorrhoids), Preparation H, sitz baths with herbal washes and/or hydrogen peroxide, along with specific treatments for parasites.

REYE'S SYNDROME occurs most frequently in young teens and usually in the fall and winter. Reye's syndrome is characterized by pneumonitis, nausea and vomiting, sudden change in mental status to deep depression, amnesia, agitation to coma and convulsions, fixed dilated pupils, and death in 42–80 percent. The cause of Reye's syndrome is thought to be consumption of aflatoxin (an exotoxin of the grain mold Aspergillus flavus). A typical liver necrosis is present on biopsy. Survivors show a 100 percent recovery of the liver tissue in twelve weeks after the attack. Treatment of Reye's syndrome include barbiturate anesthesia to lower intracranial pressure, IV fluids and electrolytes, pulmonary support, and exchange transfusions and dialysis. Take vitamin C IV at 5–10 gms per day, B-complex and B12 IV or IM, and selenium IM or IV at 250–500 mcg per day.

RHEUMATIC FEVER is caused by Streptococcus Group A infection (usually starts as a "strep throat"). Rheumatic fever is characterized by arthritis, skin rash, fever, heart valve inflammation, and brain signs (chorea). The residual valve damage is the most dangerous aspect of untreated rheumatic fever. Diagnosis of rheumatic fever is made from the typical symptoms and concurrent positive cultures of Streptococcus Group A. Treatment of rheumatic fever early in the course of the disease will prevent the heart damage. Treatment should include aspirin for joint pain and sulfadiazine orally at 500–1,000 mg/day for 1–2 years or penicillin G or V orally at 250,000 u. b.i.d. for two years.

RHEUMATISM (rheumatoid arthritis) is thought by "orthodox" rheumatologist to be a disease of the immune system. In reality, rheumatoid arthritis is caused initially by an infection by a PPLO (pleuropneumonia like organism) or Mycoplasma synovea that characteristically causes an upper respiratory infection and pneumonitis. These organisms secondarily attack the tendon sheaths, joint capsule membranes of the fingers and toes, and later, the larger joints of the shoulders and knees. This disease has been recognized and eliminated in the veterinary industry. Again the human population has been left out because the truth would eliminate an entire medical specialty. Remember the quote by the famous Dr. Arthur F. Coca: "I am a realist; as long as the profit is in the treatment of symptoms rather than in the search for causes, that's where the medical profession will go for its harvest."

Diagnosis of rheumatoid arthritis is made by biopsy of the joint membrane, x-ray, blood test (elevated SED RATE, positive for RA), and physical examination. The "orthodox" treatment is totally aimed at relieving symptoms (i.e. aspirin, gold shots, methotrexate, steroids). They claim great victory but statistics show that 75 percent of the rheumatoid arthritis patients improve in the first year without any treatment at all (up to 10 percent are disfigured and disabled despite "heroic" "orthodox" therapy).

Treatment of rheumatoid arthritis should include specific treatment for Mycoplasma synovea PPLO (Minocycline, tetracycline), for one year, IV and/or oral hydrogen peroxide, EDTA chelation, acupuncture, enterically coated bromeliad at 40 mg q.i.d., autoimmune urine therapy,

DMSO, 1-histidine at 1,000 mg t.i.d., EFA at 5 grams t.i.d., calcium and magnesium at 2,000 mg and 1,000 mg per day, selenium at 500–1,000 mcg per day, copper at 2–4 mg per day, B-6 at 100 mg t.i.d., cartilage (collogen, glucosamine sulfate, chondroitin sulfate) at 5 gm t.i.d. , acupuncture, hydrotherapy, and herbs to include topical camphor (Cinnamonum camphora), black mustard (Brassica nigra), dandelion (Taraxacum officinale), grappie (Harpagophytum procumbens), juniper (Juniperus communis), stinging nettle (Urtica dioica), and sweet vernal grass (Anthoxanthum odoratum). Dr. Wallach's Pig Arthritis Formula makes this program simple.

RICKETS is caused by a deficiency of vitamin D and is characterized by stunted growth, joint pain, and deformed long bones (i.e. bow legs, dropped wrists, "sickle shins," barrel chest, rachitic rosary, etc.).

Treatment of rickets includes supplementation with vitamin D at 400 IU orally b.i.d., calcium and magnesium at 2,000 mg and 1,000 mg per day, and exposure to sunshine for 30 minutes per day. Advanced cases will require orthotic correction and, in some cases, orthopedic surgery.

RINGING IN THE EARS (tinnitis, Miniar's disease, and Wallach's vertigo) can be caused by high blood pressure, drug side effects, and osteoporosis (fibrous connective tissue squeezing the 8th cranial nerve).

The bones of the body try to get stronger following the loss of mineral by generating connective tissue. The 8th cranial nerve can be squeezed as it passes through the skull into the inner ear. When the vestibular branch is squeezed, vertigo can be a feature; when the auditory branch is squeezed ringing in the ears occurs.

Treatment is directed toward lowering blood pressure, eliminating drug side effects, and reversing the osteoporosis with calcium 2000 mg and magnesium 1000 mg. Dr. Wallach's Pig Arthritis Formula is the treatment of choice.

RINGWORM is caused by fungi that invades the skin, nails, and hair, and the skin lesions tend to be circular thus the name "ringworm." The organisms most frequently isolated are Microsporum spp. (Tinea capitis) and Trichophyton spp. (Tinea cruris or jock itch). Cats, rabbits, and children are the most common source of infection. Diagnosis is made by seeing the characteristic lesions, culture of the fungi, and positive reaction to the Woods lamp (lesions of Microsporum will fluoresce a bright pastel green).

Treatment of ringworm should include Griseofulvin orally at 250 mg q.i.d. for four months, vitamin A at 25,000–300,000 IU/day as beta carotene, zinc at 15 mg t.i.d., vitamin E at 800–1,200 IU/day, ultra violet light directly to lesion for up to six minutes per day, and herbs topically including plantain (Plantgo major) and castor oil (Ricinus communis).

ROCKY MOUNTAIN SPOTTED FEVER (tick fever) is caused by a rickettsia (Rickettsia rickettsii) which is transmitted to man by the bite of an infected tick (i.e. the wood tick, Dermacentor andersoni, the dog tick, Dermacentor variabilis, and the lone-star tick, Amblyomma americanum). Rocky Mountain Spotted Fever occurs May through October during the tick season and affects small children who have access to heavily wooded areas directly or indirectly via the family dog who brings home the infected ticks. Ninety percent of the reported cases occur along the Eastern seaboard and only 10 percent occur in adult hunters from the mountain areas. The symptoms of RMSF follow 7–12 days after a tick bite and are characterized by headaches, chills, weakness, muscle pain, fever, and dry cough. A characteristic skin rash starts on wrists, ankles, palms, soles and forearms at first, then spreads to the neck, face, axilla, buttocks, and trunk, along with liver enlargement and pneumonitis with terminal circulatory failure in untreated cases. DO NOT WAIT FOR A POSITIVE BLOOD TEST BEFORE INSTITUTING TREATMENT AS DEATH MAY OCCUR AS QUICKLY AS 4–10 DAYS AFTER APPEARANCE OF SYMPTOMS.

Treatment of RMSF should include tetracycline at 500 mg q.i.d. orally or IV if the patient can't swallow capsules. Supportive treatment with IV fluids and electrolytes is essential to rapid and full recovery.

ROSEOLA is an acute viral disease of infants and toddlers and is characterized by high fever (up to 105° F) and a rash that predominates on the belly and chest and lightly on the face and limbs. Convulsions may occur during the high fever periods. After 3–4 days, the child will feel completely well even though the rash persists. The course of the disease and distribution of the rash are diagnostic.

Treatment of roseola is directed to reducing the fever sufficiently to prevent convulsions and topical poultices on the rash (see measles).

SCABIES (itch) is caused by an almost microscopic "mite" (Sarcoptes scabiei) that burrows into the skin. This mite is very contagious from person to person. The original infestation usually comes from an infected animal or contaminated animal bedding.

Treatment of scabies includes total body application of 1 percent gamma benzene hexachloride, 25 percent benzyl benzoate cream in adults, and 5–10 percent sulfur ointment in infants to avoid potential neurotoxicity; poke (Phytolacca decandra) may be used topically as a natural alternative.

SCARLATINA (scarlet fever) is caused by a Streptococcus Group A throat infection. The organism releases a toxin that produces a rash that is most common on the belly, sides, and skin folds and a red pulpy "strawberry" tongue. Fever in the early stages is common. Before the advent of antibiotics, deadly epidemics of scarlatina swept through the young populations. Aggressive treatment is recommended to prevent death or rheumatic fever from developing. Diagnosis is made from the characteristic lesions and positive throat cultures of Streptococcus Group A.

Treatment of scarlatina is oral penicillin V at 250 mg q.i.d. for 10–14 days.

SCHIZOPHRENIA ("split" personality): see bi-polar brain disease. There is considerable evidence to show that schizophrenia is the result of a severe niacin deficiency. The term "megavitamin" was coined to describe the large dose (4,000 mg/day) of niacin required to "cure" a schizophrenic.

SCIATICA (low back pain radiating down buttocks and legs) can be caused by "subluxations" of lumbar vertebrae, thinning of lumbar inter-vertebral disc, or even a thick wallet in one back pocket. In its most severe form, sciatica may be the result of advanced osteoporosis, bone spurs between the lumbar vertebrae, and vertebral arthritis.

Treatment of sciatica should include hydrotherapy, chiropractic, acupuncture, inversion-gravity therapy, calcium and magnesium at 2,000 mg per day and 1,000 mg per day, and the baseline nutritional supplement program. Dr. Wallach's Pig Arthritis Formula is the treatment of choice here.

SCOLIOSIS (curvature of the spine) occurs in preteens and teens (80 percent in girls) during the rapid growth stages. The patient should be examined bending over facing away from the examiner. The spine is viewed for lateral deviations. Scoliosis may be a benign disease or herald the early stages of muscular dystrophy (MD). Scoliosis is basically caused by one set of the spinal muscles being stronger than the other (i.e. right side stronger than the left) which causes an "S" curve in the spine. These changes are the result of muscle degeneration (i.e. fibromyalgia, muscular dystrophy). Prevention of scoliosis should include the religious consumption of the base line nutritional supplement program containing all 90 essential nutrients. Celiac disease type intestinal damage may be the cause of malabsorption syndromes leading to scoliosis.

Treatment of scoliosis in the early stages will result in a complete cure. Failure to aggressively take supplements will result in persistent damage requiring back braces and surgery. Treatment should include avoidance of offending food allergens, vitamin E at 800–1,200 IU per day, selenium at 500–1,000 mcg per day, calcium and magnesium at 2,000 mg and 1,000 mg per day, and the base line supplement program to include plant derived colloidal minerals. Chiropractic care can be very useful in relieving back muscle spasms associated with scoliosis.

SCURVY (bleeding gums) is caused by a vitamin C deficiency. Scurvy may occur concurrently with gingivitis (see periodontitis).

Treatment of scurvy should include vitamin C to bowel tolerance, increased green leafy vegetables and fruit intake, and herbs including dog rose (Rosa canina).

SEBACEOUS CYSTS (Wen, steatoma) are slow growing benign cystic cutaneous "tumors." They contain sebaceous material and are frequently found on the scalp (Wen), ears, back, breasts, or scrotum. The cyst ranges in size from a pea to a golf ball, is firm (like a soft-shell egg) and painless.

Treatment of a sebaceous cyst includes a "stab" incision at the lowest edge of the cyst, evacuation of the contents, and flushing the site with hydrogen peroxide. Large cysts require removal of the cyst wall to prevent refilling of the cyst, placing a sterile gauze drain in the empty cyst, and gradual removal over a period of 7–10 days.

SEBORRHEIC DERMATIS (dandruff, cradle cap) is a scaling dermatitis of the scalp and face, the composition and amount of sebum are normal. Celiac disease type intestinal lesions can be the cause of a malabsorption syndrome.

Treatment of seborrheic dermatitis should include biotin at 100 mcg t.i.d., folic acid at 15–25 mg per day, B6 at 100 mg t.i.d., vitamin E at 800–1,200 mg IU per day, EFA at 5 grams t.i.d., vitamin A at 300,000 IU per day as beta-carotene, zinc at 15 mg t.i.d., and Selsun Blue shampoo topically.

SENILE DEMENTIA (senility): see memory loss

SEXUALLY TRANSMITTED DISEASES include gonorrhea, syphilis, AIDS, Herpes II, warts, etc. SEE EACH DISEASE INDIVIDUALLY. Use condoms and select sexual partners with great care. A mistake can cost you your life.

SHARK SKIN (keratosis) is caused by a deficiency of vitamin A and zinc (usually as a result of low animal protein diets). Shark skin is characterized by cracks in the corners of the mouth (cheilosis), oral lesions that are often secondarily infected by Candida albicans (perleche), "geographic" tongue, and skin lesions characterized by hard granular plugs resulting from collections of sebaceous and keratinized material in hair follicles which gives a sandpaper-like surface (shark skin).

Treatment of shark skin and related skin problems should include B-complex at 50 mg t.i.d. and skin washes for dermatitis (see dermatitis), vitamin A at 300,000 IU per day as beta-carotene, zinc at 15 mg t.i.d., and EFA at 5 grams t.i.d.

SHINGLES (Herpes zoster) is a chronic viral infection with the chicken pox virus. The symptoms include a very painful skin lesion ("shingles").

Treatment of shingles should include Isoprinosin at 500–1,500 mg per day and American sarsaparilla (Aralia nudicaulis) as a wash or poultice.

SKIN AILMENTS (dermatitis) are caused by a variety of diseases. see dermatitis

Treatment of skin disease should include specific treatment for the underlying problem, homeopathy, EFA at 5 grams t.i.d., vitamin A at 300,000 IU per day as beta-carotene, zinc at 15 gm t.i.d., EFA at 5 gm t.i.d., and herbs including horsetail (Equisetum arvense), pansy (Viola tricolor), Quack grass (Agropyron repens), soap wort (Saponaria officinalis), stinging nettle (Urtica dioica), slippery elm (Ulmus fulva), and globe mallow (Sphaeralcea spp.).

SORE THROAT can be caused by a variety of viral and bacterial diseases. Bacterial diseases (i.e. Streptococcus Group A) tend to exhibit a higher fever than sore throats caused by viral disease (i.e. URI, cold viruses, flu, etc.).

Treatment of sore throats should include antibiotics as necessary for chronic Strep throat and herbs including flax (Linum usitatissimum), garden sage (Salvia officinalis), German chamomile (Matricaria chamomilla), marjoram (Origanum vulgare), marshmallow (Althaea officinalis), rosemary (Rosmarinus officinalis), eucalyptus (Eucalyptus globulus), myrtle (Myrica cerifera), and lobelia (Lobelia inflata).

SPRAIN is characterized by a painful stretching of ligaments of the joints. These traumas can be temporarily debilitating and locally painful. Sprains are caused by lifting, sudden stops or turns, and/or trauma.

Treatment of sprains include ice to reduce swelling as immediate first aid, then wrap with an Ace bandage for support. Fingers may be taped to the adjoining fingers for added support. Take collogen, glucosamine sulfate, and chondroitin sulfate at 5 gram t.i.d., betaine HCl and pancreatic enzymes at 75–200 mg t.i.d. in between meals, DMSO topically, pain gels topically, and herbs including arnica (Arnica montana) and comfrey (Symphytum officinale).

SPIDER BITE produces swelling, local fever, and itching. Brown recluse spider bites produce ulceration and require surgical removal.

Treatment for spider bites should include soaking bite wound in a bath prepared from 8–10 sunflowers (Helianthus annus) soaked for 30 minutes.

STOMACH DISORDERS: see dyspepsia

STRAINS are more severe than sprains and are characterized by torn ligaments and torn joint capsule with bleeding and swelling. A very painful joint trauma, emergency treatment should include ice to reduce swelling; strains frequently require a cast similar to that used for a fracture to immobilize and rest the injured joint.

Treatment of strains should include ice, DMSO, pain gels, betaine HCl and pancreatic enzymes at 75–200 mg t.i.d. between meals, and herbs including arnica (Arnica montana), comfrey (Symphytum officinale), and lavender (Lavandula spp.). A cast and crutches are appropriate to provide support and rest. Hyperbaric oxygen or oral oxygen supplements speed up the healing process.

STRESS is the body's reaction to stressors such as overwork, money problems, marriage problems, etc. The adrenals in particular suffer from chronic stress resulting in a lowering of the immune system's ability to protect you from infection and cancer, and disturbs the function of your entire endocrine system including energy management (i.e. blood sugar, blood pressure, thyroid, etc.).

Treatment of stress should include relaxation, subliminal stress relieving audio tapes, sublingual ACE drops at 5–10 drops t.i.d., vitamin C to bowel tolerance, zinc at 15 mg t.i.d., and learning to compart-mentalize time expenditure. Have 20 projects (a combination of work, family, and hobbies—remember the old saying about "giving the project to the busiest person if you want it done") so that at least one will give positive feedback.

STROKE (cerebrovascular accident, CVA) is the result of a blood clot or tumor cells blocking an artery supplying the brain. The result is local brain tissue death from the lack of oxygen and food. If the damaged area is small enough and not in a vital area, the brain will reroute the brain's functions to unused portions through a relearning and compensation process.

Treatment of stroke should include EDTA chelation and IV hydrogen peroxide as soon as possible, 5 grams t.i.d., exercise, and the base line nutritional supplement program to include hyperbaric oxygen and oral oxygen and Dr. Wallach's Pig Arthritis Formula.

SWEAT TEST a nonspecific test that measures the amount of electrolytes (i.e. sodium, chlorides, and potassium) in sweat. Originally it was thought to be a specific genetic indicator for cystic fibrosis (CF). However, today it has been found to be positive in 17 different diseases, food allergies, starvation, kwashiorkor, celiac disease, etc. The mechanism is related to EFA deficiencies and thus the lack of certain prostaglandins (short-lived hormone-like substances) which control sweat electrolyte levels in the skin.

SWIMMERS EAR is usually caused by Candida albicans growing in the external ear canal; constant dampness during the summer swimming season is thought to be the underlying cause.

Treatment for swimmers ear include hydrogen peroxide ear drops and/or Nystatin ear drops.

SYPHILIS is a sexually transmitted disease caused by the spirochete Treponema pallidum. It has been associated with 90 percent of AIDS patients in one study of homosexual males. Syphilis is characterized by active infection and by years of spontaneous remission. Symptoms of syphilis include a primary lesion or chancre sore that may persist for 3–4 months on the penis, vulva, lips, tongue, etc., skin rashes appear after 3–4 months and last for weeks to months. Eighty percent of infected people have herpes-like sores on lips, tongue, penis, or vulva. The disease may infect any organ including liver, bone, brain, eyes, heart, etc. Terminal stages of tertiary syphilis occur 10–25 years after the original infection. Diagnosis is made from a positive blood VDRL test.

Treatment for syphilis is specific in all stages with penicillin G at 2.4 million u IM with a second treatment 10–14 days later. Like AIDS, syphilis is a reportable disease to the Public Health Service.

TACHYCARDIA (rapid heartbeat) is characterized by rapid heart beat. Tachycardia can be caused by "nervous heart," hyperthyroidism, food allergies, hypoglycemia, nutritional deficiencies (i.e. B1, B3, selenium, etc.), poisons, and organic heart disease. A classic example is allergy to MSG or "Chinese Restaurant Syndrome."

Treatment of tachycardia should include the identification and treatment of the underlying cause, acupuncture, selenium at 500–1,000 mcg per day, B1 at 100 mg t.i.d., B3 at 450 mg t.i.d. as time release tablets, subliminal relaxation tapes, and herbs including English hawthorn (Crataegus oxyacantha), hops (Humulus lupulus), lavender

(Lavandula angustifolia), mother wort (Leonurus cardiaca), valerian (Valeriana officinalis), and lily-of-the-valley (Convallariana magalis).

TAPEWORMS (cestodes) can set up housekeeping in your intestines without causing any noticeable problem in a well-nourished person, but cause wasting weight loss and anemia. Tapeworms are contracted by eating contaminated watercress, raw fish, raw beef, or raw pork. The encysted larvae are released into the digestive tract and attach to the intestinal wall by suckers or hooks in their head. Diagnosis of tapeworms may be made by seeing segments on the surface of the bowel movement. They look like grains of rice that are moving. They can also be diagnosed by observing eggs in microscopic examination of the stool. See parasites in laboratory section. Prevention of tapeworms is related to cooking fish and meat before consumption and thoroughly washing vegetables.

Treatment of tapeworms requires the use of a single dose of niclosamide at 2 gm taken with a glass of water. Recheck stool in 3–6 months for reinfestation. Retreat if needed. Herbs may be helpful including garlic (Allium sativum) and male fern (Dryopteris Felixmas). Pretreating herbal remedies for tapeworms with a teaspoon of castor oil in the morning before treatment increases the efficiency.

TARDIVE DYSKINESIA (spasms of facial muscles) is on the increase as a side effect of heavy tranquilizer (phenothiazines) usage.

Treatment of tardive dyskinesia should include the discontinuation of the inducing drugs, B3 at 450 mg t.i.d. as time release tablets, phosphatidyl choline at 30 gm per day, B6 at 200 mg q.i.d., essential fatty acids at 5 gm t.i.d., manganese at 10–15 mg per day, and vitamin E at 800–1,200 IU per day.

TEETH DISCOLORATION (tetracycline) with reduced enamel thickness is a common side effect of prolonged administration of tetracyclines during the second half of pregnancy or during early tooth development. The affected teeth will be brown or gray and fluorescent orange-green in ultraviolet light. Prevention is the name of the game. Cosmetic capping is necessary if permanent teeth are affected.

TEETHING can be an uncomfortable event for infant and parents with painful local swellings, sudden fever, irritability, and diarrhea (especially irritating with severe diaper rash).

Treatment of teething includes Tylenol or aspirin drops (follow label directions) and herbs including German chamomile (Matricaria chamomilla) as teaspoon doses as needed.

TMJ (temporal-mandibular joint syndrome) is characterized by headaches, misalignment of teeth, popping the TM joints while talking or eating, etc. This syndrome is related to carpal tunnel syndrome and repetitive motion syndrome in that all three are caused by deficiencies of arsenic, manganese, and choline.

Treat for osteoporosis and be sure to include colloidal arsenic, manganese, and choline. Dr. Wallach's Pig Arthritis Formula works like a charm here.

TESTICULAR ATROPHY is not uncommon in aging men or following an episode of mumps. Testicular atrophy may result in decreased sexual drive and feminization.

Treatment of testicular atrophy should include zinc at 20 mg t.i.d., plant derived colloidal minerals, an herbal combination mixed with testosterone (Zumba), ginseng (Panax ginseng), and saw palmetto (Sarenoa serrulata).

THALLIUM POISONING (rat or insect baits) can accidentally occur when small children get into pesticides containing thallium salts. Thallium poisoning can be rapidly fatal if not treated promptly. Symptoms include bloody vomiting and diarrhea, oral irritations with severe salivation, tremors, facial palsy, and hair loss in 3–4 weeks in survivors.

Treatment for thallium poisoning should include contact with poison control centers and syrup of ipecac to induce vomiting at 15–30 ml (1–2 tbsp.) for children and adults. Follow the syrup with several pints of water until vomiting occurs. Then take one tbsp. activated charcoal in a glass of water. Control convulsions with diazepam. Chelation therapy is of no value for thallium poisoning.

THRUSH (oral candidiasis) is an oral yeast infection caused by Candida albicans. Thrush is characterized by creamy white patches that can be scraped off with a tongue depressor. Candida albicans is a ubiquitous nonpathogenic yeast under normal circumstances which becomes pathogenic and invades tissue when the host's ability to defend itself is lost through malnutrition, chemotherapy, AIDS, etc. Also occurs when the competing intestinal organisms are killed out (i.e. antibiotic therapy, etc.). Diagnosis can be made from the characteristic lesions or by looking at the exudate under the microscope.

Treatment of thrush includes the use of oral washes and gargling with hydrogen peroxide. Small infants unable to gargle may have to have topical Nystatin applied to the lesions. The underlying condition must also be dealt with to allow you to defend yourself against reinfection. Vitamin C to bowel tolerance, selenium at 25–1,000 mcg per day, vitamin E at 800–1,200 IU per day, vitamin A at 25,000–300,000 IU per day as beta-carotene, and zinc at 15 mg t.i.d. are of great value in restoring the immune status. Following extended antibiotic therapy (i.e. acne, rheumatic fever, cystic fibrosis, etc.), you can restore the competitive organisms into the bowel (to help keep yeast numbers down) by the use of Lactobacillus acidophilus. Administer Lactobacillus at ten capsules twice each day between meals for ten days each month to restore normal colon count; a retension enema with the Lactobaciilus will assure reimplantaion.

TINNITUS (ringing or buzzing in the ear) is characterized by a ringing or buzzing in the ear. "Orthodox" doctors suggest that "surgery is of no value; if you can't tolerate the ringing, play background music." In reality, there are a variety of causes of tinnitus including hypertension, lead, mercury toxicity, nutritional deficiencies, osteoporosis (connectissue squeezes the 8th cranial nerve), food allergies, and/or hypoglycemia. Do the necessary laboratory work to make a specific diagnosis including the pulse test, six-hour GTT, and hair analysis. Take the base line nutritional program.

Treatment of tinnitus should include the treatment of the underlying disease. Avoid offending food allergens, avoid sugar and all refined foods, take zinc at 15 mg t.i.d., tin from plant derived colloidal minerals, EFA at 5 grams t.i.d., vitamin A at 300,000 IU per day as beta-carotene, calcium and magnesium at 2,000 and 1,000 mg per day, and betaine HCl and pancreatic enzymes at 75–200 mg t.i.d. 15 minutes before meals. Using Dr. Wallach's Pig Arthritis simplifies the whole process.

TIREDNESS (chronic fatigue syndrome): see chronic fatigue syndrome.

TONSILLITIS is characterized by an inflamed sore throat caused by viruses or Streptococcus organisms. Treatment of tonsillitis should include hydrogen peroxide mouthwash and gargle, vitamin C to bowel tolerance, vitamin A at 25,000–300,000 IU per day as beta-carotene, zinc at 15 mg t.i.d., selenium at 25–1,000 mcg per day, herbs to include echynacia (Echynacia angustifolia), green hellebore (Veratrum viride), marshmallow (Althaea officinalis), flaxseed (Linum usitatissimum), German chamomile (Matricaria chamomilla), marjoram (Origanum vulgare), and garden sage (Salvia officinalis).

TOOTHACHE is usually caused by cavities (caries) that are stimulated to pain by sweets and cold or hot drinks.

Treatment of caries and toothache should include filling of the tooth with non-metallic composite (fiberglass). Avoid a stimulus that initiates pain. Acupuncture and herbs to include penny royal Mentha pulegium, lavender (Lavandula spp.), gelsemium (Gelsemium nitidum), and, as necessary, OTC analgesics (i.e. aspirin, Tylenol) or Tylenol-3 from your pharmacy.

TORTICOLLIS SPASMODIC (wryneck) is caused by spasms of the neck muscles and/or "subluxations" of the cervical vertebrae. Torticollis may be caused by "whiplash" injuries, calcium deficiencies, and/or muscular dystrophy.

Treatment of torticollis should include chiropractic, massage therapy, hydrotherapy, acupuncture, calcium and magnesium at 2,000 and 1,000 mg per day, selenium at 500–1,000 mcg per day, and vitamin E at 800–1,200 IU per day.

TOXIC SHOCK SYNDROME (TSS) is caused by an exotoxin produced by a Staphylococcus organism. The exotoxin is similar to if not identical to that which is produced by Staph food poisoning. Approximately 15 percent of those affected are men via food poisoning; the remainder are young women between 13–32 years of age. The syndrome is precipitated by improper use of vaginal tampons. Use of a single tampon for longer than four hours produces an ideal environment for Staphylococcus growth. TSS is characterized by high fever, sudden onset, vomiting, diarrhea, confusion, skin rash, headache, and sore throat with rapid deterioration and death within 48 hours. Prevention is the best policy with TSS, so avoid prolonged use of individual tampons, and avoid food poisoning by proper food handling. Treatment of toxic shock syndrome is a medical emergency requiring rapid emergency room care. DO NOT LET THEM MAKE YOU WAIT IN THE HALL. Treatment should include IV fluids and electrolytes, as well as penicillin to kill the Staphylococcus.

TOXOPLASMOSIS (cat coccidia) is caused by an intermediate stage of a house cat intestinal protozoa (Isospora bigemina). The intermediate stage in humans was originally named Toxoplasma gondii and the "orthodox" doctors refuse to admit that it is a cat parasite. "Toxoplasmosis" in man is characterized by a generalized brain disease. Toxoplasmosis is acquired in man from inhaling or swallowing dust from contaminated "kitty litter" boxes or outdoor sand piles or from eating rare beef. "Toxoplasmosis" is of particular danger to pregnant women as infection will cause birth defects in the fetus (i.e. brain defects, blindness, mental retardation). Symptoms in adults can mimic the flu, causing headache, rash, high fever, swollen lymph nodes, meningitis, hepatitis, pneumonitis, myocarditis, blindness, and diarrhea. Diagnosis of "toxoplasmosis" is made from a positive blood test or skin test following a high level of suspicion. Prevention of "toxoplasmosis" in pregnant women is related to avoiding cats just prior to and during, pregnancy (i.e. move cat to grandma's house temporarily), and eating well-cooked meats.

Treatment of "toxoplasmosis" should include trisulfapyrimidine orally at 25 mg (1 mg/kg for kids) daily for four weeks.

TRIGLYCERIDES (Elevated) can be a sign of diabetes, a liver disease, and deficiencies of EFA, chromium, and vanadium. Do a six-hour GTT and a full blood chemistry. Elevated triglycerides are a high risk factor for cardiovascular disease and stroke. Do a pulse test to determine if food allergies are involved.

Treatment of elevated triglycerides should include moderate exercise (walking), avoidance of sugar, avoidance of refined foods, essential fatty acids at 5 gm t.i.d., high fiber and raw foods diet and the elimination of red meat, chromium at 100–200 mcg t.i.d., selenium at 500–1,000 mcg per day, plant derived colloidal minerals, vitamin C to bowel tolerance, and the base line nutritional supplement program.

ULCER (stomach) is brought on by an infection with Helicobactor pylori. Antibiotics for 4 to 6 weeks are a preferred treatment of gastric ulcers over surgery.

Treatment of gastric ulcers should include alfalfa (Medicago sativa), for its "vitamin U" factor, bioflavonoids at 1,000 mg q.i.d., B6 at 100 mg t.i.d., vitamin A at 300,000 IU per day as beta-carotene, zinc at 20 mg t.i.d., and glutamine at 400 mg q.i.d.. Avoid alcohol, sugar, and refined foods, and consume a high fiber diet. Antibiotics are a preferred treatment of gastric ulcers over surgery. At any sign of "coffee grounds" vomiting, get to an emergency room immediately, as this is a sign of a hemorrhaging ulcer.

ULCERATIVE COLITIS see Crohn's Disease

URTICARIA (food allergy rash) see food allergies

VAGINITIS (vaginal discharge) can be caused by a great variety of diseases and syndromes ranging from panty-hose without ventilation, parasites (Trichomonas vaginalis), yeast infections (Candida albicans), venereal disease (gonorrhea, syphilis), etc. Diagnosis of the specific underlying disease is essential to correct therapy. History will be useful as well as vaginal cultures.

Treatment of vaginitis should include specific therapy following diagnostic procedures (see specific diseases). For nonspecific vaginitis you may use hydrogen peroxide douches twice weekly, vinegar douches (two tbsp./pint of warm water), yogurt douches and herbs to include myrtle (Myrica cerifera) and blue cohosh (Caulophyllum thalictroides).

VARICOSE VEINS are thought to be caused by constipation and constant vertical posture; copper deficiency may also be a contributing factor.

Treatment of varicose veins should include vitamin C to bowel tolerance, vitamin E at 800–1,200 IU per day, zinc at 50 mg t.i.d., bioflavonoids at 600 mg t.i.d., DMSO, hydrotherapy, copper at 2 mg per day (try a copper bracelet), and herbs including marigold (Calendula officinalis) topically, rue (Ruta graveolens), and yellow sweet clover (Uelilotus officinalis).

VERTIGO (dizziness, car sickness, motion sickness) see Car Sickness, Wallach's Vertigo. Take powdered peppercorns (Piper nigrum).

VITILIGO (loss of skin color) is a loss of skin color, especially in dark or black skinned people.

Treatment of vitiligo should include extracts of placenta, live cell therapy, PABA at 100 mg q.i.d., phenylalanine at 50 mg/kg/day, copper at 2 mg per day (copper bracelet), vitamin A at 300,000 IU pr day as beta-carotene, zinc at 50 mg t.i.d., Vitamin B12 at 2000 mcgs per day, folic acid 1 mg per day, and the base line nutritional supplementation program to include plant derived colloidal minerals.

WALLACH'S VERTIGO (dizziness with or without ringing in the ears) Osteoporosis of the skull. The connective tissue generated by the demineralized bones squeezes the vestibular branch of the 8th cranial nerve.

Treatment approach includes osteoporosis nutritional program— chondroitin sulfate (gelatin), calcium 200 mg, 1000 mg magnesium, boron 1 mg, and plant derived colloidal minerals containing all 60 essential minerals.

WARTS (papillomas) are contagious (viral) benign skin tumors known as warts (verrucae vulgaris), planter warts on the sole of the foot, and venereal warts (condylomata acuminata) which may be found on the vulva and penis.

Treatment of warts should include topical application of cashew nut (Anacardium occidentale), oil of yellow cedar (Thuja occidentalis), and milk-weed juice. There are commercial wart removal kits available from your pharmacy that employs salacylic acid topically.

WEIGHT LOSS: see diets

WHITE SPOTS, FINGERNAILS are caused by zinc deficiency. Treatment should include zinc at 50 mg t.i.d.; also take the base line nutritional program to include plant derived colloidal minerals.

WORMS (parasites) see parasites

Treatment may include wormwood (Artemisia absinthium) and butternut (Juglans cinerea). Levamisol is a good veterinary "wormer" that can be used very effectively in humans with minimal to no side effects.

WOUNDS (chronic ulcers) treat topically with herbs including euphorbia (Chamaesyce spp.), cliff rose (Allionia coccinea), arnica (Arnica montana), snake root (Aristolochia clematitis), German chamomile (Matricaria chamomilla), marigold (Calendula officinalis), snake root (Sanicula europaea), and witch hazel (Hamamelis virginiana)

ZITS (pimples, acne) see acne

INDEX

Dr. Joel D. Wallach, BS, DVM, ND
Dr. Ma Lan, MD, MS, LAc
Dr. Gerhard N. Schrauzer, PhD, MS, FACN, CNS

EPIGENETICS

THE DEATH OF THE GENETIC THEORY
OF DISEASE TRANSMISSION

Foreword by
Dr. Jeffrey S. Bland, PhD

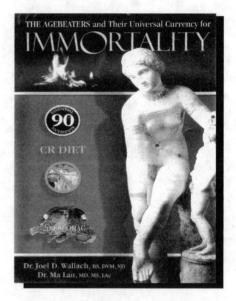

Let's Play Doctor

The Book That "Orthodox" Doctors Couldn't Kill - "How to" maximize your genetic potential for health and longevity.

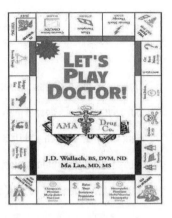

• Become your own primary health
  care provider
• Learn The Alternative Healing Arts
• Establish your own Health Clinic
• Establish a Home Pharmacy
• Home Surgery

Rare Earths Forbidden Cures
Their Secrets of Health and Longevity

The definitive home reference
on minerals, mineral deficiencies
and their relationship to:

* Degenerative Diseases
* Learning Disabilities
* Criminal Behavior
* Birth Defects
* Addition
* Food Binges
* Depression
* Infertility and More!

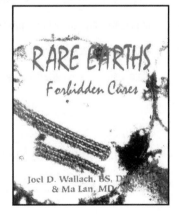

1-800-755-4656
www.drjwallach.com

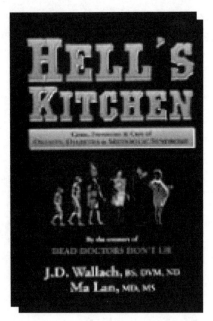

LET'S PLAY HERBAL DOCTOR

- Learn about the pharmacologilcal properties of plan herbs.

- The history of herbal medicine

- Learn how herbs work

- Active constituents of medicinal herbs

- Growing, harvesting, selecting, storage and processing of herbs

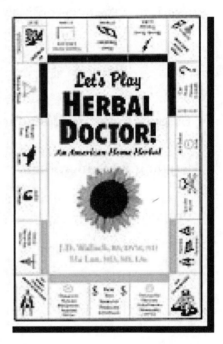

$19.95 - 10 or more $12.00 each

1-800-755-4656
www.drjwallach.com

PASSPORT TO AROMATHERAPY

Essential oils or "essences" are highly concentrated volatile oils extracted from aromatic plants

- Essential oils are legendary

  for their anti-microbial

  properties

- Essential oils are legendary

  for uplifting the emotions

$14.95 - 10 or more $8.00 each

Learn more about essential oils from this book

1-800-755-4656
www.drjwallach.com

BLACK GENE LIES

This book is a landmark expose that shows that the diseases

of the black population in

America, that the medical

community attributes to a

terrible "Black Gene", are in

fact caused by regional and

cultural eating habits and

nutritional deficiencies of trace

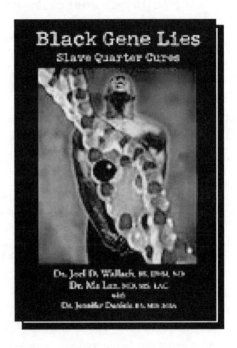

elements that are easily, safely and economically overcome

by the use of simple nutritional supplement programs and

herbal remedies

$19.95 - 10 or more $12.00 each

1-800-755-4656
www.drjwallach.com

GOD BLESS AMERICA!

- The epiphany
- American centenarians
- Medical dogmas/lies
- Health and longevity
- Weight loss
- Home defense and
- anti-terrorism plan
  Cash flow and tax plan
- Longevity recipes

$14.95 - 10 or more $8.00 each

WALLach $Treet for kids

This book is about entrepreneurship, money and business for the purpose of educating entrepreneurial kids, teens and young adults opportunities to find a "good jobs" in a changing global economy, the obvious direction for entrepreneurs is to own their business. Ownership is the true measure of power of business

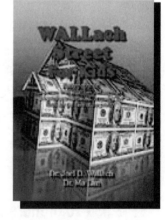

$19.95 - 10 or more $12.00 each

1-800-755-4656
www.drjwallach.com

Audio CDs

CD001	Dead Doctors Don't Lie	The origiinal tape that started it all
CD002	DDDL in Chinese, Korean, Spanish, Japanese	
CD003	Trust me, I am a Doctor	Dr.Wallach's 1996 health lecture series
CD004	Good Doctor, Bad Doctor	Dr.Wallach's 1997 health lecture series
CD005	Live Doctors Do Lie	
CD006	Medical Dogmas & Lies	Dr.Wallach's 2000 health lecture series
CD007	Medical Milking Machine	Dr.Wallach's 2000 health lecture series
CD008	What's Up Doc II	Health Products Information
CD009	Women, Athletes and Children	Menopause, ADHD and Athletes, 2003
CD010	Medical Mouse Trap	Dr.Wallach's lecture on Doctor's continue eduction
CD011	The Best of Dead Doctors Don't Lie	combination of DDDL I,II and III
CD012	Lucky Mo	Children's musical story
CD013	Hell's Kitchen	Dr.Wallach's 2004 health lecture series
CD014	God's Recipe	Health alternative to Ritalin
CD015	$10 Path to Financial Freedom	How to get your Youngevity products for free
CD016	Ferret Fat Pak 101	Weight loss product
CD017	Live Free or Die	Jonathan Emord
CD018	Healthier and Longer Life	
CD020	Dial MD for Murder	Dr.Wallach's 2004 health lecture series
CD030	Truth is Forever	Christian Songs by Dee Stocks
CD031	HE Has the Power to Heal	Christian Songs by Dee Stocks
CD033	WBA and Youngevity Opportunity	Dr.Wallach interviewed by Leroy MacMath -Athlete physical and financial health
CD034	Black Gene Lies I	interviewed by Herbalist Dirk Twine - the top killer diseases of African American
CD035	Black Gene Lies II	Dr.Wallach's lecture at World Changers Men's fellowship in Atlanta, GA
CD037	Tomato Warning	narration by Richard Dennis
CD046	Dead Athletes Don't Lie	
CD047	H5N1 Bird Flu	Dr.Ma Lan
CD048	Deadly Recipe	
CD056	Until Death Do Us Part	Outline information of Dr.Wallach's lectures
CD057	Energy Crisis	History on energy boost
CD058	Get your ACT together	Steve Wallach
CD059	New Best of DDDL	With 25 questions and answers
CD060	Tru Chocolate	Dr.Wallach , Sandy Elsberg and Elaine Lagatta
CD067	From Here To Immortality	Dr. Wallach
CD069	Aroma Therapy Oil	Dr. Wallach
CD070	Cerial Killer	Dr. Wallach
CD071	What Kills Billionaires	Dr. Wallach

order 1-10: $3.00/each, 11-20: $2.00/each, 50 and more: $1.00/each
personalized CD label is available for minimum of 50 CD order.

OTHER CDS

CD028	Selenium	Dr.Gerhard Schrauzer
CD028	Seeing is Believing	Dr.Pugh
CD032	Quality,Quality	Richard Renton
CD039	Beyond Juice	Ken Cole
CD051	Foundation for Success	Richard Stocks
CD052	Three Health Freedom Warriors	Dr.Wallach, Martin Luther King III, Jonathan Emord
CD053	Juice Cures	Jay Kordich
CD066	Who Made MD's King?	Dr. Peter Glidden
CD068	Healing is Easy	Dr. Peter Glidden
CD074	Exercise Without Supplementation is Suicide	Dirk Twine
CD075	The Secret Lives of Vegetarians!	Dirk Twine
CD076	The Truth About African American Health	Dirk Twine

PERSONALIZED CD

1) Minimum Order: 50/per title   3) Price: $1.00/per CD
2) Title: any title   4) Set-up fee: none

DVDs

		order 1-9 /	order 10
DVD001	Let's Talk Minerals	$10.00	$7.00
DVD002	Have You Heard	$10.00	$7.00
DVD005	Is It Possible to Reverse Aging (HGH)	$10.00	$7.00
DVD006	This Land Is Leached Land	$10.00	$7.00
DVD007	Take it Off, Keep it Off	$10.00	$7.00
DVD008	Undoing of Disease	$10.00	$7.00
DVD009	Live Long and Prosper	$10.00	$7.00
DVD012	Mineral Story	$10.00	$7.00
DVD013	Y Factor	$10.00	$7.00
DVD014	Dead Doctors Don't Lie	$10.00	$7.00
DVD015	Mineral Basics	$10.00	$7.00
DVD016	Health Confidence (Creflo Dollar's Church)	$25.00	$14.00

LISTEN TO DR.WALLACH'S RADIO SHOW

Talk to Dr.Wallach live on Weekdays on
his Radio Programs:

"Dead Doctors Don't Lie"
Toll free   888-379-2552
Priority line: 831-685-1080
Live 12:00 noon - 1:00 pm Pacific Time

"Let's Play Doctor"
Toll free: 877-912-7529
Live 1:00 pm - 2:00 pm Pacific Time

Listen to Dr.Wallach's radio show on line
www.kscoradio.com
click on: "pod cast"
click on: "Dead Doctors Don't Lie"

ORDER INFORMATION

1. **Order on line:**
   log on to www.drjwallach.com

2. **Order by phone:**
   800-755-4656
   8:00am - 4:30 pm , Pacific time, weekdays.

3. **Order by mail:**
   P.O. Box 1222
   Bonita CA 91908

4. **Order by fax:**
   619-420-2456 (F)

- We Accept Visa, Master, American Express and Discover Cards.
- We Accept Checks.
- Shipping: 8% Of Sub-total Or $6.00 Minimum, Which Is Greater In Continental U.S.